Bailey's
Head & Neck Surgery—
OTOLARYNGOLOGY
REVIEW

Bailey's
Head & Neck Surgery—
OTOLARYNGOLOGY
REVIEW

■ **CLARK A. ROSEN, MD**

Director, University of Pittsburgh Voice Center
Professor, Department of Otolaryngology
University of Pittsburgh Medical Center
Professor, Department of Communication Sciences Disorders
University of Pittsburgh
Pittsburgh, Pennsylvania

■ **JONAS T. JOHNSON, MD**

Chair, Department of Otolaryngology
Professor, Department of Otolaryngology and Radiation Oncology
University of Pittsburgh School of Medicine
Professor, Department of Oral and Maxofacial Surgery
University of Pittsburgh School of Dental Medicine
Pittsburgh, Pennsylvania

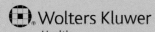 **Wolters Kluwer**
Health

Philadelphia • Baltimore • New York • London
Buenos Aires • Hong Kong • Sydney • Tokyo

Acquisitions Editor: Ryan Shaw
Product Manager: Nicole Dernoski
Production Product Manager: Bridgett Dougherty
Marketing Manager: Dan Dressler
Senior Manufacturing Manager: Beth Welsh
Design Manager: Steven Druding
Production Services: S4Carlisle Publishing Services

First Edition

© 2014 by Lippincott Williams & Wilkins, a Wolters Kluwer business

351 West Camden Street   Two Commerce Square
Baltimore, MD 21201   2001 Market Street
                              Philadelphia, PA 19103 USA
                              LWW.com

Printed in China

Library of Congress Cataloging-in-Publication Data

ISBN 978-1-45119-253-7

Cataloging-in-Publication data available on request from the Publisher.

DISCLAIMER

Care has been taken to confirm the accuracy of the information present and to describe generally accepted practices. However, the authors, editors, and publisher are not responsible for errors or omissions or for any consequences from application of the information in this book and make no warranty, expressed or implied, with respect to the currency, completeness, or accuracy of the contents of the publication. Application of this information in a particular situation remains the professional responsibility of the practitioner; the clinical treatments described and recommended may not be considered absolute and universal recommendations.

The authors, editors, and publisher have exerted every effort to ensure that drug selection and dosage set forth in this text are in accordance with the current recommendations and practice at the time of publication. However, in view of ongoing research, changes in government regulations, and the constant flow of information relating to drug therapy and drug reactions, the reader is urged to check the package insert for each drug for any change in indications and dosage and for added warnings and precautions. This is particularly important when the recommended agent is a new or infrequently employed drug.

Some drugs and medical devices presented in this publication have Food and Drug Administration (FDA) clearance for limited use in restricted research settings. It is the responsibility of the health care provider to ascertain the FDA status of each drug or device planned for use in their clinical practice.

To purchase additional copies of this book, call our customer service department at (800) 638-3030 or fax orders to (301) 223-2320. International customers should call (301) 223-2300.

Visit Lippincott Williams & Wilkins on the Internet: http://www.lww.com. Lippincott Williams & Wilkins customer service representatives are available from 8:30 am to 6:00 pm, EST.

10 9 8 7 6 5 4 3 2 1

RRS1401

DEDICATION

I dedicate this book to the amazing group of authors and editors
of the *Bailey's Head & Neck Surgery—Otolaryngology* textbook and to the authors
of the *Bailey's Head & Neck Surgery—Otolaryngology Review*.
Your energy and zeal for excellence is inspiring.

In addition, I dedicate this book to my late mother, Shirley Maureen Orr Rosen,
who always encouraged me to be the best that I could be.
Her fortitude will live on in my heart.
Clark A. Rosen, MD

I dedicate this book to the patients who have taught me so much and to the next
generation of physicians who strive to serve them.
Jonas T. Johnson, MD

AUTHORS

Basic Science/General Medicine

Shawn D. Newlands, MD, PhD, MBA, FACS
Professor and Chair
Department of Otolaryngology
University of Rochester Medical Center
Chief
Department of Otolaryngology
Strong Memorial Hospital
Rochester, New York

Karen T. Pitman, MD, FACS
Professor
Department of Otolaryngology
    and Communicative Sciences
University of Mississippi Medical Center
Jackson, Mississippi

Rhinology and Allergy

Matthew W. Ryan, MD
Assistant Professor
Department of Otolaryngology
University of Texas Southwestern
    Medical Center
Dallas, Texas

General Otolaryngology

Jonas T. Johnson, MD
Chair, Department of Otolaryngology
Professor, Department of Otolaryngology
    and Radiation Oncology
University of Pittsburgh School of Medicine
Professor, Department of Oral and
    Maxillofacial Surgery
University of Pittsburgh School of Dental
    Medicine
Pittsburgh, Pennsylvania

Shawn D. Newlands, MD, PhD, MBA, FACS
Professor and Chair
Department of Otolaryngology
University of Rochester Medical Center
Chief
Department of Otolaryngology
Strong Memorial Hospital
Rochester, New York

Laryngology

Milan R. Amin, MD
Associate Professor
Department of Otolaryngology—Head and Neck
    Surgery
New York University School of Medicine
Associate Professor
Department of Otolaryngology—Head and Neck
    Surgery
NYU Langone Medical Center
New York, New York

Michael M. Johns III, MD
Associate Professor, Otolaryngology
Director, Emory Voice Center
Emory University
Atlanta, Georgia

Clark A. Rosen, MD
Director, University of Pittsburgh Voice Center
Professor, Department of Otolaryngology
University of Pittsburgh Medical Center
Professor, Department of Communication
    Sciences Disorders
University of Pittsburgh
Pittsburgh, Pennsylvania

Trauma

Grant S. Gillman, MD, FRCS
Associate Professor
Director, Division of Facial Plastic Surgery
Department of Otolaryngology—Head and Neck
    Surgery
University of Pittsburgh School of Medicine
Pittsburgh, Pennsylvania

J. David Kriet, MD, FACS
WS and EC Jones Endowed Chair in Craniofacial
    Surgery
Associate Professor
Director, Facial Plastic and Reconstructive Surgery
Department of Otolaryngology—Head and Neck
    Surgery
University of Kansas School of Medicine
Kansas City, Kansas

Jonathan M. Sykes, MD, FACS
Professor of Otolaryngology
Director, Facial Plastic and Reconstructive Surgery
Department of Otolaryngology—Head and Neck
    Surgery
University of California Davis Medical Center
Sacramento, California

Pediatric Otolaryngology

Margaretha L. Casselbrant, MD, PhD
Eberly Professor of Pediatric Otolaryngology
Department of Otolaryngology
University of Pittsburgh School of Medicine
Director
Department of Pediatric Otolaryngology
Children's Hospital of Pittsburgh of UPMC
Pittsburgh, Pennsylvania

Charles M. Myer III, MD
Professor-Vice-Chairman
Department of Otolaryngology—Head and Neck
    Surgery
University of Cincinnati Academic
    Health Center
Residency Program Director
Department of Otolaryngology—Head and Neck
    Surgery
Cincinnati Children's Hospital Medical
    Center
Cincinnati, Ohio

Head and Neck Surgery

Christine G. Gourin, MD, MPH, FACS
Associate Professor
Department of Otolaryngology—Head and Neck
    Surgery
Johns Hopkins University
Active Staff
The Johns Hopkins Hospital
Baltimore, Maryland

Jonas T. Johnson
Chair, Department of Otolaryngology
Professor, Department of Otolaryngology and
    Radiation Oncology
University of Pittsburgh School of Medicine
Professor, Department of Oral and Maxillofacial
    Surgery
University of Pittsburgh School of Dental
    Medicine
Pittsburgh, Pennsylvania

Anna M. Pou, MD, FACS
Professor
Department of Otolaryngology—Head and Neck
    Surgery
Louisiana State University Health Sciences
    Center – New Orleans
New Orleans, Louisiana
Program Director
Department of Head and Neck Surgery
Our Lady of the Lake Regional
    Medical Center
Baton Rouge, Louisiana

Sleep Medicine

Jonas T. Johnson
Chair, Department of Otolaryngology
Professor, Department of Otolaryngology and
    Radiation Oncology
University of Pittsburgh School of Medicine
Professor, Department of Oral and Maxillofacial
    Surgery
University of Pittsburgh School of Dental
    Medicine
Pittsburgh, Pennsylvania

Otology

Barry E. Hirsch, MD
Professor, Department of Otolaryngology,
    Neurological Surgery, and Communication
    Sciences and Disorders
Eye and Ear Institute
University of Pittsburgh Medical Center
Director, Division of Otology/
    Neurotology
Department of Otolaryngology,
    Neurological Surgery, and Communication
    Sciences and Disorders
University of Pittsburgh Medical Center
Pittsburgh, Pennsylvania

Robert K. Jackler, MD
Sewall Professor and Chair
Department of Otolaryngology—Head and Neck
    Surgery
Stanford University School of Medicine
Stanford, California

Facial Plastic and Reconstructive Surgery

Grant S. Gillman, MD, FRCS
Associate Professor
Director, Division of Facial Plastic Surgery
Department of Otolaryngology—Head and Neck
    Surgery
University of Pittsburgh School of Medicine
Pittsburgh, Pennsylvania

J. David Kriet, MD, FACS
WS and EC Jones Endowed Chair in Craniofacial
    Surgery
Associate Professor
Director, Facial Plastic and Reconstructive
    Surgery
Department of Otolaryngology—Head and Neck
    Surgery
University of Kansas School of Medicine
Kansas City, Kansas

Jonathan M. Sykes, MD, FACS
Professor of Otolaryngology
Director, Facial Plastic and Reconstructive
    Surgery
Department of Otolaryngology—Head and Neck
    Surgery
University of California, Davis Medical Center
Sacramento, California

Contemporary Issues in Medical Practice

Shawn D. Newlands, MD, PhD, MBA, FACS
Professor and Chair
Department of Otolaryngology
University of Rochester Medical Center
Chief
Department of Otolaryngology
Strong Memorial Hospital
Rochester, New York

Karen T. Pitman, MD, FACS
Professor
Department of Otolaryngology
    and Communicative Sciences
University of Mississippi Medical Center
Jackson, Mississippi

Radiology

Barton F. Branstetter, MD
Professor of Radiology, Otolaryngology,
    and Biomedical Informatics
Department of Radiology
University of Pittsburgh Medical Center
Pittsburgh, Pennsylvania

PREFACE

This was the motivation for this companion book to *Bailey's Head & Neck Surgery—Otolaryngology.*

The *Bailey's Head & Neck Surgery—Otolaryngology Review* book arises from a combined effort of the individual authors of the *Bailey's* textbook and the authors of this book. The former contributed questions derived from most of the chapters of the "big book", and the latter added explanations, references, and uniformity. This collaborative effort has resulted in an outstanding resource for the young and seasoned learner to test his or her knowledge of otolaryngology—head and neck surgery.

We offer our deepest gratitude to all the authors who contributed to *Bailey's Head & Neck Surgery—Otolaryngology* and the authors of *Bailey's Head & Neck Surgery—Otolaryngology Review* for their dedication to education and advancement of the field of otolaryngology—head and neck surgery. We hope that this book assists in the reader's quest for improved knowledge of otolaryngology—head and neck surgery.

Clark A. Rosen, MD
Jonas T. Johnson, MD

ACKNOWLEDGMENT

The authors thank Dvora Konstant for her editorial and organizational efforts. She took a random list of questions and molded them into a tool for learning.

CONTENTS

Basic Science/General Medicine

1

1. All of the following are examples of absorbable suture, except which of the following?

   A. Polyglactin
   B. Poliglecaprone 25
   C. Polypropylene
   D. Polydioxanone

2. The most commonly indicated venous thromboembolic prophylaxis in otolaryngology includes which of these treatments?

   A. Early mobilization
   B. Pneumatic compression devices
   C. Pharmacologic prophylaxis in high-risk patients
   D. Calf massage
   E. None

3. Which of the following is true regarding perioperative smoking cessation therapy?

   A. The optimal timing for smoking cessation is 2 weeks before surgery.
   B. Smokers are twice as likely to have perioperative complications as nonsmokers.
   C. In smokers, lower levels of circulating oxygen are matched by a decreased rate of consumption.
   D. Nicotine replacement therapy does not lead to impaired wound healing.

4. Coblation tonsillectomy is best described by which of the following statements?

   A. Produces local temperatures much lower than those produced by electrocautery
   B. Is now used more commonly than electrocautery tonsillectomy
   C. May reduce postoperative pain and speed the return to a normal diet
   D. Both A and C
   E. All of the above

5. All of the following are immediate treatments for malignant hyperthermia developing after the induction of general anesthesia with halothane and succinylcholine except:

   A. Immediately stop halothane and succinylcholine
   B. Intravenous injection of dantrolene sodium
   C. Intravenous injection of meperidine for shivering
   D. Give 100% oxygen

6. In a diagnostic workup of headache, further radiologic evaluation with MRI or CT scan is indicated in which of the following circumstances?

   A. Pulsatile headaches
   B. Headache awakening one from sleep
   C. Onset of headache in childhood
   D. Unilateral headache

7. Which drug is most likely to be effective for the treatment of migraine-associated vertigo?

   A. Sumatriptan
   B. Meclizine
   C. Nortriptyline
   D. Diazepam

8. Hair removal prior to surgery should be completed by which of these methods?

   A. Shaving
   B. Hair clippers
   C. Chemical remover
   D. Should not be done

9. Which of the following is the *least* likely to cause tachyarrhythmias?

    A. Dopamine
    B. Epinephrine
    C. Dobutamine
    D. Norepinephrine

10. The Comprehensive Geriatric Assessment is:

    A. A prerequisite test required of all Medicare patients prior to scheduling of elective surgical procedures
    B. A rapid test that must be performed on all Medicare patients prior to all surgical procedures in order to assure appropriate reimbursement
    C. A highly formalized assessment protocol that has little effective utility for preoperative surgical assessment
    D. The only evidence-based assessment available that can reliably evaluate frailty

11. The increasing number of adults over 65 in the United States and other highly developed countries is largely due to which of these factors?

    A. Increased life expectancy due to medical and public health advances
    B. Decreasing birth rate leading to reduced total population numbers and a secondary increase in the relative percentage of older adults
    C. Earlier retirement with resultant reductions in work-related disease and death
    D. Marked improvements in data collection, particularly the recent increase in counting individuals in nursing homes and other long-term care facilities

12. Which of the following are appropriate instructions for preoperative fasting for a case scheduled for 2 p.m. the next day?

    A. No liquids after midnight
    B. Toast and milk allowed until 7 a.m.
    C. Light meal allowed until 10 a.m.
    D. No solids after midnight
    E. Coffee with milk until 12 noon

13. Chemotherapy for head and neck cancer in the palliative setting is which of the following?

    A. Requires multiagent therapy to have beneficial effect
    B. Must be weighed carefully with regard to factors such as morbidity, expected improvement in symptoms, performance status, and realistic patient/family expectations
    C. Necessarily requires significant reduction in tumor burden to have beneficial palliative effect
    D. Is rarely used

14. Surgical Care Improvement Guidelines require that preoperative antibiotics be given when?

    A. At the time of incision
    B. 2 hours before incision
    C. Within 1 hour of incision
    D. Any time during the procedure

15. A Marcus Gunn pupil is elicited with the swinging flashlight test. If positive, it is an indication of which of the following?

    A. Syphilis
    B. Amblyopia
    C. Optic nerve injury
    D. Diabetes

16. Which of the following complementary and alternative medical treatments has shown the most promise in preventing, but not treating, otitis media?

    A. Cod liver oil
    B. Osteopathic manipulation
    C. Xylitol
    D. Zinc

17. Which of the following is true of clinical outcomes research?

    A. The only outcomes measured are quality of life or functional status.
    B. Severity staging is more important than comorbidity in predicting outcome.
    C. Observational methodology is required for clinical outcomes research.
    D. Validated instruments must be used for outcomes assessment.

18. Mendelian genetics describe all of the following forms of inheritance except:

    A. Autosomal dominant inheritance
    B. Mitochondrial inheritance
    C. X-linked inheritance
    D. Autosomal recessive inheritance

19. Due to its high sensitivity and overall diagnostic performance (as compared to the gold standard of polymerase chain reaction), which of the following is the preferred method for identifying a human papillomavirus (HPV)-related carcinoma?

    A. In situ hybridization for HPV DNA
    B. Western blot analysis for the E7 protein
    C. Serum titers of anti-HPV IgG
    D. Immunohistochemical staining for p16 protein

20. Palliative care is best described by which of these statements?

    A. It is the same as hospice care and only appropriate for dying patients.
    B. It is interdisciplinary care addressing all sources of suffering for seriously ill patients and their families.
    C. It cannot be combined with disease-directed treatment, as this would interfere with the patient's need to accept that he or she is dying.
    D. It is not appropriate for patients with head and neck cancer who still want aggressive cancer treatments.

21. Perioperatively, surgeons should advise their patients to stop taking supplements such as fish oil, garlic, *Ginkgo biloba*, ginseng, and vitamin E because these may alter:

    A. The immune system
    B. Hemostasis
    C. Wound healing
    D. Fluid and electrolyte balance

22. The propagation of headache through the stimulation of the trigeminal ganglion includes all of the following except:

    A. Calcitonin gene-related peptide
    B. 5-Hydroxytryptamine
    C. Activation of the trigeminal nucleus caudalis
    D. Stimulation of the superior salivatory nucleus

23. Each line on the Snellen eye chart is meant to be read by a person with normal vision at which of the following distances?

    A. 10 feet
    B. 20 feet
    C. 30 feet
    D. 40 feet

24. Which of the following statements about the prevalence of tobacco smoking is true?

    A. Smoking is more common in women.
    B. An increase in prevalence is correlated with higher education.
    C. Prevalence increases with age.
    D. Over the last 40 years, smoking has decreased in prevalence.

25. Retinal detachment is most common in the presence of which of the following visual conditions?

    A. Hyperopia
    B. Amblyopia
    C. Optic neuritis
    D. Myopia

26. The four phases of wound healing include which of the following?

    A. Hemostasis, complement activation, proliferation, scar formation
    B. Hemostasis and coagulation, inflammation, proliferation, remodeling
    C. Complement activation, inflammation, proliferation, scar formation
    D. Complement activation, hemostasis, inflammation, proliferation

27. What is the approximate prevalence of CAM (complementary and alternative medicine) use among adults in the United States?

    A. 15%
    B. 25%
    C. 40%
    D. 70%

28. If a penetrating injury to the eye is suspected, which of the following is the safest course of action?

    A. Remove the foreign body in the emergency center.
    B. Suture the eyelids closed.
    C. Protect the eye with a metal cone.
    D. Begin topical antibiotic ointment.

29. During a radical neck dissection with your patient in the sitting position, the anesthesiologist is acutely concerned because of a sudden decrease in the patient's end-tidal CO_2 reading. Which of the following is your most appropriate immediate step?

    A. Flood the field with saline and place the patient in the Trendelenburg position.
    B. Tell the anesthesiologist to reduce the rate of ventilation as severe hypocarbia reduces cerebral blood flow.
    C. Ask the anesthesiologist to increase the percentage of nitrous oxide to allow a less-volatile agent to be used.
    D. Tell the anesthesiologist to replace the machine's leaking inspiratory valve.
    E. Place a pulmonary artery catheter and aspirate air from the pulmonary artery.

30. A 28-year-old woman presents with a long history of unilateral, pulsatile headaches that are triggered by weather changes. Her symptoms improve with over-the-counter analgesics and lying down in a quiet and dark room. What other aspects in her medical history would suggest a diagnosis of migraine headache?

    A. Unilateral headache lasting 30 minutes to 2 hours
    B. Improvement with physical activity
    C. Fully reversible loss of vision
    D. Family history of depression

31. Which of the following descriptions is characteristic of carcinoma in situ?

    A. Pushing borders with mild atypia along the basal layer
    B. Mild atypia, but with violation of the underlying basement membrane
    C. Full-thickness cellular atypia with an intact basement membrane
    D. Moderate atypia extending into the upper third of the mucosa

32. Which of these is the predominant collagen type present in the initial stages of proliferation?

    A. Type I
    B. Type III
    C. Type IV
    D. Type VII

33. All the following are true when comparing enteral nutrition to total parenteral nutrition (TPN) except:

    A. Enteral nutrition provides more nutrients.
    B. Enteral nutrition can buffer gastric acid.
    C. Enteral nutrition is less expensive.
    D. Enteral nutrition is more likely to cause hyperglycemia.

34. A 40-year-old man with a 20 pack-year smoking history complains of severe short lasting attacks of unilateral periorbital pain, nasal congestion, rhinorrhea, and eyelid edema. A CT scan and MRI of the brain reveal no abnormalities. What is the recommended initial therapy for this condition?

    A. Intranasal fluticasone
    B. Verapamil, 240 mg daily
    C. 100% oxygen via nonrebreather
    D. Subcutaneous glucocorticoids

35. Which statement below best describes the benefits of survival analysis when interpreting a cohort study on squamous cell carcinoma of the oropharynx?

    A. Survival analysis reduces bias by excluding patients with limited follow-up.
    B. Survival analysis increases precision by excluding censored observations.
    C. Kaplan–Meier survival curves are most meaningful at the far right end (long-term results).
    D. Kaplan–Meier survival curves increase precision by allowing full use of censored data.
    E. Progression-free survival is preferred over disease-specific survival for outcome reporting.

36. Which of the following are true concerning levels of individual studies?

    A. Case-control study is higher than cohort study.
    B. Randomized controlled trial is higher than case-control study.
    C. Case series is the same level as cohort study.
    D. Case series is higher than outcomes research.

37. Which of the following statements is true regarding thyroid function?

    A. Myxedema coma has a high mortality rate and often occurs in those with a concurrent illness.
    B. In a thyroid storm, propylthiouracil (PTU) or methimazole can be used to suppress thyroid hormone synthesis. Methimazole has the additional advantage of suppressing the conversion of T_4 to T_3.
    C. Potassium iodide can be used to control hyperthyroidism chronically.
    D. Glucocorticoids such as hydrocortisone are often not necessary in myxedema coma because patients have normal adrenal function.

38. All of the following are nucleotide components of DNA except:

    A. Adenine
    B. Guanine
    C. Cytosine
    D. Uracil

39. **Which of the following antibiotics inhibits synthesis of the 50S ribosomal subunit?**

    A. Neomycin
    B. Aztreonam
    C. Gentamicin
    D. Clindamycin

40. **Which of the following is true of evidence-based medicine (EBM)?**

    A. Only randomized controlled trials can be included in EBM.
    B. EBM requires the input of the clinician's experience and expertise.
    C. Evidence must include results from basic research and animal studies.
    D. The overall evidence is given a grade based on study methodology.

41. **Subarachnoid hemorrhage (SAH) is most commonly caused by:**

    A. Aneurysm
    B. Trauma
    C. Tumor
    D. Seizure

42. **Which of these are the most common pathogens found in acute otitis media?**

    A. *Streptococcus pyogenes* and *Moraxella catarrhalis*
    B. *Streptococcus viridans* and *Group A Streptococcus*
    C. *Haemophilus influenzae* and *Streptococcus pneumoniae*
    D. *Staphylococcus aureus* and *Pseudomonas aeruginosa*

43. **Which of the following is the best approach to a patient presenting for resection of a large mass at the base of the tongue?**

    A. Mask induction with desflurane, while maintaining spontaneous ventilation
    B. Rapid sequence induction with etomidate and succinylcholine
    C. Awake fiberoptic intubation
    D. Refuse to operate unless the patient agrees to an awake tracheotomy
    E. Attempt the resection with moderate sedation

44. **Robotic surgery benefits from:**

    A. 360° wristed motion
    B. Scaled motion with tremor suppression
    C. Binocular magnification
    D. Both B and C
    E. All of the above

45. Which of the following is most consistent with prerenal oliguria?

    A. Urine Na = 30
    B. Urine osmolality = 350
    C. Fractional excretion of sodium (FE_{Na}) = 0.1%
    D. Blood urea nitrogen (BUN)/creatinine ratio = 10

46. According to national surveys, the two most commonly used complementary and alternative medical products in the United States are:

    A. Xylitol and echinacea.
    B. Glucosamine and chondroitin.
    C. Echinacea and *Ginkgo biloba.*
    D. Fish oil/omega-3 and glucosamine.

47. Parathyroid cells increase in number in response to which chronic situation?

    A. Hypocalcemia
    B. Low level of $1,25(OH)_2D_3$
    C. Hypophosphatemia
    D. Uremia
    E. All of the above

48. You are asked to review a research article that compares the Epley maneuver to a sham procedure for benign, paroxysmal, positional vertigo, in which the authors present the beneficial effect of the therapy, reported as an absolute rate difference of 40% ($P < .001$) and a 95% confidence interval (CI) of 25% to 55%. Which statement below properly interprets these results?

    A. The effect is likely biased because low statistical power may be present.
    B. The 95% CI is too broad to conclude the effect is clinically important.
    C. The chance of a type 1 statistical error is significant.
    D. If 20 of 100 patients in the sham group improved, we would expect 28 of 100 to improve after the Epley maneuver.
    E. The 95% CI shows the zone of compatible results to be 25% to 55%.

49. Which of the following conditions is most likely to present with hearing loss?

    A. Migraine
    B. Vertebrobasilar insufficiency
    C. Anterior inferior cerebellar artery (AICA) occlusion
    D. Cerebellar infarction

50. What medical system is the most popular form of complementary and alternative medical (CAM) therapy in Europe?

    A. Homeopathy
    B. Chiropractic
    C. Osteopathy
    D. Naturopathic medicine

51. Which of the following is a disease that affects the outcome being measured?

    A. A comorbid condition
    B. An example of bias
    C. A dependent variable
    D. A contributor to severity

52. Which of these is the most common cause of sinus headache in a 40-year-old woman with complaints of pressure in the distribution of the sinuses, rhinorrhea, and ocular tearing?

    A. Obstruction of sinus ostia
    B. Acute rhinosinusitis
    C. A primary headache disorder
    D. Mucosal contact headache

53. Which of the following is most acceptable for an 83-year-old patient with poorly controlled hypertension presenting for middle ear surgery?

    A. Maintenance of anesthesia with isoflurane and nitrous oxide until the patient is extubated
    B. Maintenance of anesthesia with isoflurane and remifentanil
    C. Prevention of any patient movement with deep muscle relaxation from rocuronium
    D. Antihypertensives to produce deliberate hypotension (systolic blood pressure approximately 100 mm Hg) to reduce blood loss and improve operating conditions
    E. A pulmonary artery catheter to maximize the patient's intraoperative hemodynamic status

54. Genetic mutations in the 22q11.2 region of chromosome 22 are responsible for certain forms of the following syndromes except:

    A. CHARGE syndrome
    B. Velocardiofacial syndrome
    C. Pallister–Hall syndrome
    D. DiGeorge syndrome

55. Which of these is the most common inherited form of sensorineural hearing loss?

    A. Autosomal dominant syndromic sensorineural hearing loss
    B. Autosomal recessive syndromic sensorineural hearing loss
    C. Autosomal dominant nonsyndromic sensorineural hearing loss
    D. Autosomal recessive nonsyndromic sensorineural hearing loss

56. Which of the following does *not* have an active metabolite?

    A. Morphine
    B. Meperidine
    C. Fentanyl
    D. Hydromorphone

57. Outcomes in delirium are improved by identifying risk early, avoiding deliriogenic events and medications, correcting triggering pathology, and . . . (which of the following?)

    A. using physical restraints
    B. avoiding restraints
    C. administering high-dose benzodiazepines
    D. using music therapy
    E. requiring nurses to wear white uniforms and caps

58. Antineoplastic strategies in head and neck cancer are best described by which statement?

    A. Are associated with prolonged improved survival in patients with incurable, recurrent disease
    B. Can result in temporary improvement in symptoms such as pain, swelling, and dysphagia in patients with otherwise incurable disease
    C. Do not include palliative surgery in patients with incurable disease
    D. Play no role in the palliative setting

59. A 62-year-old man was treated for T3N2b carcinoma of the supraglottic larynx with chemoradiotherapy with planned posttreatment neck dissection. Combined with clinical examination, the study with the highest negative predictive value for residual disease at 10 to 12 weeks following the completion of treatment is:

    A. Contrast-enhanced neck CT
    B. MRI of neck with and without contrast
    C. CT angiography of neck
    D. Fludeoxyglucose F 18 (^{18}F-FDG) PET/diagnostic neck CT

60. **Specimen shrinkage is best described by which of these statements?**

    A. Is most marked in the immediate postresection period
    B. May be prevented by in situ fixation of the tissues
    C. Is primarily a result of formalin fixation
    D. Typically results in a 1% to 5% disparity between gross and histologic margins

61. **Which is the best description of how the evidence is graded, in the practice of evidence-based medicine?**

    A. The overall grade is a compilation of the level of the best studies.
    B. The overall grade is based on the highest level of study available.
    C. The overall grade is determined by the level of the largest number of studies.
    D. The overall grade is determined by the level of the poorest individual study.

62. **Which of the following smoking cessation regimens would have the highest rate of success?**

    A. Varenicline combined with a nicotine replacement patch
    B. Varenicline and bupropion SR
    C. Long-acting nicotine patch and short-acting nicotine gum
    D. Selective serotonin reuptake inhibitor and clonidine

63. **Which of the following is true of granulomatosis with polyangiitis?**

    A. This disease has its highest incidence in young African American women.
    B. c-ANCA is helpful in diagnosis, but the utility of the test is limited by poor specificity.
    C. This disease is self-limiting; most cases resolve without treatment.
    D. Laryngeal involvement should alert the physician that the patient is unlikely to have granulomatosis with polyangiitis, and another rheumatologic disease diagnosis should be pursued.
    E. The disease is characterized by the triad of respiratory granulomas, vasculitis, and glomerulonephritis.

64. **Which of the following fungi reveals 45° branching septate hyphae when grown on Sabouraud agar?**

    A. *Aspergillus*
    B. *Rhizopus*
    C. *Mucormycosis*
    D. *Absidia*

65. A 46-year-old woman presents with a mucosal lesion in the left hard palate. She has numbness in the left V2 distribution concerning for perineural spread of tumor. What would be the best imaging study to order?

    A. Maxillofacial CT without contrast
    B. Maxillofacial and skull base MRI without and with IV contrast
    C. Neck CT without contrast
    D. CT angiography of the neck

66. Which of the following is true concerning rheumatoid arthritis of the head and neck?

    A. Hoarseness is always due to cricoarytenoid joint involvement.
    B. Histologic examination of the cricoarytenoid joint rarely demonstrates pathology.
    C. Rheumatoid arthritis is a common cause of conductive hearing loss.
    D. Patients with rheumatoid arthritis and neck pain should have imaging of the cervical spine prior to direct laryngoscopy.
    E. The temporomandibular joint is nearly always spared in rheumatoid arthritis.

67. In a journal club, you are asked to assign a level of evidence to a study about treatment effects. In making your assignment which of the following considerations would be helpful?

    A. A systematic review of randomized trials could rank higher than a single randomized trial.
    B. A systematic review of randomized trials is preferable to a clinical practice guideline.
    C. Randomized trials, by nature of their study design, always have high methodological quality.
    D. Observational studies cannot provide a strength of evidence above level 3.
    E. Levels of evidence, in general, are not appropriate for studies of treatment effects.

68. Aminoglycoside-induced ototoxicity is caused by damage to which of the following?

    A. Inner hair cells
    B. Outer hair cells
    C. Stria vascularis
    D. Scala tympani

69. Angiogenesis is a feature of the proliferative phase of wound healing and is largely dependent upon which group of growth factors?

    A. VEGF, IL-1, EDGF
    B. VEGF, FGF, TGF-α, -β
    C. VEGF, EDGF, KGF
    D. FGF, ILGF, KGF

70. **Which of these statements best describes frailty?**

    A. It is an assessment of declining functional reserve.
    B. It is seen only in the "old-old."
    C. It has been linked to a specific mutation mapped to a locus adjacent to the Rb tumor suppressor gene.
    D. It is a standardized test.

71. **A 35-year-old woman has an MRI of the brain for headaches. The appearance of the brain is normal. A well-marginated 3-cm prestyloid parapharyngeal T2-hyperintense solid mass is incidentally seen on the study. The mass is most likely to be:**

    A. Salivary gland neoplasm
    B. Paraganglioma
    C. Hemangioma
    D. Schwannoma

72. **Which of the following statement regarding the adrenal glands is false?**

    A. Adrenal insufficiency can be diagnosed with a cosyntropin stimulation test.
    B. For patients with a recent history of adrenalectomy for Cushing disease, stress-dose steroids are necessary if patients are undergoing surgery.
    C. The best screening test for primary aldosteronism is aldosterone/renin ratio.
    D. Primary adrenalectomy is demonstrated by hyperkalemia and hypertension.

73. **General guidelines for pharmacologic treatment of chronic pain in patients with head and neck cancer include which of these statements?**

    A. Tricyclic antidepressants are the preferred medication for neuropathic pain in patients with cardiac disease.
    B. Neuropathic pain rarely responds to pharmacologic therapy.
    C. Chronic opioid therapy is necessary for most patients with moderate to severe pain.
    D. If an opioid is tolerated but ineffective at a given dose, rather than increasing the dose, a different medication should be tried.

74. **Slurred speech and tongue fasciculation are common early manifestations of:**

    A. Amyotrophic lateral sclerosis
    B. Migraine
    C. Guillain–Barré syndrome
    D. Anterior inferior cerebellar artery stroke

75. Rapamycin may improve the wound healing process by which of the following mechanisms?

    A. Phagocytosing of infiltrating bacteria
    B. Triggering apoptosis of fibroblasts
    C. Inhibiting mammalian target of rapamycin (mTOR)
    D. Promoting granulation tissue formation

76. Patients with diabetes suffer from impairment of wound healing secondary to all of the following except which of the following?

    A. Reduction in the elaboration of calcitonin gene–related peptide
    B. Dysfunctional fibroblast activity
    C. Increased levels of multiple medical problems
    D. Increased leukocyte infiltration of the wound

77. Which of the following is true of Sjögren syndrome?

    A. The primary form is associated with an increased risk of lymphoma.
    B. The secondary form is rarely associated with systemic lupus erythematosus.
    C. Primary Sjögren syndrome is a disease limited to the lacrimal and salivary glands.
    D. The diagnosis of Sjögren syndrome is made based on noncaseating granulomas on salivary biopsy.
    E. Serologic testing for Ro/SS-A and La/SS-B is highly sensitive and specific for the diagnosis of Sjögren syndrome.

78. Which of these are dermal skin substitutes?

    A. Can be divided into cellular and acellular products
    B. Remain histologically evident on a permanent basis
    C. Are rarely used
    D. Both A and B
    E. All of the above

79. A common side effect associated with phenylephrine includes:

    A. Reflex bradycardia
    B. Tachycardia
    C. Hypertension
    D. Hypotension

80. A group of investigators report superior patient satisfaction and outcomes after robotic-assisted surgery, compared with conventional surgery ($P < .0001$). The trial was randomized, but the nature of the interventions did not allow for blinding of the patients, surgeons, or outcome assessors to patient allocation. The differences between groups are *unlikely* to be caused by which of the following?

    A. Halo effect
    B. Allocation (susceptibility) bias
    C. Inadequate sample size
    D. Ascertainment (detection) bias
    E. Lack of intention-to-treat analysis

81. The recent increased emphasis on the study and management of geriatrics can be tied to:

    A. Scientific advances in the assessment and management of diseases of older adults
    B. Increased emphasis on effectiveness of medical and surgical interventions
    C. Changing demographics of the U.S. population
    D. Changing expectations of older individuals
    E. All of the above

82. A 48-year-old woman with a history of papillary thyroid carcinoma status–post–total thyroidectomy and radioactive iodine (^{131}I) ablation has a rising thyroglobulin level. Neck ultrasound and CT show no locoregional disease recurrence, and ^{131}I whole body scintigraphy is negative for iodine avid disease. What is the next best imaging study to evaluate for occult papillary thyroid carcinoma?

    A. Neck ultrasound
    B. CT angiography of the neck
    C. Whole body fludeoxyglucose F 18 PET/CT
    D. Technetium Tc 99m sestamibi single-photon emission computed tomography

83. All of the following are true of a patient who has bleeding during surgery except:

    A. The most likely cause of intraoperative bleeding is an unsecured vessel.
    B. In a bleeding patient who has a normal prothrombin time and normal activated partial thromboplastin time, the most likely deficit is impaired platelet activity.
    C. The clotting abnormality caused by heparin can be corrected with fresh frozen plasma (FFP) transfusion.
    D. The clotting abnormality caused by warfarin can be corrected with FFP transfusion.

84. Universal precautions include all of the following except:

    A. Gloves
    B. Barrier gowns
    C. Eye protection
    D. Shoe covers

85. Which of the following statements is true?

    A. Both T_3 and T_4 are produced by the thyroid gland, with more T_3 being released into the circulation.
    B. T_3 is the most active thyroid hormone as it has high binding affinity to thyroid hormone nuclear receptors.
    C. Most T_3 and T_4 in the circulation are free hormones.
    D. During illness, surgery, and trauma, there is decreased reverse T_3 production.

86. Which of the following is true concerning cat-scratch disease?

    A. The name is deceiving; cats do not appear to serve as a reservoir as this bacterium is rarely recovered from these animals.
    B. Inoculation can occur through the conjunctiva (Parinaud oculoglandular syndrome).
    C. If untreated, this disease often leads to a fulminant systemic infection.
    D. Diagnosis relies on culturing the *Bartonella henselae* organism.
    E. Multiple cervical nodes are usually found on presentation.

87. Concerning tuberculosis, which of the following is true?

    A. The worldwide incidence is falling rapidly and soon this disease will not represent a significant global health problem.
    B. Transmission occurs most efficaciously through encounters with fomites.
    C. Infectivity is especially high in the laryngeal form of the disease.
    D. Patients with positive purified protein derivative (PPD) and without a history of treatment are universally highly contagious.
    E. Treatment should not be initiated until sensitivity testing is done in culture to determine the minimal inhibitory concentration against various antituberculous drugs to pick the drug that will be most efficacious.

88. Eyelid notching after repair of a vertical marginal laceration is usually due to which of the following?

    A. Failure to close tarsal plate well
    B. Leaving sutures in too long
    C. Using absorbable sutures
    D. Not performing lateral canthotomy

89. **Which of the following statements describe oxidized cellulose topical hemostatic agents?**

    A. They provide scaffolding for clot formation.
    B. They do not have bactericidal properties.
    C. They have been shown to be less-effective hemostatic agents than microfibrillar collagen.
    D. Both A and C.
    E. All of the above.

90. **Which of the following definitions of inheritance is incorrect?**

    A. Penetrance describes whether individuals carrying a particular gene mutation also express an associated trait or phenotype.
    B. Expressivity describes the variation in phenotype among individuals carrying a particular genotype.
    C. Genetic imprinting describes a genetic process by which certain genes are expressed in a parent-of-origin–specific manner via upregulation of expression of specific alleles.
    D. Digenic inheritance or diallelic inheritance refers to coinheritance of mutation at two distinct genes or genetic loci which produce the phenotype of disease.

91. **Which of the following modifications has been shown to improve accuracy and adequacy of fine-needle aspiration (FNA) cytology specimens to the greatest extent?**

    A. Immediate assessment of adequacy by a cytopathologist/cytotechnologist
    B. Avoidance of suction during aspiration
    C. Preparation of a cell block
    D. Using a "two hand" technique of palpation with simultaneous aspiration

92. **Which of the following is the best intravenous treatment of cardiac arrest following injection of bupivacaine?**

    A. Lidocaine
    B. 20% lipids
    C. Calcium chloride
    D. Midazolam
    E. Naloxone

93. **The *mecA* gene, which is associated with methicillin resistance among *Staphylococcus aureus*, encodes for which of the following resistance mechanisms?**

    A. Enhanced penicillinase production
    B. Altered penicillin-binding protein (PBP)
    C. β-Lactamase production
    D. Decreases drug permeability by efflux pumps

94. Which of these is the most likely cause of postoperative hypotension?

    A. Inadequate pain control
    B. Hypovolemia due to inadequate fluid replacement or hemorrhage
    C. Pulmonary emboli
    D. Residual effects of intraoperative anesthetics

95. A 57-year-old woman presents with clinical signs and symptoms of primary hyperparathyroidism. Currently, the most commonly used combined imaging approach for initial preoperative localization of abnormal parathyroid tissue is:

    A. Neck CT with IV contrast and ^{131}I scintigraphy
    B. Somatostatin scintigraphy and MRI of the neck
    C. Neck ultrasound and technetium Tc 99m sestamibi single-photon emission computed tomography
    D. Somatostatin scintigraphy and neck CT with IV contrast

96. Which of the following alterations in technique will reduce the degree of artifact seen on histopathologic sectioning when the CO_2 laser is used for excision?

    A. Defocusing of the beam
    B. Using a fiber-coupled system rather than a micromanipulator
    C. Switching to the pulse-wave mode
    D. Increasing the power above 6 W

97. Patients with a Chiari type I malformation would commonly present to an otolaryngologist for the below symptoms except for:

    A. Headache
    B. Dizziness
    C. Hoarseness
    D. Unilateral hearing loss

98. Which of these statements can best describe ultrasonic shears?

    A. Present no risk to adjacent nerves
    B. Utilize ultrasonic blade vibrations at 55,000 Hz
    C. Result in electrical energy transfer to affected tissues
    D. Both A and B
    E. All of the above

99. In a thyrotoxic storm, all the following medications are used except which one of the following?

   A. Aspirin to control hyperthermia
   B. Propylthiouracil to block thyroid hormone production
   C. Iodine to prevent thyroid hormone release
   D. Propranolol to control tachycardia and tremor

100. Reading only the abstract of an original research article in an otolaryngology journal may provide an incomplete, or biased, view of study results because the abstract offers which of the following?

   A. Usually does not provide the sample size
   B. Frequently does not convey the study design
   C. Infrequently describes adverse events
   D. Provides too much information
   E. Often confuses dropouts with loss to follow-up

101. When light is shined into one eye, causing pupillary constriction, and the opposite pupil also constricts, this is known as:

   A. Consensual light reflex
   B. Direct light reflex
   C. Vergence
   D. Argyll Robertson pupil

102. For patients who have advanced head and neck cancer and are recognized to be dying, and their families, which of these statements is best?

   A. Palliative care or hospice involvement in their care has been shown to decrease the suffering and distress associated with the dying process.
   B. Resuscitation status is entirely a matter of their personal values, and no recommendation should be made by the physician.
   C. It is rare that patients have significant or distressing symptoms.
   D. Tube feedings should *not* ordinarily be discontinued in imminently dying patients who have a feeding tube.

103. Which of the following is not a manifestation of hypercalcemia?

   A. Confusion
   B. Polyuria
   C. Nephrolithiasis
   D. Tetany
   E. Constipation

104. **Which of the following is an effect of secondhand smoke exposure?**

    A. Premature death in nonsmokers
    B. Increased incidence of oral cavity cancer
    C. Development of allergies in children
    D. Hypertension

105. **Which of the following is an effect of nicotine?**

    A. Increased anxiety
    B. Slight cognitive enhancement
    C. Decreased oxygen demand
    D. Vasodilation

106. **Propofol properties are best described as:**

    A. Slow onset with decreased postoperative nausea
    B. Slow onset with hypotensive side effects
    C. Rapid onset with amnestic properties
    D. Rapid onset with analgesic properties

Chapter 1 Answers

1. **Answer: C.** Prolene (polypropylene) suture is nonabsorbable, as are silk, nylon, and polyester (Dacron, Ethibond). The other materials listed are absorbable. `PAGE 22`

2. **Answer: B.** The risk of deep venous thrombosis and pulmonary embolism in patients undergoing the majority of otolaryngologic procedures is low (<1%). Pneumatic compression devices are frequently used as a precaution. `PAGE 24`

3. **Answer: D.** Several studies suggest that nicotine replacement may not result in the complications that we have historically attributed it to. Nicotine use in the perioperative period has not been fully investigated, although current evidence suggests it does not significantly impair wound healing after surgery. `PAGE 337`

4. **Answer: D.** The temperatures generated by the coblation are between 45°C and 85°C, much lower than the 400°C and 600°C generated by electrocautery, which decreases postoperative pain and speeds recovery. However, the increased cost of the disposable parts has slowed widespread adaption. `PAGE 49`

5. **Answer: C.** Patients affected by malignant hyperthermia do not shiver. They are febrile and require measures for immediate cooling. `PAGES 45, TABLE 3.10`

6. **Answer: B.** A headache that has an onset during sleep and wakes the patient up is a red flag for a serious condition (e.g., headaches from intracranial vascular causes). Pulsatile headaches, unilateral headaches, and onset during childhood are seen in primary headache syndromes. `PAGE 310`

7. **Answer: C.** Nortriptyline is a well-tolerated tricyclic antidepressant with efficiency in treating migraine-associated vertigo. Meclizine and diazepam are not commonly used to treat migraines. Sumatriptan has limited efficiency for vestibular symptoms of migraines despite excellent results in aborting migraine headaches. `PAGE 207–208`

8. **Answer: B.** Studies have demonstrated that the infection rate is lowest when no hair removal is done prior to surgery. When hair in the operative field must be removed, it should be done by clipping only. Shaving is to be avoided as it can cause skin nicks, which can then harbor bacteria and cause wound infections. Patients also need to be instructed not to shave the operative site before surgery. `PAGE 21`

9. **Answer: D.** Epinephrine, dobutamine, and dopamine are agents most likely to cause heart rates >130 bpm. `PAGE 58`

10. **Answer: C.** The comprehensive geriatric assessment is a multifocal, expert multidisciplinary process that is time-consuming and has not been definitely shown to enhance either outcomes or cost-effectiveness and is not a current clinical standard for surgical practice. A number of frailty phenotype indicators are available. `PAGE 300`

11. **Answer: A.** The birth rate only affects the average age. Work-related death decreases are largely due to better safety standards, not earlier retirement. There is no evidence that census changes have an impact. `PAGE 299`

12. **Answer: B.** In a healthy patient, a small meal up to 6 hours before surgery is permissible; 8 hours for full meals high in fats or alcohol. Clear liquid exits the stomach within 2 hours. PAGE 248

13. **Answer: B.** Palliative chemotherapy may involve single or multiple agents; the choice depends on carefully weighing the risks and benefits. Improvement in symptoms can be observed in the absence of overt response in lesion size. PAGES 341–342

14. **Answer: C.** Prophylactic antibiotics must be given within 1 hour of incision. Studies show that antibiotic concentration in tissues is optimal when given just prior to skin incision. If administered earlier or after the incision, they lose effectiveness. PAGE 23

15. **Answer: C.** A Marcus Gunn pupil is an important physical sign in the evaluation for neurologic disease. Prompt constriction should appear if each pupil is normal. If optic nerve disease or injury is present in the affected eye, the pupil gradually dilates, indicating a decreased direct light reflex. Argyll Robertson pupil is associated with syphilis. PAGE 219

16. **Answer: C.** Common botanicals employed for the treatment of otitis media include chamomile, echinacea, marshmallow, and mullein. Xylitol is a sugar alcohol that has been found in vitro to inhibit pneumococcal growth and adhesion to nasopharyngeal walls. Xylitol in solution and as a chewing gum have been shown to reduce the number of acute otitis media episodes and the need for antibiotics in blinded randomized controlled trials. PAGE 324

17. **Answer: D.** Validity of an instrument that measures quality of life or overall health means that the instrument is measuring what it is supposed to measure. Validity is confirmed by a combination of evidence, as mentioned on PAGE 104. Many outcomes are measured in clinical research, and they are not all observational. PAGE 103

18. **Answer: B.** Autosomal dominant inheritance, X-linked inheritance, and autosomal recessive inheritance are all consequences of chromosomal inheritance. In contrast, mitochondrial DNA is derived exclusively from the egg, and thus, mitochondrial inheritance is maternal and not Mendelian. PAGE 119

19. **Answer: D.** p16 protein immunohistochemistry is the preferred test based on the combination of sensitivity and specificity. In situ hybridization is a specific test that lacks sensitivity. Western blot analysis for the E7 protein and serum titers of anti-HPV levels are not used clinically for HPV-related carcinoma. PAGE 196

20. **Answer: B.** Palliative care is a holistic approach to medical care for patients with serious illness, focused on optimizing comfort and quality of life. It is appropriate for patients receiving aggressive treatment and thus different from hospice care. PAGE 340

21. **Answer: B.** All the substances listed interfere with hemostasis. PAGE 322, TABLE 20.2

22. **Answer: B.** 5-Hydroxytrytamine (serotonin) contributes to the feeling of well-being and originates in the raphe nuclei. The other choices are related to electrical stimulation of the trigeminal ganglion. PAGE 305

23. **Answer: B.** The most important determination of general eye condition is the best-corrected-distance visual acuity and is usually assessed with a Snellen chart. Each line on the chart is meant to be read be a person with normal vision. PAGES 217–218

24. **Answer: D.** From 1965 to 2008, the percentage of the U.S. population who smoke decreased from approximately 42% to 20.6%. PAGE 329

25. **Answer: D.** Retinal detachment is more common among persons with high myopia, after cataract surgery, and following facial trauma. Optic neuritis causes loss of vision, but the retina remains intact. PAGE 222

26. **Answer: B.** The phases of wound healing are well recognized and occur in specific order, as described on PAGES 77–80 .

27. **Answer: C.** The most recent data from the 2007 National Health Interview Survey (NHIS) show that 38.3% of American adults and 11.3% of children had used a CAM in the past year. PAGE 316

28. **Answer: C.** When there is a penetrating injury, the eye should be protected and an immediate consultation requested. If foreign bodies are partially extruding from the eye, the diagnosis is evident. The foreign body should be left intact and removed in the controlled environment of an operating room. PAGES 228–229

29. **Answer: A.** The question describes a potential air embolism entering the circulation through the jugular vein and being trapped in the right atrium with immediate reduction of blood entering the pulmonary circulation. The most appropriate immediate step is to prevent further air entrainment by flooding the area with saline, placing the neck below the waist. Placing a pulmonary catheter takes time and is not an immediate step. The other choices are not appropriate for an emergency. PAGE 245

30. **Answer: C.** This story is classic for migraine headaches, especially if accompanied by an aura such as fully reversible visual symptoms. Migraine headaches last 4 to 72 hours. Physical activity aggravates the symptoms. PAGES 306–307

31. **Answer: C.** Carcinoma in situ is dysplasia (defined as disordered growth with atypia) through the full thickness of the epithelium but without breach of the basement membrane. PAGE 194

32. **Answer: B.** During the early proliferation stage, granulation tissue contains 40% type III collagen with a lower tensile strength. Unwounded dermis contains 80% type I collagen and 25% type III collagen and has maximum strength. PAGE 79

33. **Answer: D.** Several advantages to using enteral feedings versus TPN. Enteral nutrition provides more nutrients, has less chance of hyperglycemia, promotes immune function, eliminates central catheter, buffers gastric acid, and is less expensive. PAGE 26

34. **Answer: C.** This scenario describes cluster headaches. 100% oxygen is a first-line therapy for acute cluster headaches. Verapamil is a preventative therapy. Glucocorticoids have been used, with mixed results. PAGE 309

35. **Answer: D.** Survival data are measured on continuous scale, and are further classified with a graphic display to assess distribution. Numerical data that include censored data on subjects lost to follow-up or in whom a specified event has not yet occurred at the end of a study. PAGE 90, TABLE 7.5

36. **Answer: B.** See Tables 8.2 to 8.4, which define the levels of evidence and describe the meaningful use of it. PAGES 108–109

37. **Answer: A.** Myxedema coma has a high mortality despite treatment and is often precipitated by other factors. Patients with myxedema coma often have impaired adrenal reserve. PTU, not methimazole, suppresses the conversion of T_4 to T_3. The effect of potassium iodide lasts only 2 to 3 weeks. PAGE 258

38. **Answer: D.** Uracil is a component of RNA; thymine is the DNA analog. Adenine, guanine, and cytosine nucleotides are common to both RNA and DNA. PAGE 111, 113

39. **Answer: D.** Clindamycin inhibits synthesis of the 50S ribosomal subunit. Aminoglycosides such as neomycin and gentamicin bind to the 50S ribosomal subunit. Aztreonam inhibits mucopeptide synthesis in the bacterial cell wall. PAGE 132

40. **Answer: D.** In EBM, there is a fundamental principle at work: Not all evidence is equal. Studies are evaluated based on their methodology. See Tables 8.2 to 8.4, which define the levels of evidence and describe the meaningful use of it. PAGES 107–109

41. **Answer: A.** 85% of SAH are caused by aneurysms. Epidural hemorrhage is caused by trauma. Tumor-related hemorrhage is relatively rare. Seizures do not cause SAH. PAGE 204

42. **Answer: C.** Nontypeable *H. influenzae* and *Streptococcus pneumoniae* are the most common isolates in acute otitis media. Chronic supportive otitis media is polymicrobial and often involves *P. aeruginosa* and *Staphylococcus aureus*. PAGE 135

43. **Answer: C.** A tongue base mass makes for a difficult airway situation, and complete control of the airway is required for protection from loss of ventilation and aspiration of blood; thus moderate sedation is not an option. Rapid sequence induction risks creation of a paralyzed patient who cannot be ventilated, and is unsafe in this situation. Although mask induction might work without resultant obstruction, use of fiberoptic intubation while awake is preferred because it can be abandoned without consequence if the airway is not secured and it gives the anesthetist a view of the airway. Awake tracheotomy is a backup for failed fiberoptic intubation. PAGE 247

44. **Answer: E.** The da Vinci surgical system provides 360° articulated wrist motion, tremor filtration, and a binocular, magnified review. PAGE 50

45. **Answer: C.** In prerenal oliguria, urine Na is <20, urine osmolality is >500, and the BUN/creatinine ratio is >20. PAGE 64, TABLE 5.5

46. **Answer: D.** The most commonly utilized product among adults in the United States was fish oil or omega-3, which was used by 37.4% of those who reported using natural

products (in 2007). Other prevalently used natural products included glucosamine (19.9%) and echinacea (19.8%). Over 1 in 10 of those surveyed reported using *G. biloba.* PAGE 317

47. **Answer: E.** Chronic hypocalcemia, hypophosphatemia, uremia, and low level of $1,25(OH)_2D_3$ increase secretion and transcription of parathyroid hormone in addition to stimulating hypercellular parathyroid glands. PAGE 254

48. **Answer: E.** The CI describes a *zone of compatibility* with the data; for example, a 95% CI of 28% to 99% means that we do not know much about the real outcome of a treatment because the intervention is compatible with a very broad range of results. CI is a measure of the precision of a study, and the most common method to improve the CI is to increase the sample size. PAGE 98

49. **Answer: C.** The AICA supplies blood to the membranous labyrinth. Migraine and vertebrobasilar insufficiency lead to disequilibrium, while cerebellar infarction is associated with gait ataxia and paretic gaze nystagmus. PAGE 200

50. **Answer: A.** Homeopathy is a whole medical system that aims to stimulate the body's ability to heal itself by giving very small doses of diluted substances. This therapeutic system was developed by the German physician Samuel Hahnemann at the end of the 18th century. In many areas of Europe, homeopathy is the most popular form of CAM: 25% of all German physicians use homeopathy, 32% of primary care physicians use it in France, and up to 42% of physicians in the United Kingdom refer patients to homeopaths. PAGE 320

51. **Answer: A.** A comorbid condition is defined as a condition—distinct from the condition of interest—that affects the outcome being measured. PAGE 104

52. **Answer: C.** The vast majority of patients with facial pain complaints in the distribution of the paranasal sinuses do, in fact, have a primary headache disorder such as a migraine headache. Migraine referred to the trigeminal nerve distribution is often accompanied by parasympathetic symptoms of rhinorrhea, congestion, and lacrimation. PAGES 310–311

53. **Answer: B.** Muscle paralysis would inhibit facial nerve monitoring. For middle ear surgery, nitrous oxide is generally turned off 30 minutes before tympanic membrane graft placement. Central venous monitoring is not necessary for ear surgery as there is virtually no fluid shift occurring. Induced hypotension in a hypertensive, elderly patient risks hypoperfusion of critical organs. An inhalational anesthetic with a rapid-acting narcotic is a safe option in this setting. PAGE 239

54. **Answer: C.** CHARGE syndrome, velocardiofacial syndrome, and DiGeorge syndrome are due to microdeletions in the 22q11.2 region of chromosome 22. The presence of various syndromes (phenotypes) associated with deletions in the region is due to variability in the position and extent of the microdeletions. Pallister–Hall syndrome is associated with mutations within the *GL13* gene. PAGE 126

55. **Answer: D.** In hereditary hearing loss, 70% to 80% is nonsyndromic and 75% to 85% of these cases are autosomal recessive. PAGE 123

56. **Answer: C.** Of these commonly used opiates used for adults in the ICU, fentanyl is the only one that does not have an active metabolite. PAGE 65, TABLE 5.6

57. **Answer: B.** In patients with delirium, outcomes are improved by avoiding both chemical and physical restraints. Music therapy and nursing uniforms have probably not been studied in this context. PAGE 301

58. **Answer: B.** Palliative chemotherapy is associated with temporary meaningful responses in terms of survival and symptom management. Surgery can be part of the palliative approach, but the benefits must be weighed against the risks in terms of quality of life. PAGES 341–342

59. **Answer: D.** PET/CT is more accurate than conventional imaging in detecting recurrent or residual neoplasm and is useful to monitor treatment response to therapy. Following chemoradiotherapy, the high negative predictive value of FDG PET and PET/CT is useful to exclude locoregional disease and distant metastases. PAGE 160

60. **Answer: A.** There is >20% mean margin shrinkage 30 minutes after resection before formalin fixation. The overall disparity is between 30% and 47%. PAGE 182

61. **Answer: A.** Overall grade helps integrate best evidence and helps determine recommendations to integrate into a patient's management. See Tables 8.2 to 8.4, which define the levels of evidence and describe the meaningful use of it. PAGES 108–109

62. **Answer: C.** The ability to titrate the dose of nicotine can also be an issue in patients who are heavy users or continue to have cravings. Combination nicotine replacement therapy is a good practice to provide a baseline nicotine level with the patch and actively titrate levels using another source of nicotine replacement such as gum. One option for a secondary source of nicotine is nicotine gum; its major advantage is satisfying oral cravings. PAGE 333

63. **Answer: E.** Granulomatosis with polyangiitis is a rare disease affecting mostly white patients of either gender, and is characterized by Wegner triad (respiratory granulomas, vasculitis, and glomerulonephritis). The disease is fatal if untreated. c-ANCA is quite high. Subglottic stenosis occurs in 23% of patients with this disease. PAGE 276

64. **Answer: A.** A 45° branching is a hallmark of *Aspergillus*. *Rhizopus* and *Mucormycosis* have 90° branching. PAGE 134

65. **Answer: B.** Advantages of MRI are excellent soft tissue definition, multiplanar imaging, and lack of radiation exposure. Some useful applications of MRI are evaluation of skull base pathology, perineural spread of neoplasm, neoplastic marrow space involvement, neoplastic cartilage invasion, oral cavity pathology, particularly when compromised by dental amalgam artifact on CT. PAGE 148

66. **Answer: D.** Rheumatoid arthritis causes hoarseness by cricoarytenoid joint involvement, rheumatoid nodules within the cords, or involvement of the recurrent laryngeal nerve. Of patients with rheumatoid arthritis, 86% have histologic evidence of cricoarytenoid joint

involvement, and involvement of the ossicle is a rare cause of hearing loss. The temporo-mandibular joint can be severely affected. Concern for recurrent tenosynovitis involving the transverse ligament of the atlas resulting in laxity and/or odontoid process erosion, leading to instability of C1 in forward flexion with cord compression, compel one to radiographically evaluate rheumatoid arthritis patients prior to direct laryngoscopy. PAGE 270

67. **Answer: A.** In determining whether the results of a study are strong and consistent, the level of evidence generally increases as we progress from observational studies to controlled experiments (randomized trials). PAGE 99, 100, TABLE 7.12

68. **Answer: B.** Cochlear outer hair cells, particularly in patients who harbor mutation in the 12S RNA gene, are most sensitive to aminoglycoside ototoxicity. Much higher doses that cannot be given systemically are required to damage inner brain cells or the stria vascularis. PAGE 133

69. **Answer: B.** Angiogenesis restores blood flow to the wound and wound surface. The local tissue response to hypoxia is to increase the production of VEGF. In addition to VEGF, other angiogenic factors include FGF, TGF-α, and TGF-β. All promote the proliferation and growth of endothelial cells. PAGE 79

70. **Answer: A.** Frailty is the state of declining functional reserve. It may be related to epigenetic factors, but no particular genetic loci have been implicated. Frailty can exist at various ages. PAGE 299

71. **Answer: A.** The prestyloid parapharyngeal space (PPS) is anterior and lateral to the tensor-vascular-styloid fascia and contains primarily fat, minor salivary gland rests, and a small portion of the deep lobe of the parotid gland. Salivary tumors are the most common lesion of the PPS, and the MRI characteristics described are also characteristic of a pleomorphic adenoma. PAGE 171

72. **Answer: D.** Primary aldosteronism is characterized by *hypo*kalemia and hypertension. The other statements are factual. PAGES 258–259

73. **Answer: C.** Opiates are the mainstay of head and neck cancer pain therapy. Neuropathic pain does respond to pharmacologic therapy. Tricyclic antidepressants should be avoided in patients with cardiac disease. Initial opioid titration should be done with a single agent. PAGES 347–350

74. **Answer: A.** Amyotrophic lateral sclerosis is a motor neuron disease and, in the bulbar-onset form, may present with dysphagia, slurred speech, and evidence of tongue denervation. Guillain–Barré syndrome starts in the lower extremities and thus head and neck manifestations are late. Migraine does not impact motor functions, and the blood supply to the hypoglossal nucleus is from the anterior spinal artery. PAGE 208

75. **Answer: C.** There are reports of increased levels of mTOR in keloid scars. Since rapamycin inhibits mTOR, it may help to prevent hypertrophic or keloid scars and improve overall wound healing. PAGE 84

76. **Answer: D.** Diabetic wounds have dysregulated T-cell immunity; *defective leukocyte chemo-taxis*, phagocytosis, and bactericidal capacity; and dysfunctional fibroblast and epidermal cell activity. PAGE 81

77. **Answer: A.** Primary Sjögren syndrome is a diagnosis of exclusion, a progressive systemic autoimmune disease, and associated with >33% increase in the risk of lymphoma. The diagnosis of Sjögren syndrome is facilitated by testing of Ro/SS-A and La/SS-B antibodies, but these serologic tests lack sensitivity and specificity. Noncaseating granulomas are the hallmark of sarcoidosis. PAGE 271

78. **Answer: A.** The cellular dermal skin substitutes include allogenic keratinocytes and allogenic fibroblasts in addition to the acellular components (allogen and glycosaminogly-cans). Both cellular and acellular dermal skin substitutes are scaffolds that are subsequently replaced by native tissues. The acellular products are in more widespread use. PAGE 53

79. **Answer: A.** Hemodynamic effects of vasoactive agents vary among patients. Phenyleph-rine increases mean arterial and pulmonary artery occlusion pressures, may decrease or have no effect on cardiac index, and increases systemic vascular resistance. PAGE 58, TABLE 5.1

80. **Answer: B.** See Table 7.4, which provides possible explanations for positive study results. PAGE 89

81. **Answer: E.** More elderly individuals are presenting for health care, largely because of avail-ability of effective treatments. Elderly adults expect to be healthy longer, and the rise of awareness in geriatrics is tied to scientific advances in assessment and care. PAGES 298, 300

82. **Answer: C.** PET/CT has very limited utility in the evaluation of thyroid disease because ultrasound provides high-quality neck and thyroid imaging. PET/CT is reserved for patients with clinical evidence of disease recurrence and a negative posttreatment whole body ^{131}I scan and neck ultrasound. PAGE 174

83. **Answer: C.** Protamine sulfate must be used when bleeding problems occur in a heparin-ized patient. FFP will not reverse the coagulation effect caused by heparin. PAGE 30

84. **Answer: D.** Universal precautions require all methods listed except shoe covers. These are used to protect the skin and mucous membranes of the health care provider from blood and secretions. PAGE 21

85. **Answer: B.** Reverse T_3, an inactive thyroid hormone, is increased with illness, fasting, trauma, and with a variety of medicines. The thyroid releases 20 times more T_4 than T_3 into circulation. More than 99% of T_3 and T_4 are protein-bound. PAGE 257

86. **Answer: B.** *B. henselae* causes cat-scratch fever and is isolated from 50% of cats. Diagnosis is by seeing the pathogen histologically on Warthin–Starry silver staining. Inoculation is usually by scratch, but can occur via conjunctiva. The typical course is infection of an iso-lated lymph node that is self-limited. PAGE 283

87. **Answer: C.** Tuberculosis is an ongoing worldwide health problem. Transmission occurs via airborne droplets, and the laryngeal form of the disease is particularly infectious.

In contrast, after conversion of the PPD test, the disease can remain inactive. Treatment is by multidrug therapy started before drug sensitivity data are available. PAGES 284–285

88. **Answer: A.** For a lacerated eyelid, the primary repair is important because secondary scar revision and attempts to reestablish the function of a scarred eyelid or tear-drainage apparatus are difficult. Faulty primary repair, through failure to suture the tarsus well and removal of marginal sutures too soon, can produce a notch in the eyelid that interferes with its ability to spread the tear film and cause epiphora. PAGE 227

89. **Answer: D.** Oxidized cellulose topical agents, such as Surgicel (Ethicon), are knitted fabrics from oxidized cellulose that act as a scaffold for clot formation and have bactericidal properties. However, microfibrillar collagen has proven to be a superior topical hemostatic agent in randomized controlled trials. PAGE 52

90. **Answer: C.** Genetic imprinting is an epigenetic process that silences an allele derived from a specific parent such that only the genes from the other parent are expressed. The other definitions are accurate. PAGE 119

91. **Answer: A.** The availability of immediate assessment is important for maximizing yield from FNA and reduces the likelihood of repeating the procedure. Suction is commonly employed. PAGE 180

92. **Answer: B.** Treatment for cardiac arrest after overdose of local anesthetics includes management of the airway to prevent hypoxia and acidosis. A 20% lipid emulsion bolus is most helpful in treating bupivacaine overdose, although the mechanism is not well understood. Midazolam prevents seizures but does not treat cardiac arrest. Naloxone treats narcotic overdose. PAGE 237

93. **Answer: B.** mecA encodes for a PBP with low affinity for β-Lactamase antibiotics. β-Lactamase production, penicillinase production, and drug efflux pumps are other known bacterial drug resistance mechanisms. PAGE 134

94. **Answer: B.** Two studies are cited in the chapter, showing that hypovolemia secondary to inadequate fluid replacement or hemorrhage is the most likely cause of postoperative hypotension. PAGE 36

95. **Answer: C.** Sestamibi scanning is the most commonly used modality for localization of a parathyroid adenoma. Ultrasound of the neck may be an alternative for an experienced Ultrasound operator. PAGE 163, 174

96. **Answer: C.** Thermal effects of the laser may be reduced by the pulse-wave mode. Higher power will increase the thermal effect. Defocusing the beam widens the area of damage. Using a fiber does not change the energy delivered. PAGE 182

97. **Answer: D.** Chiari malformations are characterized by herniation of the contents of the posterior cranial fossa through foramen magnum, causing headaches, dizziness, and hoarseness due to involvement of the lower cranial nerves. Unilateral hearing loss is not associated with Chiari malformation. PAGE 214

98. **Answer: B.** The ultrasonic shears generate ultrasonic vibrations at 55,000 Hz (not electrical energy to denature proteins and coagulate vessels up to 2 mm). However, nearby nerves might be affected. PAGE 49

99. **Answer: A.** Tylenol is used for hyperthermia in a thyroid storm. Aspirin is contraindicated because it binds to thyroid-binding globulin and displaces T_4, increasing the available hormone. Thyrotoxic storm is treated with medications to block the production or release of thyroxine (e.g., propylthiouracil, iodides), control cardiac symptoms (e.g., propranolol if tachycardia, diuretics and digitalis if heart failure), and replace other deficiencies (e.g., hydrocortisone). PAGE 33

100. **Answer: C.** A meaningful abstract will provide a summary of the goals, methods, as well as results and significance of the research described. It is not a substitute for reading the entire article because it usually does not elaborate on the adverse events, study limitations, and dropouts or losses, and may present data that may lead to a biased conclusion. PAGE 86–87

101. **Answer: A.** A normal direct light reflex occurs when light is shined into the eye and the pupil constricts and then redilates after the stimulus is removed. The opposite pupil constricts as well with the stimulus, and this is known as the *consensual light reflex*. They should be brisk and equal. Pupillary constriction is also part of the "near-vision complex" associated with the process of accommodation. PAGE 218

102. **Answer: A.** Patients dying with advanced head and neck cancers usually have significant distressing symptoms, but their suffering can be decreased by palliative care involvement. Because cardiorespiratory arrest is the mechanism of death in these patients rather than the cause of death, resuscitation does not make sense, and this should be explained to the family. In dying patients, loss of the ability to handle tube feeds is common, so continuing tube feedings often shuts down the gastrointestinal tract, which can cause distress in the dying patient. PAGE 351

103. **Answer: D.** Confusion, polyuria, nephrolithiasis, and constipation are all manifestations of hypercalcemia. Tetany is a sign of hypocalcemia. PAGE 255, 264, TABLE 16.2

104. **Answer: A.** There is no level of secondhand smoke that is risk-free. Secondhand smoke has been proven to cause premature death and disease in both children and adults who are nonsmokers. In children, secondhand smoke results in increased risk for sudden infant death syndrome, acute respiratory infections, ear infections, and asthma. Children exposed to smoking by their parents also demonstrate slowed lung growth and suffer from respiratory symptoms. Adults exposed to secondhand smoke can develop coronary artery disease and lung cancer. PAGE 330

105. **Answer: B.** The main targets of nicotine are in the central nervous system, specifically the neuronal nicotinic acetylcholine receptors. It also acts on the mesolimbic dopamine system, resulting in reward signaling and addiction. Its effects on the brain include reduced anxiety and stress relief, in addition to slightly enhanced cognition and increased ability to fight fatigue. PAGE 329

106. **Answer: C.** Although the mechanism of action is not well understood, propofol produces sedation and amnesia with rapid onset and rapid clearance. PAGE 66

Rhinology and Allergy

1. Which of the following statements is true about the relationship of chronic rhinosinusitis and asthma?

   A. The severity of sinus symptom scores and the extent of sinus disease are directly correlated with asthma severity.
   B. Medical and surgical treatment of chronic rhinosinusitis in asthmatic patients does not seem to improve asthma symptoms.
   C. Sinus surgery does not lead to improvement of asthma symptoms in patients with Samter triad/aspirin-exacerbated respiratory disease (AERD).
   D. Almost no patients with cystic fibrosis show radiologic evidence of sinus disease.

2. A pregnant (20 weeks, primiparis) woman presents to your clinic complaining of severe nasal congestion for the past month, which has made it difficult for her to sleep. On examination she has a straight septum, bilateral boggy inferior turbinates, and no additional nasal abnormalities on endoscopy. What is the best initial recommendation?

   A. Trial of saline irrigations.
   B. Loratadine (Claritin) and a medrol dose pack.
   C. Loratadine (Claritin) and steroid nasal sprays.
   D. Do nothing, as there are no safe medications for the developing fetus.

3. Retaining a "periorbital sling" over the medial rectus during orbital decompression can prevent which complication?

   A. Diplopia
   B. Epistaxis
   C. Retro-orbital hematoma
   D. Overrecession of the globe

4. Which one of these cytokines is secreted by eosinophils and is responsible for their function and survival?

   A. Interleukin (IL) 2
   B. IL-4
   C. IL-5
   D. IL-12

5. During septoplasty, what maneuver should be avoided when addressing the bony septum?

   A. Grasp the perpendicular plate with forceps and use a twisting motion to remove the fragments of bone.
   B. Use a double action instrument to make a superior cut in the bony septum, followed by removal of the deviated portion of the septum.
   C. Use an osteotome to fracture the bony septum; then remove the fragments of bone.
   D. Use through-cutting instruments to remove the bony septum in a piecemeal fashion.

6. Which of these is the most commonly identified organism in intracranial abscesses due to sinusitis?

   A. *Pseudomonas aeruginosa*
   B. *Haemophilus influenzae*
   C. *Streptococcus pneumoniae*
   D. *Streptococcus viridans*

7. Which of the following is true for iatrogenic cerebrospinal fluid (CSF) leaks resulting from endoscopic sinus surgery?

   A. Most commonly occur at the posterior ethmoid roof.
   B. Leaks more commonly occur on the right side.
   C. Majority of leaks manifest in a delayed fashion.
   D. Leaks are equally common in the hands of novice and experienced surgeons.

8. A 52-year-old man complains of fluctuating smell loss and nasal obstruction. Which of these would be your first line of treatment to prescribe?

   A. Zinc supplements and α-lipoic acid
   B. Immunotherapy for allergic rhinitis
   C. Gabapentin with nasal saline drops
   D. Tapered dose of oral steroids, followed by topical nasal steroids

9. Within which suture line is the anterior ethmoid canal found?

    A. Nasofrontal
    B. Zygomaticosphenoid
    C. Frontoethmoidal
    D. Zygomaticofrontal

10. What is the most common location of the ophthalmic artery in relation to the optic nerve as it runs through the optic canal?

    A. Lateral
    B. Superior
    C. Inferior
    D. Medial

11. A cerebrospinal fluid leak during ethmoidectomy is most likely to occur at:

    A. The junction of fovea ethmoidalis and lamina papyracea
    B. The medial fovea ethmoidalis
    C. The insertion of the uncinate process
    D. The planum sphenoidale

12. Which of the following is felt to be the primary effector cell type in nasal polyp inflammation?

    A. T lymphocyte
    B. IgE-producing plasma cell
    C. Epithelial cell
    D. Eosinophil

13. Which of the CD markers is present on all T cells?

    A. CD3
    B. CD6
    C. CD16
    D. CD33

14. Which of the following is most true regarding allergic fungal rhinosinusitis?

    A. It should be treated with surgical removal of mucin and polyps.
    B. Fungal stains and cultures are not necessary.
    C. Postoperative oral corticosteroids are not as important as preoperative administration.
    D. Topical antifungal medications reduce postoperative mucosal inflammation.

15. To best determine whether the lamina papyracea is intact, which test or procedure should be used?

    A. Intraoperative CT scan
    B. Fat float test
    C. Bulb press test
    D. Endoscopic dissection and search for orbital fat

16. At which location is the anterior ethmoidal artery found?

    A. Behind the anterior face of the ethmoid bulla unless a suprabullar recess exists
    B. Between the agger nasi cell and the ethmoid bulla
    C. Running posteromedially to anterolaterally in a mesentery across the skull base
    D. In a bony mesentery running across the skull base

17. Which of the following has been demonstrated for environmental control of allergic disease?

    A. Complete elimination of allergen alleviates symptoms.
    B. Dehumidifiers are superior to HEPA filters for dust mite control.
    C. Mattress/pillow covers reduce dust mite-induced allergy symptoms.
    D. Dehumidifiers reduce allergy symptoms but cause more nasal dryness.

18. An appropriate initial management option for patients with intermittent allergic rhinitis characterized by itchy, sneezy, runny nose includes:

    A. Oral corticosteroids
    B. Surgical turbinate reduction
    C. Antihistamines
    D. Allergen-specific immunotherapy

19. What postoperative complication may occur with excessive manipulation of the posterior aspect of the inferior turbinate during reduction surgery?

    A. Rhinitis
    B. Sinusitis
    C. Cerebrospinal fluid rhinorrhea
    D. Epistaxis

20. Which of these is the most commonly identified organism in subperiosteal orbital abscess due to sinusitis?

    A. *Pseudomonas aeruginosa*
    B. *Haemophilus influenzae*
    C. *Streptococcus pneumoniae*
    D. *Streptococcus viridans*

21. Patients with Pott's puffy tumor do not typically have:

    A. Purulent rhinorrhea
    B. Osteomyelitis of the frontal bone
    C. Frontal sinusitis
    D. Epidural abscess

22. Comprehensive sinus dissection prior to orbital decompression will usually prevent postobstructive sinusitis. What additional maneuver is recommended to prevent frontal outflow tract obstruction?

    A. Perform a Draf III.
    B. Leave postoperative packing for 4 weeks.
    C. Do not dissect anterior to the bulla ethmoidalis.
    D. Retain 1 cm of lamina papyracea.

23. Occupational rhinitis can be caused by low-molecular-weight or high-molecular-weight compounds. Which of the following is true of low-molecular-weight compounds?

    A. Animal dander is an example of a low-molecular-weight compound.
    B. Low-molecular-weight compounds more commonly cause occupational rhinitis.
    C. Skin allergy testing is readily performed with standardized extracts of low-molecular-weight compounds.
    D. Low-molecular-weight compounds must be coupled with a protein to form a hapten–protein complex in order to elicit an IgE-mediated response.

24. What is the most common cause of epiphora for a woman in her 70s?

    A. Dacryolith
    B. Lacrimal duct stenosis
    C. Trauma related
    D. Dacryocyst

25. MRI is most appropriate in evaluating:

    A. Extent of sinus disease in chronic sinusitis
    B. Determining normal anatomic structures in cases of extensive nasal polyposis
    C. Suspected orbital or intracranial extension of tumor
    D. Location of the anterior ethmoidal artery

26. Which of these is an intracranial complication with the most favorable outcome?

    A. Epidural abscess
    B. Meningitis
    C. Subdural abscess
    D. Intracerebral abscess

27. A patient undergoing endoscopic sinus surgery has proptosis, chemosis, and a firm globe despite attempts to treat with medical therapy. Which one of the following is the next best treatment at this time?

    A. Stat CT scan
    B. Lateral canthotomy and orbital decompression
    C. Re-treat with a higher dose of mannitol and dexamethasone
    D. Transfer to ophthalmology service for ocular paracentesis

28. Which of the following is *not* an indication for computer-image-guided surgery according to the American Academy of Otolaryngology-Head and Neck Surgery consensus statement guidelines?

    A. Revision sinus surgery
    B. Extensive nasal polyposis
    C. Cases involving cerebrospinal fluid (CSF) leak repair
    D. Cases involving concha bullosa takedown

29. Which of the following irrigations has proven to be effective at breaking up biofilm while at the same time preserving greater than 90% ciliary function in clinical trials?

    A. Manuka honey
    B. Baby shampoo
    C. Citric acid zwitterionic surfactant
    D. None of the above

30. Which of the following is the most common complication of endoscopic sinus surgery (ESS)?

    A. Synechia formation
    B. Cerebrospinal fluid leak
    C. Orbital violation
    D. Epistaxis

31. What is the purpose of preserving the "keystone area" during septoplasty?

    A. To maintain appropriate support of the nasal dorsum to prevent postoperative saddle nose deformity
    B. To keep cartilage available for future rhinoplastic procedures
    C. To support the lower lateral cartilages
    D. To prevent postoperative epistaxis

32. For which reason is Fel d 1 a "major allergen" from cats?

    A. More than 50% individuals sensitized to cat are sensitized to Fel d 1.
    B. Fel d 1 sensitization is associated with more symptoms than other cat allergens.
    C. Fel d 1 is the most common protein found in cat dander.
    D. Fel d 1 is the only cat allergen with which sIgE can bind.

33. Which of the following bacteria is not commonly seen in chronic sinusitis?

    A. *Pseudomonas aeruginosa*
    B. *Staphylococcus aureus*
    C. *Chlamydia trachomatis*
    D. Coagulase-negative Staphylococcus

34. What is the recommended first-line antibiotic in a patient with acute sinusitis and no medication allergies?

    A. Penicillin
    B. Azithromycin
    C. Amoxicillin
    D. Levafloxacin
    E. Amoxicillin-clavulanate

35. What postoperative complication may occur as a result of resection of the inferior turbinate or injury to the inferior turbinate mucosa?

    A. Sinusitis
    B. Nasal septal perforation
    C. Empty nose syndrome
    D. Samter's triad

36. Which of the following laboratory studies is most specific for suspected cerebrospinal fluid (CSF) rhinorrhea?

    A. Glucose strip test
    B. Protein analysis of fluid
    C. Albumin level of fluid
    D. β2-transferrin analysis

37. What is the most common attachment site for the uncinate process?

    A. Lamina papyracea
    B. Skull base
    C. Bulla ethmoidalis
    D. Middle turbinate

38. Which of the following drugs is *not* recommended for the treatment of methicillin-resistant *Staphylococcus aureus* (MRSA) in monotherapy?

    A. Rifampin
    B. Linezolid
    C. Tetracycline
    D. Clindamycin

39. In patients with cerebrospinal fluid (CSF) rhinorrhea after skull base fracture, the use of prophylactic antibiotics is associated with:

    A. Decrease in frequency of meningitis
    B. Reduction in meningitis-related mortality
    C. Less need for surgical repair of CSF leakage
    D. No apparent therapeutic benefit

40. All of the following are advantages of MR imaging for sinonasal disease, *except*:

    A. Lack of radiation exposure
    B. Excellent bony anatomy definition
    C. Multiplanar reconstruction
    D. Detailed soft tissue definition
    E. Differentiation between secretions and soft tissue

41. Which of these are the most common pathogens associated with acute bacterial rhinosinusitis?

    A. *Streptococcus pneumoniae, Haemophilus influenzae, Staphylococcus aureus,* and *Moraxella catarrhalis*
    B. *Streptococcus pneumoniae, H. influenzae,* Enterobacteriaceae, and *M. catarrhalis*
    C. *Streptococcus pneumoniae, H. influenzae, Staphylococcus aureus,* and Enterobacteriaceae
    D. Enterobacteriaceae, *H. influenzae, Staphylococcus aureus,* and *M. catarrhalis*

42. In cases of acute invasive fungal rhinosinusitis in which *Pseudoallescheria boydii* is identified, which of the following management steps is recommended?

    A. Medical therapy with voriconazole.
    B. Limit surgical resection outside the paranasal sinuses.
    C. Repeat the fungal culture in diabetic patients.
    D. Amphotericin use should be limited to topical nasal irrigations.

43. What is the most characteristic skin lesion of sarcoidosis?

    A. Erythema nodosum
    B. Lupus pernio
    C. Subcutaneous nodules
    D. Ulcerative lesions

44. Which of these is the main IgG subclass that is increased during maintenance immunotherapy?

    A. IgG1
    B. IgG2
    C. IgG3
    D. IgG4

45. **For which of the following reasons is CT favored over MR for routine sinonasal imaging?**

    A. CT better demonstrates the bony walls of the sinuses.
    B. CT provides better soft tissue detail compared to MR.
    C. CT differentiates between soft tissue and fluid.
    D. CT is ideal for evaluating the brain and orbit.

46. **Which of the following is true about the relationship between allergic rhinitis and asthma?**

    A. There is no evidence of inflammation in both the upper and lower airways in patients who have either allergic rhinitis or asthma.
    B. Medical treatment of allergic rhinitis in patients with concurrent asthma has no effect on asthma symptoms.
    C. Allergic rhinitis is an independent risk factor for the development of asthma.
    D. Targeted/specific immunotherapy in patients with allergic rhinitis without asthma does not seem to slow or prevent the subsequent development of asthma.

47. **Hereditary hemorrhagic telangiectasia is best described by:**

    A. Most commonly presents on the turbinates
    B. Requires screening for endocarditis
    C. Is treated in the perioperative period with amino caproic acid
    D. Results from dysregulation in the transforming growth factor beta (TGF-β) and vascular endothelial growth factor (VEGF) pathways

48. **Chronic sinusitis is differentiated from acute sinusitis on CT imaging based on the presence of:**

    A. Frothy secretions within the paranasal sinuses
    B. Ostial obstruction
    C. Bony sclerosis
    D. Mucosal thickening

49. **What structure marks the posterior limit of the frontal recess?**

    A. Agger nasi
    B. Basal lamella
    C. Anterior ethmoid artery
    D. Bulla ethmoidalis

50. The natural os of the maxillary sinus is identified in what orientation?

    A. Parasaggital plane
    B. Coronal
    C. Axial
    D. Variable

51. A patient presents in the office with a history of smell loss that occurs intermittently and with varying degrees. During the evaluation and testing, you would expect to find:

    A. Absent olfactory bulbs on MRI
    B. Frontal contusions on contrast-enhanced CT of the brain
    C. Opacified ethmoid sinuses on noncontrast CT of the sinuses
    D. Areas of demyelination on contrast-enhanced MRI of the brain

52. What is the mechanism of action of vasoconstriction by topical decongestants?

    A. α-Adrenergic stimulation of the nasal mucosa and blood vessels
    B. Release of exogenous norepinephrine
    C. Parasympathetic stimulation of the nasal mucosa
    D. Release of endogenous acetylcholine

53. In which form do bacteria most commonly exist?

    A. 10% planktonic, 90% in biofilm
    B. 30% planktonic, 70% in biofilm
    C. 90% planktonic, 10% in biofilm
    D. 1% planktonic, 99% in biofilm

54. Which of these is the pattern of auricular inflammation in relapsing polychondritis?

    A. Lobule-sparing
    B. Conchal bowl only
    C. Helical sparing
    D. Total auricle

55. During an anterior transmaxillary approach, the anterior wall of the maxillary sinus should be reconstructed with:

    A. Bone graft
    B. Cartilage graft
    C. Titanium mesh
    D. No need for reconstruction

56. The term "allergy" refers to which of the following?

    A. An elevated total serum IgE level
    B. Demonstrable IgE reaction to an allergen
    C. Presence of corresponding symptoms upon allergen exposure
    D. In vitro demonstration of an allergen-specific IgE

57. The anterior transmaxillary approach provides access to:

    A. Pterygopalatine fossa
    B. Lateral recess of the sphenoid sinus
    C. Infratemporal fossa
    D. All are correct

58. Which surgical landmark indicates the posterior limit of bone dissection in the endo-scopic modified Lothrop procedure (EMLP)?

    A. Middle turbinate
    B. Posterior table of frontal sinus
    C. Posterior border of septectomy
    D. First olfactory neuron

59. The sphenopalatine artery is a branch of:

    A. Facial artery
    B. Ascending palatine artery
    C. Superficial temporal artery
    D. Internal maxillary artery

60. A patient has nasal congestion when in his basement apartment. A specific IgE (sIgE) panel is positive only for a mold, *Helminthosporium*. He seeks a second opinion, and his skin prick test is negative for *Helminthosporium*. Which is the best explanation?

    A. sIgE testing is more sensitive and less specific than skin prick tests.
    B. His mold sensitization changed in the week between tests.
    C. *Helminthosporium* testing may vary between manufacturers.
    D. His nasal congestion is not caused by mold allergy.

61. Which of these is the most effective pharmacological treatment for children and adults with AR?

    A. Intranasal antihistamines
    B. Intranasal steroids
    C. Oral antihistamines
    D. Leukotriene inhibitors

62. What are the indications for imaging in acute sinusitis?

    A. Any patient who has a child in day care or works in a health care environment
    B. Any patient who has had exposure to antibiotics within the previous 6 weeks
    C. Any patient suspected of complications of acute sinusitis or who is immunocompromised and at high risk for such complications
    D. Any patient who has a history of recurrent acute sinusitis presenting with an acute flare

63. All structures have a relation with the sphenoid sinus, *except*:

    A. Anterior cranial fossa
    B. Posterior cranial fossa
    C. Meckel's cave
    D. Optic nerve
    E. External carotid artery

64. The creation of a middle meatus antrostomy includes removal of:

    A. Anterior pole of middle turbinate
    B. Inferior concha bone
    C. Uncinate process
    D. Agger nasi

65. What is the proper initial work-up for a patient status post bone marrow transplant who complains of a change in sensation in left trigeminal distribution, left facial pressure, and headache but no fever nor nasal discharge?

    A. CT scan of the sinuses
    B. CT scan of the sinuses and otolaryngology consultation for sinonasal endoscopy
    C. CT scan of the sinuses, otolaryngology consultation for sinonasal endoscopy, MRI of brain and sinuses
    D. CT scan of the sinuses, otolaryngology consultation for sinonasal endoscopy, MRI of brain and sinuses, neurology consultation

66. What additional therapy or work-up is indicated if a patient diagnosed with acute rhinosinusitis has been treated with nasal saline irrigations, topical decongestant sprays, and acetaminophen, but has persistent congestion, purulent nasal discharge, low-grade fever, and headache on day 4 of illness?

    A. Add an antibiotic
    B. Culture the maxillary sinus contents
    C. Obtain a CT scan of the sinuses
    D. Adjust analgesic medication for improved pain control
    E. Add an antihistamine

67. Eosinophilic mucin is characterized by all of the following *except*:

    A. Accumulations of pyknotic and degranulated eosinophils
    B. Clumps of fungal debris
    C. Sheets of lightly eosinophilic mucin
    D. Charcot–Leyden crystals

68. What is the condition called when a patient complains of excessive tearing that runs on to their cheek?

    A. Watery eye
    B. Conjunctivitis
    C. Epiphora
    D. Dacryocystitis

69. Which of the following is a significant limitation of endoluminal embolization for control of epistaxis?

    A. High incidence of facial necrosis.
    B. Inability to safely embolize contributions from the internal carotid artery.
    C. Few agents are available to occlude the small internal maxillary branches.
    D. Requires inguinal artery catheterization.

70. Which of the following forms the medial boundary of the frontal recess?

    A. Septum
    B. Middle turbinate
    C. Lamina papyracea
    D. Ethmoid bulla

71. Toxic shock syndrome results from the exotoxin of which bacteria?

    A. *H. influenzae*
    B. *M. catarrhalis*
    C. *S. aureus*
    D. *P. aeruginosa*

72. Which of the following are indications for obtaining a CT scan of the sinuses during the evaluation of sinonasal pathology?

    A. Clinical deterioration on medical therapy for acute bacterial rhinosinusitis
    B. Failed medical management of chronic rhinosinusitis
    C. Preoperative planning of sinonasal neoplasm resection
    D. Frontal sinus fracture
    E. All of the above

73. What is the most common complication of acute sinusitis?

    A. Meningitis
    B. Orbital subperiosteal abscess
    C. Pott's puffy tumor
    D. Subdural abscess
    E. Epidural abscess

74. A teenage patient seen in your office has a runny nose, sneezing, and tired-looking eyes on examination. When questioned, he reports that his grades at school have dropped off, and he "always feels tired." He reports that the symptoms have been constant "for about the last 5 months, and they are worse in the spring." According to the 2008 ARIA (the Allergic Rhinitis and its Impact on Asthma) guidelines, what classification of allergic rhinitis would this patient have?

    A. Moderate/severe seasonal
    B. Mild intermittent
    C. Mild seasonal
    D. Moderate/severe persistent
    E. Moderate/severe intermittent

75. Which of the following classes of medications are effective for chronic rhinosinusitis with nasal polyps, as demonstrated by multiple randomized placebo-controlled trials?

    A. Nasal steroid spray
    B. Antibiotics
    C. Montelukast
    D. Guaifenesin

76. Underlying factors that may contribute to the development of chronic rhinosinusitis (CRS) include all of the following except:

    A. Smoking
    B. Allergy
    C. Biofilms
    D. Alcohol intake

77. Which of the following is a useful anatomic relationship to find the sphenoid sinus?

    A. The sphenoid sinus is 1 cm distal to the skull base.
    B. The posterior wall of the maxillary sinus is in the same plane as the anterior wall of the sphenoid sinus.
    C. The distance from nasal spine to sphenoid ostium is 6 cm.
    D. The sphenoid ostium lies lateral to the superior turbinate just behind the last posterior ethmoid cell.

78. The carotid artery and optic nerve are dehiscent in the lateral aspect of the sphenoid sinus in what percentage of patients?

    A. 50% / 25%
    B. 5% / 15%
    C. 25% / 6%
    D. 10% / 1%

79. What is the initial radiographic study of choice in a patient with suspected cerebrospinal fluid (CSF) leak from accidental trauma?

    A. High-resolution CT scan
    B. MR imaging
    C. CT cisternogram
    D. Radionuclide cisternogram
    E. MR cisternogram

80. Our ability to identify specific odors depends on:

    A. The one receptor–one odor theory
    B. Visual collateral input to the entorhinal cortex
    C. Intact taste receptors
    D. Differential activation of different olfactory receptors

81. Regarding the external ethmoidectomy, which statement is *correct*?

    A. An incision in the periorbita facilitates the dissection posteriorly and exposure of the lamina papyracea.
    B. The anterior ethmoidal artery is encountered in the frontoethmoidal suture line approximately 24 mm posterior to the anterior lacrimal crest.
    C. The distance between the anterior ethmoidal artery and the posterior ethmoidal artery is constant (10 mm).
    D. The dissection beyond the posterior ethmoidal artery is safe if performed up to 8 mm from the artery.

82. Which of the following is the most important reason to identify Onodi cells on preoperative CT?

    A. They allow identification of the posterior limit of the ethmoid cavity.
    B. When present, they alter the level of the ethmoid skull base.
    C. When present, the opticocarotid recess resides in the ethmoid cavity.
    D. When present, they alter the location of the sphenoid ostia.

83. Which sphenoid pneumatization pattern is the most common?

    A. Conchal
    B. Presellar
    C. Sellar
    D. Onodi cell

84. A 38-year-old woman presents with olfactory loss of one-month duration after a severe upper respiratory tract infection. She is particularly disturbed by a constant foul odor seemingly occurring from the right side. Which of the following would you advise the patient to do?

    A. To undergo a craniotomy and resection of the olfactory bulbs to completely eliminate the foul smell
    B. To start gabapentin to decrease the severity of the smell
    C. To use saline drops and wait for the smell to diminish over time
    D. To undergo endoscopic resection of the right olfactory epithelium

85. A false-positive sweat test can occur with all the following diseases, *except*:

    A. Hypoparathyroidism
    B. Dehydration
    C. Adrenal insufficiency
    D. Skin edema
    E. Lab error

86. Which one of the following conditions is *not* a risk factor for the development of fungal balls of the paranasal sinuses?

    A. Age >49 years
    B. Prior extractions of maxillary dentition
    C. Endodontic treatment of the maxillary dentition
    D. Zinc-oxide–containing amalgam materials in endodontic surgery

87. Which of the following is not considered part of the nasal valve?

    A. Head of the inferior turbinate
    B. Bony piriform aperture
    C. Nasal floor
    D. Membranous septum

88. What is the thinnest part of the anterior skull base?

    A. Ethmoid roof (fovea ethmoidalis)
    B. Lateral lamella
    C. Sella turcica
    D. Planum sphenoidale

89. Which of these cells are responsible for the regenerative capacity of the olfactory neuroepithelium?

    A. Basal cells
    B. Microvillar supporting cells
    C. Olfactory neurons
    D. Ensheathing cells

90. If nasal lymphoma is suspected, the otolaryngologist should:

    A. Feel comfortable taking exclusive patient care
    B. Obtain biopsies of sample tissue sent fresh
    C. Obtain biopsies of ample tissue sent in formaldehyde
    D. Obtain a sparing biopsy sent fresh or in formaldehyde

91. A patient complains of nasal allergies during the spring season. A multiprick device is used to apply eight skin prick tests consisting of a positive and negative control and six local antigenic trees. At 20 minutes, all eight skin sites have developed 7-mm wheals. Which is the best interpretation?

    A. The patient has allergic sensitivity to all six trees tested.
    B. The patient is exhibiting a hypersensitivity to the glycerin.
    C. The patient has recently taken an antihistamine, which interferes with the results.
    D. Although the patient denies any previous skin conditions, he or she likely has psoriasis.

92. Which of these branching patterns does the most recent classification of chronic rhinosinusitis (CRS) use?

    A. Eosinophilic vs. noneosinophilic, then polypoid vs. nonpolypoid
    B. Polypoid vs. nonpolypoid, then eosinophilic vs. noneosinophilic
    C. Polypoid vs. nonpolypoid, then neutrophilic vs. nonneutrophilic
    D. Neutrophilic vs. nonneutrophilic, then polypoid vs. nonpolypoid

93. A 43-year-old man presents with a 3-week history of facial pain, nasal congestion, and purulent nasal drainage. Symptoms are slowly improving after being placed on antibiotics for 10 days, but are persistent. Which of the following statements is the most correct?

    A. A CT scan at this time is necessary to determine the sites of involvement.
    B. An MRI would be appropriate to determine the potential for complicated sinusitis.
    C. A CT with contrast would be helpful to assess for nasal polyposis.
    D. Imaging is not indicated at this time.

94. Which of the following methods is most commonly used to make the diagnosis of nasal polyp disease?

    A. Biopsy
    B. MR imaging
    C. History and examination
    D. Flow cytometry

95. Which of the following is most true about the relationship of allergy and chronic rhinosinusitis (CRS) with nasal polyposis?

    A. Studies have consistently found that nasal polyp patients with allergy have more severe disease.
    B. Allergen-specific immunotherapy has been shown to induce nasal polyp regression.
    C. Dysregulated IgE metabolism in nasal polyps is demonstrated by elevated antigen-specific and total IgE within nasal polyp tissue.
    D. Eosinophils in nasal polyps are a result of late-phase allergic inflammation.

96. Which of the following etiologies of cerebrospinal fluid (CSF) rhinorrhea is associated with highest risk of recurrence?

    A. Tumor
    B. Traumatic
    C. Spontaneous
    D. Congenital

97. Th2 cells secrete all of the following cytokines except:

    A. INF-γ
    B. IL-4
    C. IL-6
    D. IL-13

98. Which of the following is an imaging characteristic of most malignancies?

    A. CT high density
    B. T1 hyperintense
    C. T2 hypointense
    D. Orbital invasion

99. The agger nasi cell is identified on a coronal CT scan as:

    A. Cell extending into the frontal sinus
    B. Cell attached to the lamina papyracea
    C. Cell anterior to the attachment of middle turbinate
    D. Cell pneumatizing into middle turbinate

100. What is the best explanation for the pathophysiologic link between chronic rhinosinusitis and asthma?

    A. Nasobronchial reflex
    B. Pharyngobronchial reflex
    C. Posterior nasal drainage of inflammatory mediators
    D. Shared (systemic) inflammation

101. A 25-year-old man presents to you with severe nasal pruritus, sneezing, and profuse watery rhinorrhea. He had previous skin allergy testing, which showed no significant reactions. You perform a nasal smear, which shows 27% eosinophils. Which of the following is true of this patient's clinical syndrome?

    A. His symptoms were likely preceded by a history of aspirin sensitivity.
    B. The presence of nasal eosinophilia is generally regarded as a good prognostic indicator for his response to topical nasal steroids.
    C. The pathophysiology of this syndrome is well documented to be via COX-2 inhibition and leukotriene excess.
    D. Saccharin clearance test in this patient will likely be normal.

102. A patient presents for allergy testing using skin prick tests. The positive control of histamine shows no response. Which is the most likely explanation?

    A. The allergy nurse forgot to add the histamine to the diluent.
    B. The patient has no allergies, not even to histamine.
    C. The patient has anergic skin and should be evaluated for an immune deficiency.
    D. The patient has taken a medication that suppresses the response.

103. Which of the following is characteristic of the inflammatory response in allergic rhinitis?

    A. Mast cells degranulate upon the first/initial exposure to antigen/allergen.
    B. There is a predominance of Th2 cytokines like interleukin (IL) 4, IL-5, and IL-13.
    C. The late-phase allergic response occurs 30 minutes after exposure to antigen/allergen.
    D. There is a predominance of Th1 cytokines like interferon gamma, IL-2, and tumor necrosis factor beta.

104. Which is *not* a symptom used to make the diagnosis of chronic sinusitis?

    A. Mucopurulent drainage
    B. Nasal obstruction
    C. Facial pressure
    D. Headache

105. The diagnosis of allergic rhinitis is primarily based on:

    A. Allergy skin testing
    B. Specific IgE levels in serum
    C. Thorough history and physical examination
    D. Total IgE levels in serum

106. Side effects from long-term use of oral glucocorticoids include:

    A. Cataracts
    B. Avascular necrosis of the hip
    C. Glaucoma
    D. All of the above

107. Which of the following agents for the treatment of aspirin-exacerbated respiratory disease (AERD) targets the primary disease pathway?

    A. Oxymetazoline
    B. Fluticasone
    C. Montelukast
    D. Diphenhydramine

108. Chronic invasive fungal rhinosinusitis is clinically distinguished from acute invasive fungal rhinosinusitis by:

    A. Time course of disease
    B. Degree of tissue inflammation
    C. Causative fungal organism
    D. Presence of immunocompromise

109. Which of the following is not a technique to address the internal nasal valve?

    A. Spreader grafts
    B. Park sutures
    C. Splay graft
    D. Batten graft

110. When comparing subcutaneous immunotherapy (SCIT) to sublingual immunotherapy (SLIT), which of the statements below is true?

    A. SCIT has a lower rate of anaphylaxis than SLIT.
    B. SLIT efficacy is superior to SCIT.
    C. Sublingual therapy is an option for patients with an aversion to needles.
    D. SCIT requires daily injections.

111. Which of the following cell types are not found in normal olfactory neuroepithelium?

    A. Olfactory neurons
    B. Microvillar sustentacular cells
    C. Goblet cells
    D. Pseudostratified columnar epithelial cells

112. The prevalence of olfactory dysfunction in people older than 20 years is around which percentage?

    A. 1%
    B. 40%
    C. 20%
    D. 5%

113. The most common site of epistaxis is:

    A. Inferior turbinate
    B. Middle turbinate
    C. Anterior septum
    D. Sphenopalatine artery

114. The bony ridge that extends between the maxillary antrostomy inferiorly and the lamina papyracea superiorly allows which anatomic relationship to be noted?

    A. Posterior ethmoid air cells will be superior and the sphenoid sinus inferior.
    B. Sphenoid sinus will be superior and the posterior ethmoid air cells inferior.
    C. Frontal sinus outflow tract.
    D. Identification of the skull base posteriorly.

115. The Riedel procedure consists of which of these procedures and results?

    A. Removal of the entire anterior table of the frontal sinus and its floor. The frontal scalp stays in direct contact with the posterior table of the frontal sinus or dura and obliterates the frontal sinus, resulting in forehead concavity.
    B. Removal of the frontal sinus floor from orbit to orbit. The interfrontal septum and the superior nasal septum are resected to create a common outflow pathway for both frontal sinuses.
    C. Complete removal of the posterior table of the frontal sinus. The frontal recesses are covered with a pericranial flap to separate the nasal cavity from the intracranial space.
    D. The use of pericranium as an osteoplastic flap to obliterate the frontal sinus. A gap in the anterior table should remain along the inferior aspect of the osteotomy to provide space for the transposition of the pericranial flap into the frontal sinus and avoid compression of the flap pedicle.

116. A 30-year-old woman complains that her nose runs, she sneezes, and her eyes itch during the local ragweed season only. She has a cat, but denies her cat provokes any symptoms. Skin prick tests are positive for both ragweed and cat allergen with appropriate control responses. Which is the best interpretation of the positive cat allergen skin prick test?

    A. She is clinically allergic to cats, with poor symptom awareness.
    B. She is sensitized to cat allergen, but does not exhibit a clinical allergic response.
    C. The skin prick test is usually positive in cat owners.
    D. She is only clinically allergic to her cat during ragweed season.

117. Which of the following methods is used to diagnose aspirin-exacerbated respiratory disease (AERD)?

    A. Urinary leukotriene levels
    B. History of gastrointestinal discomfort after taking aspirin
    C. Aspirin challenge
    D. Genetic testing

118. A type 4 frontoethmoidal cell is defined as:

    A. A single cell above the agger nasi cell
    B. A tier of cells above the agger nasi cell not extending above the frontal beak
    C. A tier of cells above the agger nasi cell extending above the frontal beak
    D. A cell extending more than 50% of the vertical height of the frontal sinus

119. Which of the following factors argues most strongly against the "fungal hypothesis" to explain chronic sinonasal inflammation?

    A. Fungi are ubiquitous and can be cultured from almost all healthy noses.
    B. Randomized trials have failed to show a benefit from antifungal treatment.
    C. Staphylococcal enterotoxins are more common than fungi in nasal mucus.
    D. Allergy to fungi has not been consistently demonstrated in clinical studies.

120. Which of the presenting symptoms of an intracranial complication of sinusitis, in the order of most to least common, is listed below?

    A. Purulent rhinorrhea > Fever > Headache > Altered mental status
    B. Fever > Altered mental status > Purulent rhinorrhea > Headache
    C. Headache > Fever > Altered mental status > Purulent rhinorrhea
    D. Altered mental status > Purulent rhinorrhea > Headache > Fever

121. All the following medications can impair allergy skin testing, *except*:

    A. Leukotriene receptor antagonist
    B. Tricyclic antidepressants
    C. Systemic corticosteroids
    D. H_1-receptor antagonists
    E. H_2-receptor antagonists

122. A 7-year-old boy presents with frequent upper respiratory tract infections. On auscultation, he is found to have rales, and after chest x-ray, bronchiectasis is suspected. He was referred by his primary care physician for evaluation of nasal polyps. What additional examination should be performed?

    A. MRI
    B. Sweat chloride
    C. Erythrocyte sedimentation rate
    D. Lip biopsy
    E. Flow cytometry

123. Which of the following most commonly causes nasal valve obstruction?

    A. Previous rhinoplasty
    B. Turbinate hypertrophy
    C. Nasal polyposis
    D. Congenital

124. Which of the following is a minor symptom of chronic rhinosinusitis (CRS)?

    A. Purulence
    B. Facial pressure
    C. Nasal obstruction
    D. Headache

125. A 66-year-old woman with epistaxis. Among the diagnoses provided, which is most likely?

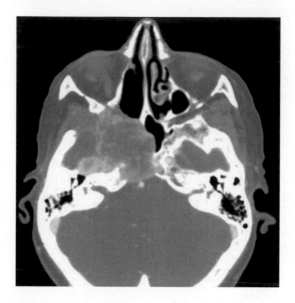

    A. Juvenile nasal angiofibroma (JNA)

    B. Hemangiopericytoma

    C. Meningioma

    D. Esthesioneuroblastoma

    E. Primary brain tumor

126. An 87-year-old woman with confusion. What is the duration of her sinusitis?

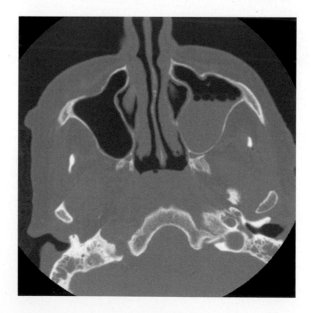

    A. Acute

    B. Subacute

    C. Chronic

    D. Lifelong

    E. There is no definite evidence of sinusitis

127. A 67-year-old man with nasal congestion. The most likely diagnosis is:

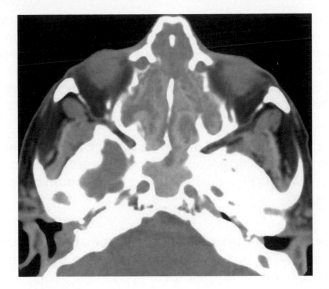

   A. Nasal polyposis
   B. Esthesioneuroblastoma
   C. Acute bacterial sinusitis
   D. Invasive fungal sinusitis (IFS)
   E. Allergic fungal sinusitis

128. A 66-year-old man being evaluated before endoscopic sinus surgery. What is the most worrisome complication of functional endoscopic sinus surgery in this patient?

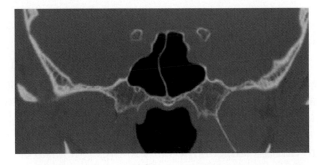

   A. Cerebrospinal fluid leak
   B. Empty nose syndrome
   C. Meningitis
   D. Carotid artery injury
   E. Encephalocele

Chapter 2 Answers

1. **Answer: A.** In patients with chronic rhinosinusitis and asthma, there is a positive correlation between the severity of sinus disease and the severity of asthma. Most patients with cystic fibrosis have radiologic evidence of sinus inflammatory disease. Treatment of rhinosinusitis improves asthma symptoms. Finally, patients with AERD obtain the same degree of symptomatic improvement after endoscopic sinus surgery as other patients with chronic rhinosinusitis. PAGE 554–555

2. **Answer: A.** Saline nasal sprays and irrigations are safe for pregnant women with rhinitis. Other medications may be considered "allowed" at various stages of pregnancy—for example, Loratadine (Claritin) is a category B drug—but should be approved by the patient's OB-GYN. PAGE 480–481

3. **Answer: A.** Leaving a strip of periorbita over the medial rectus during endoscopic orbital decompression will reduce prolapse of the muscle into the ethmoid compartment and reduce the incidence of diplopia. PAGE 633

4. **Answer: C.** IL-5 is secreted by Th2 cells, activated eosinophils, and mast cells. It functions as a growth and survival factor for eosinophils and is one of the cytokines that appear to be upregulated in eosinophilic inflammatory disease. PAGE 384

5. **Answer: B.** During septal bone removal, it is important not to apply strong torqueing forces to the bone attached to the skull base. Doing so may cause a cerebrospinal fluid leak. For this reason, through-cutting instrumentation should be used, or the septal bone should be incised superiorly, allowing the inferior bony septum to be removed with greater force. PAGE 615

6. **Answer: D.** The viridans group streptococci are the most common cause of complicated sinusitis with intracranial extension. PAGE 577–578

7. **Answer: B.** Iatrogenic CSF leaks occur more commonly on the right side. Most should be recognizable intraoperatively. Studies have shown that surgeon experience determines the rate of complications such as CSF rhinorrhea. Why do most CSF leaks occur on the right? Most surgeons are right handed. The natural angle of view and vector of surgical instrumentation tends to direct a surgeon medially in the right nasal cavity. The thinnest portion of the anterior skull base is the lateral lamella of the cribriform plate, along the medial aspect of the ethmoid roof. This location is a common site for iatrogenic CSF leak. PAGE 664

8. **Answer: D.** Fluctuating loss of smell, accompanied by nasal obstruction points to inflammatory sinonasal disease as the etiology. Although immunotherapy might be beneficial for patients with allergic rhinitis, it is not first-line therapy. PAGE 373, 376

9. **Answer: C** While performing external ethmoidectomy, the anterior ethmoid artery may be reliably found in the frontoethmoidal suture line. PAGE 506

10. **Answer: C.** The ophthalmic artery courses inferior to the optic nerve, as demonstrated in the figure. PAGE 624

11. **Answer: B.** The thinnest portion of the anterior skull base is at the medial aspect of the fovea ethmoidalis (the lateral lamella of the cribriform plate). PAGE 656

12. **Answer: D.** Most chronic rhinosinusitis with nasal polyposis is characterized by a pronounced eosinophilic inflammation. The eosinophils secrete a variety of substances which cause tissue damage and perpetuate a cycle of inflammation. PAGE 530

13. **Answer: A.** CD3 is known as the pan–T cell marker. PAGE 385

14. **Answer: A.** The treatment approach for allergic fungal rhinosinusitis includes surgical removal of mucin and polyps, systemic corticosteroids administered perioperatively and as needed for polyp recurrence, and long-term topical steroids. Detection of fungus in sinus secretions is required for the diagnosis. Both pre- and post-op systemic steroids are considered to be important. Topical antifungal agents are not recommended. PAGES 570–571

15. **Answer: C.** Frequent reassessment of the bony integrity of the lamina papyracea during ethmoidectomy and frontal sinusotomy is recommended, especially if using powered instrumentation. This is best accomplished with the bulb press test. PAGE 651

16. **Answer: A.** If a suprabullar recess does not exist, the anterior wall of the bulla serves as a valuable landmark to identify the anterior ethmoid artery at the skull base. The anterior ethmoidal artery courses along the skull base in a posterolateral-to-anteromedial orientation. PAGE 683

17. **Answer: A.** Most environmental control efforts are incompletely successful because single measures do not adequately reduce allergen exposure. The relative efficacy of individual measures is not known. However, complete elimination of allergen exposure (as can occur with a geographic change) will alleviate symptoms. PAGE 463

18. **Answer: C.** For patients with intermittent allergic rhinitis, antihistamines are first-line therapy. Immunotherapy is reserved for patients with persistent allergic rhinitis. Surgery and oral steroids are used only in select circumstances. PAGE 464

19. **Answer: D.** The inferior turbinate receives most of its blood supply from sphenopalatine branches that enter the turbinate posteriorly. Surgery on the posterior portion of the inferior turbinate increases the risk of large-volume epistaxis postoperatively. PAGE 618

20. **Answer: D.** The viridans group of streptococci is the most common cause of orbital subperiosteal abscess. These organisms are also the most common cause of intracranial complications. PAGES 577–578

21. **Answer: A.** Patients with Pott's puffy tumor present with frontal swelling and pain due to infection of the frontal sinus and frontal bone. They may develop epidural abscess. However, purulent rhinorrhea is not common. PAGE 583

22. **Answer: D.** Although most of the lamina papyracea needs to be removed to accomplish an effective medial orbital decompression, retaining 1 cm of anterior lamina in the region of the frontal outflow tract is important to prevent frontal obstruction. PAGE 633

23. **Answer: D.** Some rare allergens are too small to function as an epitope. These low-molecular-weight substances can function as an allergen only when conjugated to another protein (called a hapten). PAGE 474

24. **Answer: B.** The most common cause of epiphora in elderly women is lacrimal duct stenosis. PAGE 624 Epiphora in middle-aged women is generally caused by a dacryolith formed in the lacrimal sac.

25. **Answer: C.** MR imaging is not appropriate for most rhinosinusitis, and is not as helpful as CT for defining sinonasal anatomy. However, MR imaging is superior for the evaluation of soft tissue processes in the anatomic compartments adjacent to the paranasal sinuses. PAGES 422–425

26. **Answer: A.** Of all the intracranial complications listed here, epidural abscess has the best prognosis. PAGES 580–581

27. **Answer: B.** This patient has signs of an orbital hematoma. Failed medical management should prompt immediate decompression, which can be accomplished endoscopically and via lateral canthotomy/inferior cantholysis. PAGE 651

28. **Answer: D.** Image guidance is neither appropriate nor required for simple nasal surgeries such as a concha bullosa resection. Image guidance *is* indicated for sinus surgery in the setting of neoplasm, CSF leak, nasal polyp disease, or revision surgery. PAGE 601

29. **Answer: D.** Although a variety of substances have the ability to disrupt bacterial biofilms, these often have damaging effects on the nasal mucosa and can disrupt mucociliary clearance. PAGE 546

30. **Answer: A.** Synechia formation is the most common complication of ESS. Often these synechiae do not have functional significance. On the other hand, they may impair endoscopic access to the sinuses, cause mucus recirculation, limit access for topical therapy, or cause sinus obstruction. PAGE 657

31. **Answer: A.** The perpendicular plate and quadrangular cartilages just underneath the upper lateral cartilages should be preserved to avoid external nasal deformity. PAGE 614

32. **Answer: A.** A major allergen is defined as an antigen to which >50% of allergic individuals are sensitive. Most "allergens," such as dust mites, contain multiple potentially allergenic proteins. PAGE 413

33. **Answer: C.** Culture studies of patients with chronic sinusitis have shown *Pseudomonas* and *Staphylococcus* to be common bacteria in chronic sinusitis. *C. trachomatis* is a sexually transmitted pathogen that affects the urogenital tract. PAGE 589

34. **Answer: C.** Despite high rates of antibiotic resistance in the current era, amoxicillin is still considered to be first-line therapy for acute bacterial sinusitis. In uncomplicated cases there is little additional benefit to be gained from the use of more expensive broader-spectrum antibiotics. PAGE 518

35. **Answer: C.** Overaggressive surgery on the inferior turbinates may result in excessive nasal drying or phantom (paradoxical) nasal obstruction. PAGE 618

36. **Answer: D.** The most specific laboratory test to detect CSF is the β-transferrin assay. β-Transferrin is not present in sinonasal secretions. PAGES 665–666

37. **Answer: A.** In the most common variation, the anterosuperior portion of the uncinate process inserts onto the lamina papyracea so that the uncinate process separates the ethmoidal infundibulum from the frontal recess. In this setting, the frontal recess opens into the middle meatus medial to the ethmoidal infundibulum, between the uncinate process and the middle turbinate. When the uncinate process inserts onto the ethmoid roof or the middle turbinate, the frontal recess opens directly into the ethmoidal infundibulum. The frontal sinus opens into the middle meatus medial to the uncinate process in 88% of patients and lateral to the uncinate in the remaining 12% of patients. PAGE 360

38. **Answer: A.** MRSA may rapidly develop resistance to rifampin if it is used as monotherapy. PAGE 589

39. **Answer: D.** The use of prophylactic antibiotics in traumatic CSF leaks is controversial. Studies have not shown a clear therapeutic benefit, and antibiotics may select out resistant organisms. PAGE 668

40. **Answer: B.** MR imaging is superior to CT imaging for soft tissue pathology and characterization of opacified sinuses. However, CT provides superior definition of sinonasal bony anatomy. PAGE 449

41. **Answer: A.** Enterobacteriaceae are uncommon pathogens in acute bacterial sinusitis. PAGES 535, 536

42. **Answer: A.** *P. boydii* is resistant to amphotericin B; however, this fungus is susceptible to voriconazole. PAGE 562

43. **Answer: B.** A variety of skin lesions may develop in sarcoidosis, but lupus pernio is the most characteristic of the disease. It occurs more commonly in sarcoidosis with sinonasal fibrosis. PAGE 491

44. **Answer: D.** During immunotherapy, antigen-specific IgG4 levels increase in the serum. Induction of this antibody may be one immunologic mechanism by which immunotherapy exerts its beneficial effects in allergic disease. PAGES 386, 403

45. **Answer: A.** Clear delineation of bony sinonasal anatomy is a distinct advantage of CT imaging. In general, MR is better able to differentiate soft tissue mass from retained secretions, and at imaging soft tissues. PAGE 422–442, TABLE 27.1

46. **Answer: C.** Allergic rhinitis has been shown to be a risk factor for the subsequent development of asthma. Patients with asthma almost universally have sinonasal inflammation, though it may be subclinical. Treatment of upper respiratory disease can improve patients' asthma. Finally, allergen-specific immunotherapy in rhinitis patients may prevent the subsequent development of asthma. PAGES 553–554

47. **Answer: D.** The nasal hereditary hemorrhagic telangiectasias (HHT) most commonly develop on the nasal septum. These patients need to be screened for pulmonary and intracranial arteriovenous malformations. The genetic aberrations in HHT involve the TGF-β and VEGF genes. PAGE 497

48. **Answer: C.** The clinical differentiation of acute and chronic sinusitis is usually made clinically. However, the finding of bony sclerosis in sinus walls suggests a chronic inflammatory process. PAGE 426

49. **Answer: C.** The anterior ethmoid artery originates from the ophthalmic artery in the orbit and passes through the anterior ethmoidal foramen to enter the anterior ethmoidal cells. The artery typically crosses the ethmoids very near the skull base at the ethmoid roof and marks the posterior border of the frontal recess. PAGE 360

50. **Answer: A.** The natural os of the maxillary sinus lies in a somewhat oblique parasagittal plane. PAGE 596

51. **Answer: C.** A history of intermittent smell loss suggests that inflammatory sinonasal disease is the cause. PAGE 373

52. **Answer: A.** Topical decongestants act via α-adrenergic receptors. PAGE 479

53. **Answer: D.** Most bacteria exist in the form of a biofilm. (PAGE 537) Biofilms appear to be the preferred form of bacterial existence, with only approximately 1% of bacteria existing in the free-floating planktonic form. The Centers for Disease Control and Prevention estimates that around 65% of all human infections are caused or persist due to biofilms.

54. **Answer: A.** One characteristic of relapsing polychondritis of the ear is the lobule-sparing pattern of inflammation. PAGE 494

55. **Answer: D.** Removal of the anterior wall of the maxillary sinus does not weaken the structural integrity of the midface, nor does it result in cosmetic deformity. Therefore reconstruction is not required. PAGE 605

56. **Answer: C.** Clinical allergy is defined by symptoms after exposure to a specific allergen. A positive allergy test does not define allergic disease. Some individuals may demonstrate "hypersensitivity" or "sensitization" via testing, yet have no allergic symptoms. This is one reason that allergy testing should be performed only when there is a clinical suspicion of allergy. PAGE 452

57. **Answer: D.** The anterior transmaxillary approach provides broad access to the skull base anatomic compartments. PAGE 604

58. **Answer: D.** During EMLP, the anterior poles of the middle turbinates are resected up to the skull base. A valuable landmark to facilitate safe posterior dissection is the first olfactory nerve (or filum). Once this is reached, no further posterior resection of the middle turbinates should be performed. PAGE 684

59. **Answer: D.** The sphenopalatine artery is a terminal branch of the internal maxillary artery.
    PAGE 503

60. **Answer: C.** Nonstandardized allergens such as *Helminthosporium* may yield conflicting results if multiple testing modalities are used. There are multiple variables that affect test results for nonstandardized and especially mold allergens. Differences between manufacturers may be clinically important. PAGE 413

61. **Answer: B.** As also discussed in the chapter on allergic rhinitis, the most effective pharmacologic class used for treatment of allergic rhinitis is the intranasal steroid sprays. PAGE 402

62. **Answer: C.** Sinus imaging is appropriate in complicated acute sinusitis. CT is the preferred imaging modality. Plain films have limited value in contemporary medicine. PAGE 516

63. **Answer: E.** The sphenoid sinus is anatomically related to many important structures and compartments, including the internal carotid artery (not the external carotid). PAGE 610

64. **Answer: C.** In general, a middle meatus antrostomy requires neither resection of the middle turbinate nor disruption of the inferior concha. The agger nasi cell does not obstruct access to the maxillary sinus. However, visualization of the natural maxillary ostium usually requires removal of at least part of the uncinate process. PAGE 598

65. **Answer: B.** In this scenario, a patient with immune compromise develops some of the cardinal symptoms of acute invasive fungal sinusitis. The appropriate management includes CT sinus imaging and diagnostic nasal endoscopy by otolaryngology. If fungal sinusitis is diagnosed and there is suspicion of extension out of the paranasal sinuses, MR imaging may further delineate the extent of disease. PAGES 512–513

66. **Answer: D.** Conservative management of acute upper respiratory infection includes saline, decongestants, and analgesics. The typical clinical course will last a week, with some symptoms persisting up to a month. This patient most likely has a viral rhinosinusitis based on the time course of illness, and continued symptomatic treatment is appropriate. PAGE 517

67. **Answer: B.** Eosinophilic mucin is composed of eosinophils, mucin, and Charcot-Leyden crystals, which are a product of eosinophils. Fungal hyphae may be present, but are not definitional. PAGE 568

68. **Answer: C.** Epiphora is distinguished from watery eye by the physical dripping of tears down the cheek. Conjunctivitis is characterized by vascular injection and irritative symptoms. Dacryocystitis is an inflammation of the lacrimal sac that causes pain, redness, and swelling inferior to the medial canthus. PAGES 625–626

69. **Answer: B.** Embolization for control of epistaxis carries significant risks, though complications are rare. An additional limitation of embolization is that feeding vessels from the internal carotid circulation cannot be safely embolized. PAGE 507

70. **Answer: B.** The middle turbinate forms the medial boundary of the frontal recess. In the majority of cases the frontal sinus outflow tract will be found just lateral to this structure. PAGE 675

71. **Answer: C.** Staphylococcal exotoxins are responsible for toxic shock syndrome. PAGE 505

72. **Answer: E.** All of these are plausible scenarios where CT imaging may aid in management. CT imaging is not indicated in uncomplicated acute sinusitis. PAGE 449

73. **Answer: B.** Orbital and intracranial complications of acute bacterial sinusitis are rare. The most common of these complications is orbital subperiosteal abscess. PAGE 520

74. **Answer: D.** Allergy symptoms that interfere with sleep or affect quality-of-life factors like school performance denote "moderate/severe" disease in the ARIA classification system. PAGE 462

75. **Answer: A.** A variety of commercially available nasal steroid sprays have been shown to be effective at reducing symptoms in patients with polypoid chronic rhinosinusitis. Some of these randomized placebo-controlled trials have shown a reduction in nasal polyp size. There is no such body of evidence for antibiotics, leukotriene modifiers, or guaifenesin. PAGE 588

76. **Answer: D.** A variety of extrinsic or environmental influences may serve as risk factors or co-factors for the inflammation in CRS. Alcohol consumption thankfully is not among them. PAGE 537

77. **Answer: B.** When visualized endoscopically (coronal view) or on axial CT images, the anterior wall of the sphenoid sinus is in the same plane as the posterior wall of the maxillary sinus. The sphenoid ostium is medial to the superior turbinate. PAGES 641–642

78. **Answer: C.** The high rates of bony dehiscence over these important structures serve as a reminder that the surgeon should be vigilant and use safe technique when working in their close proximity. PAGE 600

79. **Answer: A.** In patients with suspected CSF rhinorrhea, the skull base should be evaluated first with a high-resolution CT scan. MR imaging is appropriate if meningoencephalocele is suspected. Cisternograms can assist in localizing the leak site. A radionuclide cisternogram is sometimes the only way to confirm a low-flow leak. PAGE 666

80. **Answer: D.** The process of olfaction is complicated and does not rely on specific odorant-receptor pairing. Rather, multiple receptors are activated to varying degrees by a specific odorant. This differential activation is responsible for the wide variety of perceived smells. PAGE 373

81. **Answer: B.** During an external ethmoidectomy, the periorbita should be left intact. The anterior ethmoid artery is reliably located in the frontoethmoidal suture line at approximately 24 mm from the anterior lacrimal crest. Dissection 8 mm beyond the posterior ethmoid artery may result in significant optic nerve injury. PAGE 609

82. **Answer: C.** Large Onodi cells may cause the surgeon to become disoriented and put anatomic structures such at the optic nerve and carotid at risk. `PAGE 434`

83. **Answer: C.** The degree of sphenoid pneumatization is classified into three types: sellar (86%), presellar (11%), and conchal (3%). A sellar-type sphenoid sinus is pneumatized inferior to the sella turcica and the pituitary gland. `PAGE 362`

84. **Answer: C.** Most phantosmias due to upper respiratory tract infection will resolve with time, but simple remedies such as nasal saline may be helpful in some patients. Neurologically active medications and surgery to remove olfactory neurons are treatments reserved for refractory cases in special circumstances. `PAGES 376–377`

85. **Answer: D.** A variety of factors may make sweat tests for CF unreliable. Skin edema is not one, however. `PAGE 450`

86. **Answer: B.** Fungus balls are more common in older patients. Endodontic surgery on the maxillary dentition may increase the odds of developing a fungus ball of the maxillary sinus. `PAGE 567`

87. **Answer: D.** The membranous septum is the portion of the septum that is anterior to the quadrangular cartilage. The cartilaginous septum *does* form the medial boundary of the nasal valve, and septal deviation is a significant cause of nasal valve narrowing. `PAGE 363`

88. **Answer: B.** The thinnest part of the anterior skull base is the lateral lamella of the cribriform plate, and therefore a common site of skull base violation. `PAGE 360`

89. **Answer: A.** The horizontal and globose basal cells have the ability to differentiate into other cell types to repair and replace lost olfactory cells. `PAGE 372`

90. **Answer: B.** The diagnosis of lymphoma is facilitated by biopsies for flow cytometry. This requires nonfixed tissue, so specimens should be sent to a pathology lab in saline. The treatment for sinonasal lymphoma includes chemotherapy and radiation, so the appropriate specialists need to be involved in their care. `PAGE 490`

91. **Answer: B.** Some patients develop a wheal response and skin erythema from glycerin, which is used as a preservative and diluent for allergen extracts. Multiple uniform-sized wheals in this patient suggest glycerin sensitivity. This case highlights the value of using a negative glycerin control in all skin testing. `PAGE 415`

92. **Answer: B.** The current classification of CRS distinguishes between polypoid and nonpolypoid disease. A further subdivision distinguishes between cases with eosinophilic or noneosinophilic inflammation. There are important treatment implications to this subdivision. `PAGE 536`

93. **Answer: D.** Imaging is not indicated in uncomplicated acute sinusitis. `PAGE 422`

94. **Answer: C.** The definitive diagnosis of nasal polyp requires histologic examination of a tissue biopsy. However, in practice the diagnosis is usually made based on the patient's history and examination or endoscopy findings. The finding of unilateral polyp disease should raise the suspicion of neoplasm. PAGE 526

95. **Answer: C.** The importance of allergy in CRS with nasal polyps is unclear. Allergy may be a disease-modifying factor, but is not considered a "cause" of nasal polyp disease. Immunotherapy is not a proven treatment for nasal polyp disease. Some nasal polyps have high levels of antigen-specific IgE, and dysregulated IgE metabolism may play a role in the disease. PAGES 530–531

96. **Answer: C.** Spontaneous CSF leaks are often due to elevated intracranial pressure. Patients with elevated intracranial pressure may develop delayed recurrent leaks or develop new sites of CSF leak over time. PAGE 665

97. **Answer: A.** IFN-γ is one of the characteristic Th1 cytokines. PAGE 385

98. **Answer: C.** Solid tumors are hypointense on T2-weighted MR images and often isointense on T1 images. With contrast administration, malignancies may appear hyperintense on T1-weighted images. CT cannot reliably differentiate soft tissue and secretions; however, high density on CT is often a sign of dense inspissated secretions or a fungus ball. PAGE 437

99. **Answer: C.** The agger nasi cell is intimately related to the nasolacrimal sac and the anterior attachment of the middle turbinate to the lateral nasal wall. PAGE 677

100. **Answer: D.** Upper and lower respiratory inflammatory diseases like allergic rhinitis and asthma worsen and improve in tandem. The most likely explanation for this connection is that these two conditions are separate manifestations of a systemic inflammatory disease. PAGE 554

101. **Answer: B.** Nonallergic rhinitis with eosinophilia (NARES) is a poorly understood eosinophilic inflammatory disease of the nose and sinuses. NARES may be a precursor to aspirin-exacerbated respiratory disease. As an eosinophilic respiratory disease, corticosteroids are the recommended treatment. PAGE 473

102. **Answer: D.** A lack of skin response to the histamine positive control prick suggests that histamine receptors are not functioning normally. The usual culprit is unknown or accidental antihistamine use. PAGE 415

103. **Answer: B.** Allergic rhinitis is characterized by "Th2" inflammation. Mast cells will degranulate on repeated exposure to allergen, not initial exposure. The late-phase allergic response occurs within hours of exposure. PAGE 551

104. **Answer: D.** Headache is not considered to be a cardinal symptom of chronic sinusitis. The other choices are. PAGES 586–587

105. **Answer: C.** A thorough history is still considered the best way to make a diagnosis of allergic disease. Testing serves a confirmatory role. PAGES 461–463

106. **Answer: D.** Both acute and long-term toxicities of oral glucocorticoids limit their use. All of the side effects listed may result from chronic use. PAGE 588

107. **Answer: C.** All of these agents may be used in the treatment of AERD; however, montelukast, a CysLT1 receptor antagonist, directly targets the primary metabolic derangements in this disease process (namely, overproduction of leukotrienes). PAGE 479

108. **Answer: A.** The time course of disease separates acute from chronic invasive fungal sinusitis from a clinical standpoint. There are a variety of clinicopathologic differences between these two conditions, but none of the other answers provides a distinguishing difference. PAGE 558

109. **Answer: D.** Alar batten grafts support the weak portion of the nasal ala that contains only fibrofatty tissue. The ala is the lateral border of the *external* nasal valve. The other techniques address internal nasal valve narrowing. PAGES 619–620

110. **Answer: C.** SLIT almost never causes anaphylaxis and is a treatment option for patients who do not want repeated injections. The relative efficacy of SCIT vs. SLIT is inadequately studied. SCIT utilizes injections every 1 to 4 weeks. PAGES 465–466

111. **Answer: C.** Normal olfactory epithelium does not contain goblet cells, though these may be present in patients with chronic rhinosinusitis. PAGE 367

112. **Answer: C.** Olfactory dysfunction in adults is a common problem, affecting up to 20% of people over 20. PAGE 371

113. **Answer: C.** The vast majority of epistaxis problems originate on the anterior septum. PAGE 501

114. **Answer: A.** The chapter describes "the ridge" as a landmark coming off the lamina that may reliably be used to separate the posterior ethmoid sinuses superiorly and the sphenoid sinus inferiorly. PAGE 601

115. **Answer: A.** Now largely abandoned because of the success of the osteoplastic flap approach to the frontal sinus, the Reidel procedure entailed removal of the anterior table of the frontal sinus, resulting in a very obvious contour deformity of the forehead. Choice B describes a Lothrop procedure. Choice C describes frontal sinus cranialization. Choice D describes an osteoplastic frontal obliteration. PAGE 609

116. **Answer: B.** It is possible to have allergic sensitivity indicated by testing, but no clinically significant hypersensitivity to an allergen. PAGE 413

117. **Answer: C.** The diagnosis of AERD may be strongly suggested by the patient's history. However, definitive diagnosis requires aspirin challenge (to trigger signs and symptoms of disease). PAGES 532–533

118. **Answer: D.** A former classification described the type 4 frontal cell as an ethmoid cell "completely within the frontal sinus." However, by definition, a frontoethmoidal cell must have some component in the ethmoid space. The Wormald classification of the type 4 cell uses the height of the cell within the frontal sinus as the key distinguishing feature. PAGE 677, TABLE 46.2

119. **Answer: B.** Multiple clinical trials have failed to demonstrate a clinical benefit with topical intranasal amphotericin B treatment. PAGE 531

120. **Answer: C.** Interestingly, purulent rhinorrhea, a cardinal symptom of acute sinusitis, is rare in patients who present with intracranial complications of sinusitis. Headache is the most common presenting symptom, followed by fever and altered mental status. PAGE 579

121. **Answer: A.** Leukotriene modifiers have been shown *not* to impair allergy skin test responses. The antihistamines and other medications with antihistaminic properties can weaken the skin response seen with allergy testing. Systemic steroids may theoretically impair skin test responses. PAGE 453

122. **Answer: B.** A child with nasal polyps and bronchiectasis should be evaluated for cystic fibrosis. A sweat chloride test is the first step in this process. PAGES 489–490

123. **Answer: B.** All of the above may be potential sources of nasal valve obstruction; however, an enlarged anterior pole of the inferior turbinate is the most common culprit. PAGE 364

124. **Answer: D.** Headache is not considered to be a cardinal (major) symptom of CRS. The other choices are. PAGE 551

125. **Answer: B.** This patient is the wrong demographic group for JNA. The tumor is in the wrong location for esthesioneuroblastoma. Meningiomas and primary brain tumors are not as destructive and do not cause epistaxis. PAGES 437–441

126. **Answer: A.** This image demonstrates frothy fluid within the left maxillary sinus. The presence of sinus fluid in a nonintubated atraumatic patient indicates acute bacterial sinusitis. PAGE 425

127. **Answer: E.** The image shows a characteristic cascading pattern of thickened mucosa and high-density secretions completely filling the sinuses and nasal cavity, indicating allergic fungal sinusitis. This is a noncontrast scan; the high density of the secretions should not be confused with enhancement that might suggest IFS or tumor. PAGE 435

128. **Answer: D.** There is a dehiscence of the bone overlying the left carotid artery, which predisposes this patient to carotid injury during endoscopic sphenoid sinus surgery. The other complications could also occur, but there is nothing on the image that would put the patient at above-average risk. PAGE 434

General Otolaryngology

1. Which stimuli use ion channels for taste transduction?

   A. Sweet
   B. Sour
   C. Salty
   D. Bitter
   E. A, B, C
   F. B, C

2. Which of the following symptoms of chronic rhinosinusitis would be least improved by endoscopic sinus surgery?

   A. Postnasal discharge
   B. Facial pain
   C. Hyposmia
   D. Nasal congestion

3. A 44-year-old woman with diabetes presents with a 2-day history of painful swelling of the submandibular gland. Her symptoms are exacerbated by eating. Purulence is expressible from Wharton duct. A CT scan demonstrates enlargement of the submandibular gland with surrounding fat stranding, and a 3-mm intraductal sialolith is present. Her blood glucose is 320 mg/dL. The next appropriate step in management would be:

   A. Sialendoscopy and removal of the obstructing sialolith
   B. Admission to the hospital, intravenous antibiotics, and tight blood glucose control
   C. Oral antistaphylococcal antibiotics, sialagogues, and gland massage
   D. Transoral removal of the sialolith

4. The Agency for Healthcare Research and Quality (AHRQ) offers a number of health care effectiveness resources for clinicians. Which of the following is one among them?

   A. Health-related quality-of-life instruments
   B. Technology assessments
   C. Meta-analysis tutorials
   D. Links to patient interest group sites

5. A 45-year-old woman presents to the emergency room with a 2-day history of progressive swelling of the floor of mouth, firm induration of the submandibular region, trismus, and dyspnea. Which of the following is the most appropriate next step in management?

   A. Awake tracheotomy
   B. Conventional endotracheal intubation
   C. Close observation and monitoring in the intensive care unit
   D. Thoracic surgery consultation

6. Which of the following is the most common etiology of acute pharyngitis in children and adults?

   A. Bacterial
   B. Viral
   C. Fungal
   D. Inflammatory
   E. Autoimmune

7. Which is the most robust taste sensation?

   A. Sweet
   B. Salty
   C. Sour
   D. Bitter
   E. A and C

8. Severe complications of Kawasaki disease include:

   A. Acute renal failure
   B. Coronary artery aneurysm
   C. Pulmonary hemorrhage
   D. Ascending neuropathy
   E. Hepatic dysfunction

9. A 7-year-old boy presents with a 5-week history of a parotid mass. The boy was evaluated by his pediatrician and completed a 14-day course of amoxicillin without improvement. There is a 2-cm fluctuant mass with a violaceous hue to the closely adherent overlying skin. Fine-needle aspiration (FNA) demonstrated acid-fast bacilli in the aspirate. Resolution of the patient's disease would be most effectively achieved by:

   A. Incision and drainage of the abscess and culture
   B. Incision and drainage of the abscess and clarithromycin
   C. FNA, culture, and clarithromycin
   D. Superficial parotidectomy

10. A 3-year-old boy presents with an abscess of the retropharyngeal space. What is the most likely etiology for this infectious process?

    A. Sialadenitis
    B. Upper respiratory tract infection
    C. Tooth decay
    D. Surgical instrumentation trauma

11. Which of the following is the most consistent landmark for the localization of the facial nerve?

    A. 1 cm lateral and inferior to the tragal pointer
    B. 6 mm to 8 mm deep to the tympanomastoid suture
    C. Anterolateral aspect of the styloid process
    D. Lateral to the posterior belly of the digastric muscle

12. Which of the following statements is true regarding treatment of disorders of the temporomandibular joint (TMJ)?

    A. Clinical evidence supports the use of open surgical intervention over arthroscopy for intracapsular disorders of TMJ.
    B. Nonsteroidal anti-inflammatory drugs (NSAIDs) have been shown to reduce discomfort from myofascial pain, symptomatic intracapsular disorders, and otalgia associated with temporomandibular disorder (TMD).
    C. Restorative dental procedures prevent worsening of TMD in the presence of mild TMD.
    D. Comminuted, laterally displaced segments in fractures of the mandibular condyle should be treated nonoperatively.

13. A 27-year-old otherwise healthy man is admitted to the hospital for a fever of unknown origin. The next morning he presents with a right-sided jugular vein thrombosis, ptosis, anhidrosis, and miosis. The infection is most likely located in which deep neck space?

    A. Prestyloid parapharyngeal space
    B. Poststyloid parapharyngeal space
    C. Retropharyngeal space
    D. Anterior visceral space

14. Which of the following organisms are common sources of infection in acute bacterial sialadenitis?

    A. Gram-positive cocci
    B. Aerobic gram-negative rods
    C. Anaerobic gram-negative rods
    D. All of the above

15. An 81-year-old woman presents on postoperative day 6 following a hemicolectomy with swelling and severe tenderness over the right preauricular region, purulent fluid from Stensen duct, and no trismus. In addition to hydration, antimicrobials targeting which organism should be administered?

    A. *Klebsiella pneumoniae*
    B. *Streptococcus viridians*
    C. *Streptococcus pyogenes*
    D. *Staphylococcus aureus*

16. Sensory innervation of the temporomandibular joint is from:

    A. Facial nerve
    B. Auriculotemporal, deep temporal, and masseteric nerves
    C. Great auricular nerve
    D. Superficial temporal nerve

17. A 25-year-old woman is diagnosed with Crohn disease. Which characteristic oral manifestation of Crohn disease might you expect to see in this patient?

    A. Strawberry gingivitis
    B. Ulcers that heal with scarring
    C. Fissuring of the tongue
    D. Buccal mucosal cobblestoning

18. Odontogenic infections are more prevalent in which demographic?

    A. Children
    B. Elderly men
    C. Middle age men
    D. Elderly women

19. Which of the following medications has demonstrated efficacy in preventing chemoradiation-related mucositis?

    A. Topical triamcinolone
    B. Palifermin
    C. Hydroxyurea
    D. Second-generation cephalosporins

20. Which of the following odontogenic space infections do not commonly have trismus at presentation?

    A. Buccal space infection
    B. Masseteric space infection
    C. Temporal space infection
    D. Pterygoid space infection

21. Where are taste buds located?

    A. Fungiform papillae
    B. Filiform papillae
    C. Foliate papillae
    D. Circumvallate papillae
    E. A, C, D

22. Which of the following statements is true regarding pemphigus vulgaris (PV)?

    A. Direct immunofluorescence shows linear deposition of IgG and C3 along the basement membrane.
    B. Oral involvement is rare in PV.
    C. The pathogenesis of PV is loss of cell-to-cell adhesion due to damaged desmosomal proteins.
    D. PV has not been associated with other autoimmune disorders.

23. Which of the following properties allow saliva to act as a good lubricant and biofilm barrier?

    A. High solubility
    B. Low viscosity
    C. High elasticity
    D. Weak adhesiveness

24. Which of the following glands produce the majority of the unstimulated saliva?

    A. Parotid glands
    B. Minor salivary glands
    C. Sublingual glands
    D. Submandibular glands

25. Which of the following attributes of a health-related quality-of-life instrument would be particularly important in planning a study to evaluate the effect of an intervention?

    A. Construct validity
    B. Interobserver reliability
    C. Face validity
    D. Responsiveness

26. Which of the following is important in the evaluation of burning mouth syndrome?

    A. Punch biopsy of the tongue
    B. Patch testing of oral mucosa
    C. Trial of α-lipoic acid
    D. Serum ferritin and B vitamin levels

27. Based on the multicellular theory of tumorigenesis, mucoepidermoid carcinoma arises from:

    A. Excretory duct cells
    B. Acinar cells
    C. Striated duct cells
    D. Intercalated duct cells

28. **Appropriate management of an 18-year-old patient with infectious mononucleosis with a positive monospot test includes:**

    A. Rest, hydration, antipyretics, and analgesics
    B. A single dose of intramuscular ceftriaxone
    C. Oral penicillin
    D. Intravenous penicillin
    E. Oral acyclovir

29. **How many cell types are there in a taste bud?**

    A. Five
    B. One
    C. Three
    D. More than 10

30. **Which of the following antibiotics represents the most appropriate empiric treatment of an odontogenic infection?**

    A. Amikacin
    B. Clindamycin
    C. Erythromycin
    D. Doxycycline

31. **Temporomandibular disorders (TMDs) are associated with:**

    A. Depression
    B. Irritable bowel
    C. Fibromyalgia
    D. All of the above

32. **Tasters and nontasters are identified based on the individual's ability to perceive:**

    A. Capsaicin
    B. Alcohol
    C. Sucrose
    D. 6-*n*-Propyl-thiouracil (PROP)

33. **Which of the following statements regarding juvenile recurrent parotitis is false?**

    A. The disease typically resolves by the end of adolescence.
    B. Treatment during acute parotitis episodes is similar to acute bacterial sialadenitis.
    C. Ligation of Stenson duct and tympanic neurectomy have been shown to be effective treatment options.
    D. Sialendoscopy with dilation, saline irrigation, or steroid irrigation has been shown to improve symptoms.

34. **Which cells are responsible for producing the primary salivary secretion?**

    A. Myoepithelial cells
    B. Ductal cells
    C. Acinar cells
    D. Basal cells

35. **Which of the following statements best describes concurring occlusal appliance (splint) therapy?**

    A. The type of appliance is of critical importance.
    B. Use of the device repositions the displaced articular disc over time.
    C. This therapy is effective for temporomandibular joints (TMJs)-related myofacial pain.
    D. This therapy slows the progression of arthritis in the TMJ.

36. **Which structure directly contributes to the borders of the retropharyngeal space?**

    A. Pharyngobasilar fascia
    B. Pharyngeal constrictor musculature
    C. Buccopharyngeal fascia
    D. Prevertebral fascia

37. **Which muscle attachment helps predict the spread of odontogenic infections into the submandibular space?**

    A. Anterior digastric muscle
    B. Genioglossus muscle
    C. Mylohyoid muscle
    D. Stylohyoid muscle

38. Which of these salivary glands are most sensitive to injury from radiation treatment?

    A. Submandibular glands
    B. Parotid glands
    C. Sublingual glands
    D. Minor salivary glands

39. According to the World Health Organization's International Classification of Functioning, Disability, and Health (ICF) definitions, tinnitus would be classified as a(n):

    A. Disorder
    B. Handicap
    C. Disability
    D. Impairment

40. Generic health-related quality-of-life instruments are usually divided for measurement into three core domains. They are:

    A. Physical, social, and psychological
    B. Physical, emotional, and self-help
    C. Physical, role functioning, and mood
    D. Physical, interpersonal interactions, and vocational

41. Odontogenic infections are most likely to arise from:

    A. Maxillary central incisor
    B. Mandibular lateral incisor
    C. Maxillary first molar
    D. Mandibular second molar

42. Which of the following disorders can be confused with oral mucosa drug eruptions, contact allergies, and lupus?

    A. Lichen planus
    B. Behçet disease
    C. Recurrent aphthous stomatitis
    D. Orofacial granulomatosis

43. Which of the following statements is *not true* regarding temporomandibular disorder (TMD) pathology?

    A. Studies have shown abnormal pain processing in patients with chronic myofascial pain.
    B. Cytokines, metalloproteinases, free radicals, and reperfusion injury likely all contribute to intracapsular pathology and symptoms in TMD.
    C. The disc of the temporomandibular joint has a central, abundantly neurovascular zone which contributes to pain when it is damaged.
    D. Disc displacement in intracapsular disorders moves the disc anteriorly, and may be followed by reduction and accompanied by joint noise, or may be nonreducing and have an absence of joint noise.

44. After a positive rapid antibody detection test (RADT) for group A β-hemolytic streptococcus (GABHS) in a 4-year-old patient, which of the following is the next appropriate step in management?

    A. Confirmation with GABHS culture on blood agar
    B. Symptomatic therapy
    C. Treatment with amoxicillin
    D. Treatment with azithromycin
    E. Treatment with acetaminophen

45. In a patient with suspected acute retroviral syndrome pharyngitis, initial diagnostic testing for human immunodeficiency virus (HIV) is performed by:

    A. Western blot
    B. Southern blot
    C. Culture on chocolate agar
    D. Enzyme-linked immunosorbent assay (ELISA)
    E. Monospot test

46. A 34-year-old man with drooling and fever. What is the most likely source for the abscess seen on this CT?

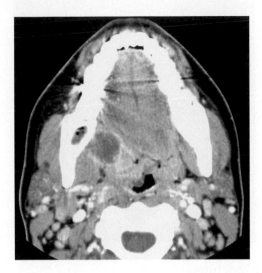

   A. Hematologic
   B. Palatine tonsils
   C. Odontogenic
   D. Suppurative node
   E. Osteomyelitis

47. A 19-year-old girl with deep space neck infection. What is the most likely complication that should be sought through further imaging?

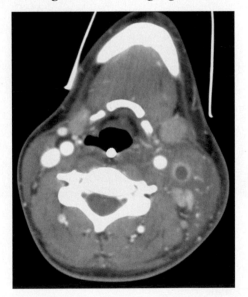

   A. Retropharyngeal abscess
   B. Danger space extension to the mediastinum
   C. Osteomyelitis
   D. Intracranial infection
   E. Lung abscess

48. A 29-year-old with neck swelling. The key finding on this CT is:

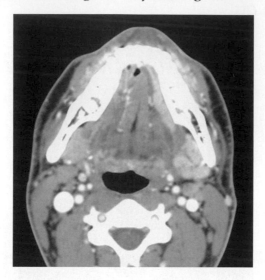

   A. Submandibular sialadenitis
   B. Sublingual sialadenitis
   C. Sialolithiasis
   D. Cellulitis
   E. All of the above

49. A 68-year-old woman with headaches and facial pain. What is the most likely cause?

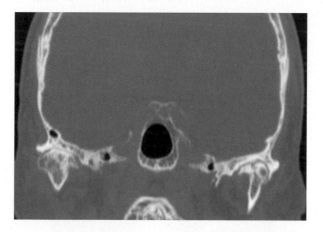

   A. Sinusitis
   B. Paget disease
   C. Cervical spondylopathy
   D. Cerebrospinal fluid leak
   E. Temporomandibular osteoarthropathy

50. A 38-year-old woman with sinus pain. What is the most likely source of maxillary sinusitis?

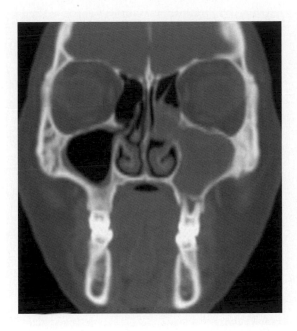

A. Odontogenic
B. Isolated nasal polyp
C. Nasal polyposis
D. Cystic fibrosis
E. Nasal cavity malignancy

51. A healthy, nonsmoking 48-year-old man with painless neck mass. What is the most likely diagnosis?

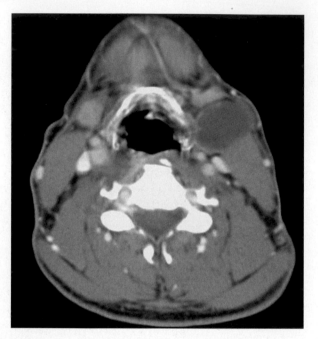

   A. Branchial cleft cyst
   B. Thyroglossal duct remnant
   C. Mycobacterial infection
   D. Bacterial abscess
   E. Squamous cell carcinoma (SCC)

Chapter 3 Answers

1. **Answer: F.** Salts and sour acidic stimuli use ion channels, while sweet and bitter substances react with protein compounds. PAGE 730

2. **Answer: C.** A series of systematic reviews conclusively demonstrate that endoscopic sinus surgery relieves nasal obstruction, drainage, and facial pain. This surgery has less effect on headache and the sense of smell. PAGE 725

3. **Answer: B.** In the setting of acute toxicity, admission and stabilization is the first obligation. Sialendoscopic extraction of this stone may be considered after control of sepsis and hyperglycemia. PAGE 703

4. **Answer: B.** In the United States, health technology assessments are undertaken by the AHRQ to determine the benefit or added value of new technology for the purpose of reimbursement and pricing decisions. PAGE 719

5. **Answer: A.** The patient has Ludwig angina. Asphyxia is the leading cause of death with this disease, so airway management is paramount. Intubation is difficult in this setting; attempts at intubation can lead to loss of the airway and emergent tracheotomy. Surgical drainage is required. Observation is not appropriate. PAGE 808

6. **Answer: B.** In adults and children, viral infections are the primary cause of acute pharyngitis; though in children 30% to 40% of acute pharyngitis is bacterial compared to 5% to 15% in adults. The other listed items make up a small percentage of cases. PAGE 757

7. **Answer: A.** Sweet taste, present even in utero, is the most robust taste sensation. PAGE 730

8. **Answer: B.** Sudden death can result from Kawasaki disease-related coronary artery aneurysms if not recognized and treated. The other choices are not associated with this disease. PAGE 762

9. **Answer: D.** This clinical presentation suggests infection with atypical mycobacteria. These organisms are commonly encountered in soil, water, and food and are carried by both domestic and wild animals. FNA may help confirm the presence of acid-fast bacilli. Culture is unreliable, and antibiotics often fail, while excision is usually curative. PAGE 704

10. **Answer: B.** Retropharyngeal space infections are usually seen in children younger than 5 years and result from upper respiratory tract infections spreading to nodes of Rouvière. These lymphatics involute with age. In older children and adults, trauma may lead to infections in this space. Salivary and dental infections do not spread to the retropharyngeal space. PAGE 806

11. **Answer: B.** The facial nerve emerges 6 mm to 8 mm deep to the tympanomastoid suture. The nerve is on the posterolateral aspect of the styloid and is medial to the tragal pointer. The nerve is superior posterior and deep to the posterior belly of the digastric muscle. PAGE 694

12. **Answer: B.** NSAIDs are the mainstay of initial TMD treatment. There is no evidence that restorative dentistry worsens or improves TMD. The clinical evidence is weak that supports any particular approach to TMJ surgery. Lateral displaced comminuted condyle fractures are an indicator for open reduction. PAGES 788–789

13. **Answer: B.** The poststyloid compartment houses the carotid sheath and cranial nerves IX and X. Involvement of the sympathetic ganglion leads to Horner syndrome (ptosis, anhidrosis, and miosis). Prestyloid parapharyngeal space infections present with trismus, medial bulging of the pharyngeal wall, and systemic toxicity. The retropharyngeal and anterior visceral spaces do not involve the affected structures. PAGE 809

14. **Answer: D.** Historically *Staphylococcus aureus* was the most commonly encountered organism in acute bacterial sialadenitis. More recently, polymicrobial infections, including bacteroides and β-lactamase-producing organisms, have been observed. PAGE 703

15. **Answer: D.** The patient described has acute parotitis, which is common in postoperative patients. The bacteria involved are almost always *Staphylococcus aureus*. PAGE 810

16. **Answer: B.** The auriculotemporal, deep temporal, and masseteric nerves are all branches of the mandibular nerve (V3). The facial nerve is a motor nerve. The superficial temporal nerve is a bunch of the auriculotemporal nerve to the anterolateral scalp. The greater auricular nerve arises from the cervical plexus (C2-C3) and innervates the shin over the parotid, mastoid, and auricle. PAGE 783

17. **Answer: D.** 40% of patients with Crohn disease have oral symptoms at presentation, including cobblestoning of the buccal mucosal, angular cheilitis, or deep linear ulcerations in the gingivalbuccal sulcus. Strawberry gingivitis is a manifestation of granulomatosis with polyangiitis. Ulcers that heal with scarring are typical of Behçet disease. PAGE 747

18. **Answer: C.** Odontogenic infections peak in third and fourth decades of life. They are not more common in either gender. PAGE 770

19. **Answer: B.** Palifermin is a recombinant human keratinocyte growth factor 1 that is thought to offer mucosal protection by inducing epithelial hyperplasia. Triamcinolone treats stomatitis symptoms. Hydroxyurea can cause mucositis. Cephalosporins are antibiotics and not useful in this scenario. PAGE 738

20. **Answer: A.** The masseteric, temporal, and pterygoid spaces house the large muscles of mastication which can spasm with infection. The buccal space does not. PAGES 773–774

21. **Answer: E.** Taste buds are contained within the fungiform, foliate, and circumvallate papillae. The filiform papillae are nongustatory. PAGE 729

22. **Answer: C.** PV is an autoimmune mucocutaneous bullous disease caused by IgG antibodies to desmoglein 3 and 1 which lead to loss of cell-to-cell adhesion. Oral involvement is seen in 90%, and PV is associated with autoimmune disorders such as rheumatoid arthritis and

systemic lupus erythematosus. Direct immunofluorescence shows *intracellular* deposits of IgG and C3. PAGE 745

23. **Answer: C.** Mucin has high elasticity, high viscosity, low solubility, and strong adhesiveness, all properties that improve lubrication. PAGE 697

24. **Answer: D.** Average daily salivary flow is 1,000 to 1,500 mL. The parotid glands produce about 20%, while the paired submandibular glands produce about 65%, and the sublingual glands produce about 8%. PAGE 698

25. **Answer: D.** Responsiveness of an instrument indicates the extent to which changes in value correlate with true changes in status. Validity is the extent to which an instrument measures what it claims to measure. Reliability is a measure of the reproducibility of the results. PAGE 723

26. **Answer: D.** There is no clinical feature, pathologic finding, or drug response that is diagnostic of burning mouth syndrome. Since there is no treatment for this disorder, evaluation for alternative diagnosis such as nutritional deficiency of iron or B vitamins is important. PAGE 753

27. **Answer: A.** The excretory duct cells can give rise to either mucoepidermoid or, perhaps, squamous cell carcinoma. The intercalated duct cells are supposed to give rise to pleomorphic adenoma, Warthin tumor, and adenocarcinoma. PAGE 697

28. **Answer: A.** Mononucleosis is treated supportively. Antibacterial pharmacotherapy is not helpful for this viral infection. Clinical data do not support the use of acyclovir in acute mononucleosis, despite the good virologic activity demonstrated by this drug against the Epstein–Barr virus. PAGE 763

29. **Answer: C.** The life span of a taste cell is about 10 days. The taste bud contains sensory cells, supporting cells, and basal cells. As the sensory cells die, the basal cells differentiate into new receptor cells. PAGE 730

30. **Answer: B.** The prevalent bacteria in odontogenic infections are gram-positive anaerobic cocci and gram-negative anaerobic rods. The usual empire choice is clindamycin or amoxicillin–clavulanate. Amikacin, erythromycin, and doxycycline are not as effective against anaerobic bacteria. PAGE 779

31. **Answer: D.** Depression, irritable bowel, and fibromyalgia are all associated with TMD. Trauma to the joint is also associated with TMD. PAGE 782

32. **Answer: D.** Tasters can be distinguished from nontasters based on the ability to perceive PROP. Compared with supertasters, nontasters experience less-negative (e.g., bitterness) and more-positive (e.g., sweetness) sensations from certain foods and beverages like alcohol. PAGE 731

33. **Answer: C.** This idiopathic, but difficult, problem is sometimes self-limiting, but when active causes a tremendous burden on the patient and family. Attempts to use duct ligation and neurectomy have failed to produce good results. PAGES 707–708

34. **Answer: C.** The acinar cells produce serous secretions which are protein rich. The myoepithelial cells contribute to moving the saliva toward the excretory duct. Basal cells are capable of differentiating into ductal epithelium. PAGE 697

35. **Answer: C.** The utility of TMJ splints is in the improvement of myofacial pain and protection of dentition against parafunctional habits (bruxism). The splints do not reposition the disc or arrest progression of degenerative or inflammatory disease. PAGE 788

36. **Answer: C.** The retropharyngeal space is medial to the carotid sheath, anterior to the danger space, and posterior to the buccopharyngeal fascia. The constrictor muscles are anterior to the buccopharyngeal fascia and the prevertebral fascia is the posterior border of the danger space. The pharyngobasilar fascia is anterior to the visceral musculature. PAGE 797

37. **Answer: C.** Many odontogenic infections initially spread to the sublingual space from mandibular teeth. Only dental infections from the second and third molars, where the tooth roots extend below the mylohyoid line of the mandible, generally spread directly to the submandibular space. PAGE 774

38. **Answer: B.** The parotid glands are more susceptible to radiation injury. Damage is severe when exposed to 20Gy to 30Gy. PAGE 711

39. **Answer: D.** Tinnitus is most commonly perceived as impairment. If truly severe, it could be considered a handicap that prevents an individual from carrying out his/her life role or, for a few, a disability leading to a restriction in performing some or all of life's duties. PAGE 719-SEE FIGURE 49.1

40. **Answer: A.** The core of health-related quality-of-life assessment is the perception that physical, emotional (psychological), and social well-being are factors that affect satisfaction with life. PAGE 718

41. **Answer: D.** In adults, most infections arise from mandibular molars. Children have fewer odontogenic infections, but are more likely to occur in maxillary teeth. PAGE 770

42. **Answer: A.** Lichen planus drug eruptions, allergic reactions to dental restorative materials, graft-versus-host disease, and discoid lupus, all cause oral lichenoid lesions. The other choices cause oral aphthous ulcers, and in the case of orofacial granulomatosis, lip enlargement and lymphatic obstruction. PAGE 751

43. **Answer: C.** Trauma to the vascular and richly-innervated retrodiscal tissues can cause effusion and pain. The central disc is thin and avascular. Various theories of TMD pathology

implicate free radicals, cytokines, metalloproteinases, and reperfusion injury. Deviation of the jaw towards the affected site without joint sounds is a sign of disc displacement without reduction. PAGE 784

44. **Answer: C.** Because of the time required to obtain culture and the desire to treat GABHS infections to prevent late complications of rheumatic heart disease, the RADT is recommended for the initial office visit with immediate treatment of patients with positive results using amoxicillin for patients who are not allergic to this antibiotic. Penicillin-allergic patients can be treated with azithromycin. PAGE 759

45. **Answer: D.** The initial testing for the diagnosis of acute HIV infection is by ELISA, followed by Western blot analysis for confirmation. The viruses cannot be cultured on chocolate agar; this media is used to grow fastidious respiratory bacteria. The monospot test is for Epstein–Barr virus. PAGE 764

46. **Answer: C.** Abscess that arises along a mandibular surface is most likely from an odonotogenic source. The unhealed tooth socket confirms that there was a recent extraction in this case. Although the tonsil is inflamed, this is not the usual location and spread for a peritonsillar abscess. There are no lymph nodes in this location. PAGE 773

47. **Answer: E.** This image demonstrates jugular thrombophlebitis. The most likely complication is Lemierre syndrome (lung abscesses from septic emboli from jugular thrombophlebitis). Although there is edema in the retropharyngeal space, there is no abscess in that location, so the danger space is not at risk. Intracranial infection and osteomyelitis would be less commonly seen in this scenario. PAGES 804–805

48. **Answer: E.** This CT depicts a stone lodged at the puncta of Wharton duct, causing enlargement and increased enhancement of both the sublingual and submandibular glands. Stranding of the surrounding fat and thickening of the platysma muscle are indicators of cellulitis. PAGE 708

49. **Answer: E.** This coronal CT shows marked narrowing of both temporomandibular joints (TMJs), with large osteophytes and remodeling of the glenoid fossa. The skull base is otherwise intact, and the skull is normal. There is no sinusitis in this limited view of the sphenoid sinuses. TMJ disease is an often-overlooked cause of facial pain. PAGE 785

50. **Answer: A.** The eroded bone overlying the apical abscess makes an odontogenic source most likely. Nasal polyposis and cystic fibrosis would affect both sides. The nasal polyp is secondary to the odontogenic infection. PAGE 772

51. **Answer: E.** This is a classic location for a branchial cleft cyst; but in an adult, a cystic neck mass at this location is most likely SCC, often from an oropharyngeal primary. This is the wrong location for a thyroglossal duct remnant, and the wrong age group for mycobacterial infection. The surrounding fat lacks the inflammation that would be associated with an abscess. PAGE 1902

4

Laryngology

1. Which is *not* a component of the lamina propria of the vocal fold?

   A. Middle layer
   B. Superficial layer
   C. Vocalis muscle
   D. Deep layer

2. A patient is sent to you with dysphagia and dysarthria and demonstrates an exaggerated jaw jerk and gag, a spastic tongue, and emotional lability. Which of the following terms refers to this constellation of symptoms?

   A. Amyotrophic lateral sclerosis (ALS)
   B. Bulbar palsy
   C. Pseudobulbar palsy
   D. Botulism from improperly canned food

3. In essence, voice therapy does which of the following?

   A. Strengthens the vocal folds
   B. Balances the systems of respiration, phonation, and resonance
   C. Instructs patients in good vocal hygiene
   D. Instructs patients not to yell and scream

4. Workup for a new diagnosis of vocal fold paralysis does not routinely include:

   A. CT scan
   B. Laryngeal electromyography (LEMG)
   C. Swallowing assessment
   D. Serology

5. Pill dysphagia without solid food dysphagia suggests a problem in which phase of swallowing?

    A. Anticipatory

    B. Oropharyngeal

    C. Pharyngeal

    D. Esophageal

    E. Gastric

6. Which of the following lasers cannot be used in both contact and noncontact modes?

    A. KTP

    B. CO_2

    C. Omniguide™ delivery method

    D. PDL

    E. Thulium

7. Use of a Passy-Muir speaking valve is contraindicated in the presence of:

    A. Cognitive dysfunction

    B. Presence of a cuffed tracheostomy tube

    C. Upper airway obstruction

    D. Severe tracheal stenosis

    E. All of the above

8. Which of the following is the most common cause of unilateral vocal fold paralysis (UVFP)?

    A. Lung cancer

    B. Iatrogenic injury

    C. Idiopathic cause

    D. Endotracheal intubation

    E. Infections

9. The most commonly affected site for laryngeal sarcoid is:

    A. Postcricoid region

    B. Subglottis

    C. Glottis

    D. Supraglottis

    E. Anterior Commissure

10. Which of the below muscles is *not* an intrinsic muscle of the larynx?

    A. Interarytenoid
    B. Lateral cricoarytenoid
    C. Thyrohyoid
    D. Thyroarytenoid

11. What are the three component parts of any voice therapy program?

    A. Manage laryngopharyngeal reflux, increase hydration, and decrease screaming
    B. Increase vocal hygiene, decrease phonotrauma, and increase coordinated voice production
    C. Relaxation, breath support, and articulation
    D. Psychosocial counsel, increase hydration, and increase voice rest
    E. Decrease vocal hygiene, increase phonotrauma, and decrease balanced voice production

12 Which of the following best describes botulinum toxin injection?

    A. It can only be used for the parotid gland.
    B. It is an effective one-time intervention for sialorrhea.
    C. It can be injected safely with ultrasound guidance.
    D. It should be used as a first-line therapy for mild sialorrhea.

13. Which is the incorrect choice regarding vocal fold nodules?

    A. They are bilateral.
    B. They cause minimal disruption to the mucosal wave.
    C. They require surgical excision.
    D. They are fairly symmetric.
    E. They resolve with voice rest/voice therapy.

14. Which of the following is a potential complication of awake injection laryngoplasty?

    A. Injection is too superficial in the vocal fold
    B. Failure to completely correct the glottal gap
    C. Hematoma formation within the vocal fold
    D. Injection material placed too far lateral in paragottic space
    E. All of the above

15. Which of the following histologic features must be included in the diagnosis of Barrett esophagus?

    A. Intestinal metaplasia
    B. Columnar mucosa
    C. Dysplasia
    D. Immotile cilia
    E. Leukoplakia

16. What is the first-line treatment for recurrent respiratory papillomatosis?

    A. Surgical removal
    B. Inhaled cidofovir
    C. High-dose oral steroid burst
    D. Azathioprine
    E. Radiation therapy

17. Which laryngeal muscle is bilaterally innervated?

    A. Thyroarytenoid
    B. Interarytenoid
    C. Cricothyroid
    D. Lateral cricoarytenoid
    E. Posterior cricoarytenoid

18. What is the singer's formant?

    A. Clustered third, fourth, and fifth formant regions which amplify harmonic sound frequencies between 2,800 and 3,500 Hz
    B. Clustered third, fourth, and fifth formant regions which amplify harmonic sound frequencies between 1,000 and 2,500 Hz
    C. Clustered first, second, and third formant regions which amplify harmonic sound frequencies between 1,000 and 2,500 Hz
    D. Clustered first, second, and third formant regions which amplify harmonic sound frequencies between 2,800 and 3,500 Hz

19. Which of the following is *not* a contraindication to percutaneous tracheotomy?

    A. High innominate artery
    B. Body mass index (BMI) > 30
    C. Large midline neck mass
    D. Unprotected airway
    E. Inability to palpate the cricoid cartilage

20. **Which voice disorder would be the least amenable to voice therapy?**

    A. Primary muscle tension dysphonia
    B. Secondary muscle tension dysphonia
    C. Nodules
    D. Functional aphonia
    E. Paradoxical vocal fold motion dysfunction

21. **Which of the following is true of diagnostic testing of laryngopharyngeal reflux (LPR)?**

    A. A 24-hour dual-probe pH testing is highly effective at identifying those with acid reflux.
    B. Presence of esophagitis on esophagoscopy is necessary to diagnose LPR.
    C. A positive response to acid-suppressive therapy is diagnostic of LPR.
    D. A reflux symptom index (RSI) of 20 is diagnostic of LPR.
    E. Demonstration of abnormal lower esophageal sphincter (LES) pressures on manometry is diagnostic of LPR.

22. **Which of the following is *not* routinely included in the treatment options for bilateral true vocal fold paralysis?**

    A. Tracheostomy
    B. Suture lateralization
    C. Botulinum toxin injections
    D. Vocal fold augmentation
    E. Transverse cordotomy
    F. Arytenoidectomy

23. **Which statement is *incorrect* regarding microflap surgery of the vocal fold?**

    A. A conservative surgical approach for submucosal benign pathology.
    B. Involves complete removal of vocal fold mucosa for the treatment of dysphonia.
    C. Surgical precision and patience are required.
    D. Microinstrumentation with various angulations is involved.
    E. Saline or epinephrine submucosal infusion can help with the microflap elevation.

24. **You have been consulted repeatedly for aspiration pneumonia occurring in long-term patients at a local long-term facility. Which of the following might you consider?**

    A. Meet with the facility leadership to discuss infection control strategies
    B. Meet with the facility leadership to discuss formation of a dysphagia team
    C. Offer to begin teaching nurses and respiratory therapists about swallowing function
    D. B and C
    E. Eliminate thin liquids from the diet of all of the residents.

25. A 45-year-old patient had no return of swallowing function 12 months after his stroke and is trach dependent and has severe aspiration. He has a percutaneous endoscopic gastrostomy and desires to be discharged to home. Which of the following is probably the most appropriate for this patient?

    A. Laryngotracheal separation
    B. Place a laryngeal stent and change it monthly
    C. Replace his tracheostomy tube with a tube with a foam cuff
    D. B and CE. Discharge home without any intervention

26. What connotes success in voice therapy?

    A. Lesion size decreases
    B. Return to functional vocal abilities
    C. Better sounding voice
    D. Better feeling voice
    E. A happy patient

27. Which of the following is true about bile salts?

    A. Bile salts are incapable of causing epithelial inflammation.
    B. Bile salts are inactivated at low pH.
    C. Bile salts are inactivated at high pH.
    D. Bile salts can enter laryngeal epithelial cells at both acid and neutral pH and induce damage.
    E. Bile salts are produced by the lining of the stomach.

28. Signs commonly associated with laryngopharyngeal reflux (LPR) include:

    A. Anterior rhinorrhea
    B. Posterior laryngeal granuloma
    C. Vocal fold paralysis
    D. Cervical osteophytes
    E. Vocal fold atrophy

29. Stroboscopy allows assessment of the following *except*:

    A. Vocal fold closure
    B. Vocal fold mobility
    C. Mucosal pliability
    D. Vocal fold level during phonation
    E. Vocal fold sub-epithelial pathology

30. Which of the following statements applies to Hunsaker tube?

    A. It provides excellent exposure for microlaryngeal surgery.
    B. It is laser-safe.
    C. It is associated with a low complication rate.
    D. It is versatile.
    E. All of the above.

31. In a dysphagic patient who had previously undergone treatment for advanced laryngeal cancer, impaired laryngohyoid elevation would be most readily detected by:

    A. Videofluoroscopic swallow study (VFSS)
    B. High-resolution manometry
    C. Fiberoptic endoscopic evaluation of swallowing (FEES)
    D. Clinical bedside swallow evaluation
    E. Narrow band imaging

32. Which muscle does a singer use to keep the vocal folds approximated when using a chest voice mechanism?

    A. Thyroarytenoid
    B. Interarytenoid
    C. Lateral cricoarytenoid
    D. Cricothyroid
    E. Thyrohyoid

33. Which of the following is most descriptive of the esophageal B ring?

    A. A mucosal narrowing at the gastroesophageal junction usually associated with a hiatal hernia
    B. A thickening of the lower esophageal sphincter (LES) muscle
    C. Esophageal trachealization
    D. The narrowing in the lower esophagus associated with the diaphragm
    E. A mucosal narrowing located at the upper esophageal sphincter

34. A 67-year-old man with a progressive neuromuscular disorder requires a permanent tracheostomy. The attending surgeon will use the technique described by Eliachar. Which of the following statements is true?

    A. The technique involves complete laryngotracheal separation by suturing the subcricoid trachea and exteriorizing the remaining trachea.
    B. The technique involves removing the anterior portion of tracheal rings 2, 3, 4, and 5 in order to create a large opening which is unlikely to close.
    C. The technique involves suturing a superiorly based tracheal flap to the superior skin flap and suturing the inferior and lateral tracheal edges to the inferior skin flap.
    D. The technique requires fewer steps than a standard surgical tracheotomy and heals more rapidly, usually in 5 to 7 days.
    E. None of the above.

35. A helpful hint to avoid catching the endotracheal tube (ETT) on the arytenoid cartilages during fiberoptic intubation is to:

    A. Place the ETT bevel *down* on the fiberoptic scope for oral intubations and bevel *up* for nasal intubations.
    B. Place the ETT bevel *up* on the fiberoptic scope for oral intubations and bevel *down* for nasal intubations.
    C. Cut off the bevel on the ETT *prior* to placement.
    D. Rotate the fiberoptic scope *prior* to advancing the endotracheal tube through the larynx.
    E. Extend the endotracheal tube beyond the tip of the endoscope *before* entering the larynx.

36. On a modified barium swallow study, the epiglottis does not invert during the pharyngeal phase of swallowing. Which of the following does this suggest?

    A. Paresis of the aryepiglottic folds
    B. Pharyngeal delay
    C. Preferential filling of only one pyriform sinus
    D. Tongue base weakness
    E. Esophageal achalasia

37. A patient demonstrates aspiration *after* the swallow on a modified barium swallow study. This could be the result of:

    A. Inadequate hyolaryngeal elevation
    B. Glottal incompetence
    C. Incomplete mastication
    D. Reduced labial closure
    E. Reduced tongue mobility

38. Which of the following mechanisms is *not* used to manipulate the vibratory source in voice production?

    A. Subglottic pressure
    B. Vocal fold approximation
    C. Thyrohyoid tension
    D. Vocal fold tension
    E. Tongue tension

39. Sequelae of radiation to the larynx can include:

    A. Erythematous, edematous mucosa
    B. Decreased mucosal clearance of secretions
    C. Decreased vibration of phonatory mucosa
    D. Decreased vocal fold range of motion
    E. All of the above

40. Distal esophageal spasm is characterized by:

    A. Nonperistaltic low amplitude contractions
    B. Peristaltic low amplitude contractions
    C. Nonperistaltic normal or high amplitude contractions
    D. Peristaltic normal or high amplitude contractions
    E. Aperistalsis with low amplitude contractions

41. Our ability to safely swallow different consistencies and volumes of food and liquid is based on:

    A. Autonomic response
    B. Involuntary response
    C. Patterned motor response
    D. Voluntary response
    E. Cognitive processing

42. A 67-year-old man with terminal lung cancer is unable to eat due to aspiration. He would like an opportunity to eat. Examination demonstrates left vocal cord paralysis. Which of the following is probably the most appropriate recommendation?

    A. Make patient NPO (nil per os) and place an nasogastric tube
    B. Recommend laryngotracheal separation
    C. Since it is terminal, no treatment is warranted
    D. Vocal fold augmentation
    E. Targeted radiotherapy

43. The rate of failed emergency department intubations and subsequent surgical airway management is approximately between:

    A. 0% and 0.5%
    B. 0.5% and 1%
    C. 1% and 1.5%
    D. 1.5% and 2%
    E. 2% and 2.5%

44. A patient with Parkinson disease is referred to you for hypophonia. On examination you see vocal fold bowing. The next appropriate step would include:

    A. Referral for placement of a deep brain stimulator
    B. Referral for LSVT (Lee Silverman Voice Therapy)
    C. A MRI scan
    D. Sleep study
    E. Audiologic assessment

45. Which of the following statements is correct regarding keratosis of the vocal folds?

    A. Change in size and nature of keratosis should prompt surgical excision.
    B. Erythroplakia is a worse prognosis than leukoplakia.
    C. Leukoplakia is a worse prognosis than erythroplakia.
    D. All keratotic lesions must be completely surgically removed at all times.
    E. Observation is appropriate because this is solely a benign process

46. Which of the following is *not* one of the most common causative bacteria for bacterial laryngitis?

    A. *Haemophilus influenzae*
    B. *Staphylococcus* species
    C. *Klebsiella pneumoniae*
    D. *Streptococcus* species
    E. Enterococcus species

47. Voice therapy usually requires:

    A. 1 to 2 sessions of indirect voice therapy and 4 to 6 sessions of direct voice therapy
    B. 4 to 6 sessions of indirect voice therapy and 1 to 2 sessions of direct voice therapy
    C. 12 weekly sessions
    D. 6 sessions of indirect voice therapy
    E. 6 sessions of direct voice therapy

58. Antoni A and Antoni B areas are classically seen in which of the following laryngeal pathologies?

    A. Chondroma
    B. Schwannoma
    C. Recurrent respiratory papillomatosis
    D. Systemic lupus erythematous
    E. Amyloid deposits

59. What is the mixed voice range?

    A. The register between head and chest voice
    B. The register between falsetto and passagio voice
    C. The register between bass and tenor voice
    D. The register between alto and soprano voice
    E. The register between tenor and baritone voice

60. Continuous positive airway pressure (CPAP) is effective for obstructive sleep apnea (OSA) because it:

    A. Supports the soft palate
    B. Compresses the tongue base
    C. Stimulates activity of dilating muscles
    D. Prevents pharyngeal collapse during expiration
    E. Forces the pharynx open after obstruction

61. An elderly patient is referred for a bedside swallow evaluation. A shortcoming particular to this examination is:

    A. The need for trained personnel and specialized equipment
    B. Its inability to detect silent aspiration
    C. Radiation exposure
    D. Its contraindication in patients following acute stroke
    E. The need for a team of dysphagia experts

62. Elastin fibers are most numerous in which layer of the vocal fold?

    A. Quadrangular ligament
    B. Superficial lamina propria
    C. Intermediate lamina propria
    D. Deep lamina propria
    E. Vocal ligament

63. **Which measures can improve dysphagia as a result of pulmonary compromise?**

    A. Chest muscle conditioning through physiotherapy
    B. Large volume food bolus ingestion
    C. Promoting eating when patients are tachypneic
    D. Not encouraging good oral hygiene
    E. Placement of a nasogastric feeding tube

64. **A 45-year-old man with hypercoagulopathy suffers a severe brainstem stroke. He is cognitively intact, but is aspirating continuously. What is an appropriate early intervention?**

    A. Make patient NPO (nil per os) and pass NGT (nasogastric tube)
    B. Perform tracheostomy, percutaneous endoscopic gastrostomy (PEG), and place laryngeal stent
    C. Perform laryngotracheal separation
    D. Chemodenervate his cricopharyngeal muscle
    E. A and then B

65. **Proton pump inhibitors (PPIs) reduce symptoms of laryngopharyngeal reflux (LPR) by:**

    A. Combining with inactivating bile salts
    B. Irreversibly blocking the conversion of pepsinogen to pepsin
    C. Lowering the pH of gastric secretions
    D. Raising the pH of gastric secretions
    E. Binding with neural receptors and altering the cough reflux

66. **Which of the following best describes the sulcus vocalis?**

    A. Involves a predisposition for vocal fold cancer
    B. A derangement of the vocal fold lamina propria
    C. Related to problems with the neuromuscular status of the vocal fold
    D. Is solely a congenital disorder
    E. Always occurs bilaterally

67. **In addition to diabetes, other established risk factors for failure in open airway surgery include:**

    A. Inflammation
    B. Age
    C. Multilevel stenosis
    D. A and C
    E. A, B, and C

68. Which compensatory posture presents the greatest risk for aspiration of food contents?

    A. Chin tuck
    B. Head rotation
    C. Head back
    D. Head tilt
    E. Shoulder elevation

69. Temporary vocal fold augmentation materials include:

    A. Silastic
    B. Hyaluronic acid
    C. Titanium
    D. Gore-Tex
    E. Teflon

70. The sensitivity of fiberoptic endoscopic evaluation of swallowing with sensory testing (FEESST) is improved by including assessment of:

    A. Gag reflex
    B. Pharyngeal squeeze
    C. Laryngeal adductor reflex
    D. Intrabolus pressure in the upper esophageal sphincter
    E. Vocal fold motion

71. Which of the following is an absolute contraindication to an awake laryngeal procedure?

    A. Patient is unable to stop anticoagulant medications.
    B. Patient anxiety.
    C. Patient is unable to tolerate endoscopic visualization of larynx despite maximal anesthesia due to intense gag reflex.
    D. Cervical dystonia.
    E. Large tongue

72. Reflux of gastric contents is best treated by:

    A. Three months of histamine (H_2) blocker therapy
    B. Three months of proton pump inhibitor therapy
    C. Laparoscopic fundoplication
    D. Three months of sucralfate therapy
    E. Three months of prokinetic agent therapy

73. **When should permanent treatment for vocal fold paralysis be undertaken?**

    A. At 1 month after onset
    B. No earlier than 6 months after onset
    C. When laryngeal electromyography (LEMG) demonstrates poor prognosis for recovery
    D. Only for severe symptomatology
    E. After resolution of dysphagia symptoms

74. **The upper motor neurons involved in laryngeal control descend:**

    A. In the extrapyramidal system
    B. In the corticobulbar tract, decussate and synapse on neurons in bilateral nucleus ambiguus
    C. In the corticobulbar tract and synapse on neurons in the spinal trigeminal nucleus
    D. In the carotid sheath, the right looping around the subclavian and the left around the arch of the aorta
    E. In the corticobulbar tract, decussate, and synapse in the nucleus tractus solitarius.

75. **Which of the following muscles abducts the vocal fold?**

    A. Cricothyroid muscle
    B. Thyrohyoid muscle
    C. Lateral thyroarytenoid muscle
    D. Lateral cricoarytenoid muscle
    E. Posterior cricoarytenoid muscle

76. **A patient is referred to you with Parkinson disease. His voice is dysphonic. On examination you see a vocal fold paralysis. What would the next appropriate step be?**

    A. Sleep study and sleep medicine referral
    B. Tracheotomy
    C. Vocal fold injection
    D. Referral for placement of a deep brain stimulator
    E. Testing for tuberculosis with a PPD test

77. **Which of these is *not* a potential side effect of systemic steroids?**

    A. Change in mental status
    B. Aseptic necrosis of the hip
    C. Predisposition to vocal fold hemorrhage
    D. Tendon rupture
    E. Sleep disturbance

78. **Permanent vocal fold augmentation materials include:**

    A. Silastic
    B. Carboxymethylcellulose
    C. Hyaluronic acid
    D. Collagen
    E. Gelatin sponge

79. **An *exit* procedure refers to which of these?**

    A. A procedure that allows for relief of airway obstruction by creating an "exit" for airflow.
    B. A procedure whereby the airway of a newborn is secured while maintaining uteroplacental circulation with only partial delivery.
    C. A method of extubation that involves the use of specialized equipment for visualization of the airway prior to removal of the tube.
    D. An intubation technique that involves the use of X-ray technology for identifying the airway.
    E. An emergency airway technique that is useful in situations where facemask ventilation is not possible.

80. **Which of the following statements best describes Bullard laryngoscopies?**

    A. It was originally designed for obese patients.
    B. It is placed through the nasal cavity.
    C. It has an attached stylet.
    D. It is an inexpensive disposable device.
    E. It relies primarily on transillumination for intubation.

81. **Zenker diverticula develop in:**

    A. Between the cricopharyngeus muscle and the inferior pharyngeal constrictor muscle
    B. Between the inferior and middle pharyngeal constrictor muscles
    C. Between the cricopharyngeus and the circular muscle of the esophagus
    D. Between the circular and longitudinal muscles of the esophagus
    E. Between the cricopharyngeus and the superior constrictor muscle.

82. Which of the following is the most common cause of iatrogenic bilateral vocal fold paralysis?

    A. Cervical spine surgery
    B. Lung surgery
    C. Thyroid surgery
    D. Carotid surgery
    E. Mediastinoscopy

83. In a normal swallow, passage of the bolus through the relaxed upper esophageal sphincter (UES) is the result of which of these responses?

    A. Bolus pressure exerted on the inferior constrictor muscle
    B. Hyolaryngeal elevation with traction on the UES
    C. Relaxation of the cricopharyngeus muscle
    D. Response to glottic closure
    E. All of the above

84. Transnasal esophagoscopy (TNE) affords many advantages over conventional per oral esophagoscopy, though traditional esophagogastroduodenoscopy (EGD) remains the preferred choice for which of these situations?

    A. Complication profile
    B. Patient tolerance
    C. Barrett esophagus screening at the gastroesophageal junction
    D. Interventional procedures requiring sedation
    E. Patient on anti-platelet therapy

85. A healthy 33-year-old woman is now 2 months s/p (status post) total thyroidectomy complicated by bilateral vocal fold motion impairment and symptomatic airway obstruction. Of the following, which one is a reasonable option for her treatment at this time?

    A. Artificial larynx for speech/voice
    B. Suture lateralization
    C. Total arytenoidectomy
    D. Posterior cricoid grafting
    E. Interarytenoid botulinum toxin injection

86. You are injecting botulinum toxin in a patient with vocal tremor. Which of the following statements describes the disease and treatment options?

    A. With the correct dose, the tremor will completely disappear.
    B. Toxin injections will dampen but not eliminate the tremor.
    C. Patients injected for vocal tremor never get dysphagia as a side effect.
    D. Medications work well for vocal tremor and should be used instead of toxin injections.
    E. A single treatment is effective for dysphagia

87. A classic LMA (laryngeal mask airway) does which of the following?

    A. Protects the airway from regurgitation or aspiration.
    B. Can be utilized in situations of subglottic obstruction.
    C. Can be used with airway pressures greater than 20 to 25 cm H_2O.
    D. Is inserted under direct visualization into the hypopharynx.
    E. Is a supraglottic device consisting of an inflatable mask fitted against the periglottic tissues, to form a seal above the glottis.

88. A patient demonstrates premature spillage on a videofluorographic study. This indicates:

    A. Poor preparation of the bolus
    B. Premature glottal closure
    C. Reduced posterior oral control
    D. Velopharyngeal competence
    E. Velopharyngeal incompetence

89. A 52–year-old man with a history of prior chemoradiation for stage III squamous cell carcinoma of the oropharynx is to undergo a left neck dissection for persistent disease. On examination, he has trismus (can open his mouth 2 fingerbreadths), poor dentition, a Malampatti Class 4 view, a shortened thyro-mental distance, and a very indurated neck. At the time of surgery, the safest way to establish an airway on the patient would be to:

    A. Proceed directly to awake tracheotomy
    B. Proceed to orotracheal intubation with a MacIntosh blade following administration of propofol and succinylcholine
    C. Proceed to blind nasotracheal intubation
    D. Consider percutaneous tracheotomy
    E. Establish a plan with the anesthetist, starting with awake fiberoptic nasotracheal intubation, with the surgeon on standby, ready to perform an awake tracheotomy if intubation fails.

90. 65-2. Which structure of the larynx contributes to the convergent shape of the subglottis?

  A. Cricoid cartilage
  B. Conus elasticus
  C. Cricothyroid membrane
  D. Inferior pharyngeal constrictor muscle
  E. Arytenoid cartilage

91. Which of the following best describes vocal fold granuloma?

  A. Is often related to recent endotracheal intubation
  B. Occurs at the vocal process of the arytenoid cartilage
  C. Involves caseating nodules on histology
  D. Can often be a recurrent problem
  E. A, B, D

92. Which of the following is a property of an ideal laser for laryngeal surgery?

  A. Superficial tissue penetration with minimal collateral tissue injury
  B. Ability to cut and coagulate
  C. Deliverable through a flexible fiber that can be passed through a flexible endoscope
  D. Hemostatic properties
  E. All of the above

93. Wegener disease has a predilection for which part of the larynx; and emerging therapy includes the use of what treatment?

  A. Glottis; augmentative cartilage grafts
  B. Glottis; monoclonal antibodies
  C. Subglottis; augmentative cartilage grafts
  D. Subglottis; monoclonal antibodies
  E. None of the above

94. A 68-year-old man with treated right tonsillar squamous cell carcinoma and long-stranding left vocal cord paralysis. What is the source of the asymmetric FDG (fluoro-2-deoxyglucose) uptake on this fused PET (positron emission tomography)/CT image?

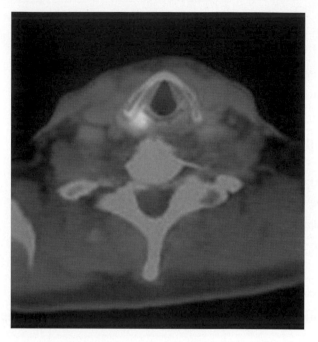

A. Recurrence at the primary site
B. Recurrence in cervical lymph nodes
C. Infection
D. Chondroradionecrosis
E. Vocal fold paralysis

95. An 81-year-old man with submucosal laryngeal mass. What is the most likely diagnosis?

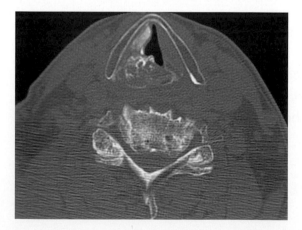

A. Osteosarcoma
B. Chondrosarcoma
C. Squamous cell carcinoma (SCC)
D. Hemangioma
E. Polyp

96. A 76-year-old woman with difficulty swallowing. What is the cause of her dysphagia?

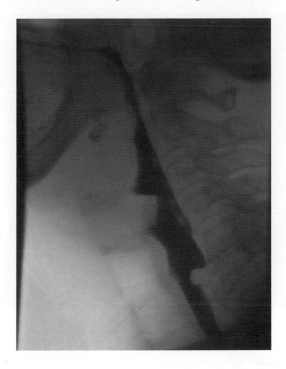

   A. Laryngeal tumor
   B. Cricopharyngeal achalasia
   C. Hypopharyngeal tumor
   D. Pharyngeal denervation
   E. Gastroesophageal reflux

97. A 50-year-old woman with stridor. What is the most likely cause?

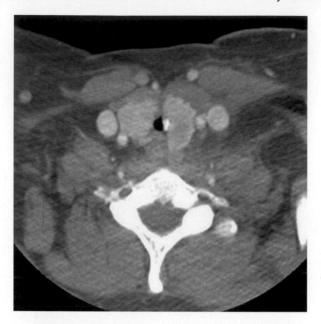

  A. Prior tracheostomy causing tracheomalacia
  B. Multinodular goiter
  C. Thyroid carcinoma
  D. Congenital anomaly
  E. The tracheal diameter is within normal limits

98. To evaluate complaints of dysphagia following ischemic stroke, videofluoroscopic swallow study (VFSS) offers what advantage over fiberoptic endoscopic evaluation of swallowing (FEES)?

  A. Assessment of vocal fold mobility
  B. Detection of frank aspiration
  C. Evaluation of hyolaryngeal elevation
  D. Assessment of laryngeal and pharyngeal mucosal pathology
  E. Assessment of pharyngeal mucosal pathology

Chapter 4 Answers

1. **Answer: C.** The vocalis muscle is not a part of the lamina propria layer, but it is deep to it. PAGE 950

2. **Answer: C.** This constellation is seen in pseudobulbar palsy. ALS and bulbar palsy often do not lead to emotional lability. Tongue fasciculations are seen associated with tongue weakness. Botulism presents more systemically. PAGE 1030

3. **Answer: B.** The goal of voice therapy is to rebalance the coordination of breathing, phonation, and resonance. Answers C, D, and E describe means to that goal. Voice therapy is not intended to strengthen the vocal folds. PAGE 1050

4. **Answer: D.** Serology has been found to be largely unhelpful at determining the etiology of new-onset unilateral vocal fold paralysis and does not help guide treatment. The other studies mentioned can contribute information on possible etiology or can help with management decisions. PAGE 1011

5. **Answer: A.** A patient who can swallow normal-size solid boluses should be able to swallow pills of the same caliber. Patients often have a harder time anticipating a swallow of a pill, which may lead to pill dysphagia in the absence of solid food dysphagia. PAGE 817

6. **Answer: B.** The CO_2 laser is traditionally a "line of site" laser and thus is directed with the use of mirrors. The OmniguideTM is a fiber-based CO_2 laser delivery method. The laser energy is conducted by the use of a hollow core tube (fiber), within which the laser bounces around until it reaches its target. Because of the heat generated by the laser, gas is typically pumped through the hollow fiber. Due to this, the fiber cannot be placed in contact with the tissue. The other lasers can be used in a contact or non contact method. PAGES 1087–1088

7. **Answer: E.** Passy-Muir valves allow for speaking by inhalation through the tracheotomy tube and exhalation through the native airway. Answers B, C, and D will prevent air egress into the native upper airway. Cognitive dysfunction may impair speech and management of the valve, precluding the value of the Passy-Muir. PAGES 932–933

8. **Answer: B.** A recent large review showed that iatrogenic injury is the most common cause of UVFP. PAGE 1004

9. **Answer: D.** Laryngeal sarcoid is an infiltrative disease that can result in supraglottic scarring and distortion of the normal supraglottic structures. PAGE 982

10. **Answer: C.** The thyrohyoid muscle is involved in gross laryngeal movement during swallowing and during certain vocal tasks. It is external to the larynx and a strap muscle. PAGE 945

11. **Answer: B.** The answer highlights the essential components of voice therapy and focuses on the three broad categories of voice therapy. The other answers contain elements of each of these larger categories, but do not list all three components as described in the text. PAGES 1048–1050

12. **Answer: C.** Answer A is wrong because botulinum toxin is most useful for nonstimulated salivary flow produced by the submandibular gland. Answer B is wrong because it can be injected serially as the effect wears off. Answer C is correct, in that ultrasound may give more accuracy in injection guidance, though it might not be necessary. Answer D is wrong. Medical therapy should be initiated first. PAGE 846

13. **Answer: C.** Nodules respond favorably to rest/therapy, are symmetric, disrupt mucosal wave minimally, and are always bilateral/midmembranous. Surgery is rarely required. PAGE 990

14. **Answer: D.** All the above answers have been described in the literature. PAGE 1086

15. **Answer: A.** Intestinal metaplasia is the hallmark of Barrett esophagus. Dysplasia may or may not be present within this metaplastic tissue. PAGE 853

16. **Answer: A.** Surgical removal remains the mainstay of therapy, though there are a variety of adjunctive treatments that have been described. Cidofovir is injected intralesionally, not inhaled, and is not indicated for early treatment. Oral steroids and azathioprine have not been described as effective treatments. PAGE 983

17. **Answer: B.** The interarytenoid muscle is the only unpaired laryngeal muscle and has bilateral innervation. PAGE 873

18. **Answer: A.** Formant clustering in this range leads to harmonic amplification and the ability for a singer to be heard over significant background noise, such as an orchestra. PAGE 1062

19. **Answer: B.** BMI > 30 is not a contraindication for percutaneous tracheotomy. However, the other choices are demonstrated contraindications for safe performance of percutaneous tracheotomy. High innominate artery poses high risk of severe hemorrhage. Midline neck masses that are large preclude safe dilational tracheotomy. Airway protection (oral exercise tolerance test in place) is mandatory, and if the cricoid cartilage cannot be palpated, safe placement of the tracheotomy tube cannot be ensured. PAGE 936

20. **Answer: B.** Secondary muscle tension dysphonia refers to a condition where the muscle tension is in response to an underlying glottal incompetence. In these cases, voice therapy is less successful, as the glottal incompetence may need to be surgically corrected before the patient can eliminate the muscle tension behaviors. The other listed conditions often have a favorable response to voice therapy. PAGE 1055

21. **Answer: A.** A 48-hour pH testing with a pharyngeal probe, often combined with impedance testing for fluid flow, is the best present test for the diagnosis of LPR. LPR can occur in the absence of esophagitis. Positive response to acid-suppression therapy may be related to placebo effect. The RSI is not specific for LPR. A high RSI score can occur in other disorders not related to LPR. LPR may occur within the setting of normal LES pressures. PAGE 967

22. **Answer: D.** The goal of treatment for bilateral vocal fold paralysis (which usually results in airway compromise) is to widen the glottis airway or bypass it (tracheostomy). All of the listed treatment options, except vocal fold augmentation, are designed to improve the glottic opening. PAGES 1020–1022

23. **Answer: B.** Answer B refers to vocal fold stripping, a historical procedure involving complete removal of vocal fold mucosa. Microflap surgery is a conservative resection of submucosal pathology, limiting dissection of normal lamina propria and preserving normal tissue. Patience and specialized microinstrumentation are required. PAGE 999

24. **Answer: D.** Education is required in this situation for the facility leadership and on-site clinicians to improve systemwide practices to prevent this recurrent problem. PAGE 859

25. **Answer: A.** A. This procedure is the best next step to prevent aspiration-related complicationsfrom severe loss of swallow function. Laryngectomy could be considered as well. Discharging the patient without reducing the aspiration is likely to lead to recurrent pneumonia. PAGES 864–865

26. **Answer: B.** Success in voice therapy is difficult to quantify, but is based in patient outcome measures, generally. The most important outcome is typically judged to be a return to functional abilities, as opposed to changes in lesions size (which does not often correlate with voice quality), or other more subjective measures such as a better sound, better feel, or happiness. PAGE 1056

27. **Answer: D.** Bile salts enter epithelial cells and may cause damage at both acid and neutral pH. PAGE 960

28. **Answer: B.** Vocal process granulomas are highly associated with LPR. Rhinorrhea, paralysis, cervical spine disease, and adenotonsillar hypertrophy are not. PAGES 964–965

29. **Answer: B.** Stroboscopy is performed during vocal fold adduction and therefore does not assess vocal fold movement. The other features mentioned can be assessed by this examination. PAGE 955

30. **Answer: E. Hunsaker tube** is slim-line and is minimally obstructive in the airway. It is laser-safe. When used appropriately with allowance of airway egress, complications are low. Thus, it is versatile. PAGE 914

31. **Answer: A.** VFSSs allow for precise measurement of laryngohyoid movement (PAGE 831). Manometry and FEES do not assess this parameter. Although a clinical bedside evaluation can detect laryngohyoid movement, it is difficult to reliably measure.

32. **Answer: B.** Interarytenoid activity maintains vocal fold approximation, while thyroarytenoid muscle activity is largely responsible for pitch adjustment in chest voice mechanism. PAGE 1065

33. **Answer: A.** An esophageal B ring, also known as a Schatzki ring, represents a mucosal stricture rather than a thickening of muscle at the LES (A ring) or external compression from the diaphragm. (PAGE 856) Epithelial trachealization is typical of eosinophilic esophagitis. This type of ring is found in the distal esophagus.

34. **Answer: C.** This procedure requires more steps than conventional tracheostomy, yet provides a mature stoma that often can be managed without a stent or tube. The other choices are incorrect. PAGE 931

35. **Answer: A.** The tip of the ETT can often get caught on the arytenoids during fiberoptic intubation. Rotating the bevel can help avoid this and allow for easier advancement of the tube. PAGE 900

36. **Answer: D.** Epiglottic inversion is largely passive based on laryngeal elevation and anterior motion during swallowing. PAGE 821

37. **Answer: A.** Based on the choices provided, A is the best choice. Reduced hyolaryngeal excursion impairs emptying of the hypopharynx of bolus residue, leading to increased risk of postswallow aspiration. More important to prevent postswallow aspiration is the presence of adequate laryngeal sensation. PAGE 821

38. **Answer: C.** Thyrohyoid tension has no effect on the vibratory source (vocal fold vibration). Thyrohyoid tension acts as antagonist to cricothyroid muscle action and can limit vocal range capabilities. PAGES 1063–1064, 1071

39. **Answer: E.** Radiation has multiple fibrotic effects on the larynx, including all those mentioned above. PAGE 982

40. **Answer: C.** This disorder results in frequent simultaneous rather than peristaltic contractions. This is considered a hyperkinetic disorder, since the contractions are generally normal or high amplitude. PAGE 854

41. **Answer: C.** Swallowing function is only voluntary in the oral phase. The pharyngeal phase and esophageal phase are a function of patterned motor response—neither voluntary, nor involuntary, nor autonomic. PAGE 817

42. **Answer: D.** Vocal fold augmentation is the best initial choice of management. It is minimally invasive and may provide the ability for this patient to eat. Although Answer B would also be helpful, it is a much more aggressive intervention and not the first line of treatment. PAGE 862

43. **Answer: B.** The rate of failed intubations is quite low. PAGE 905

44. **Answer: B.** LSVT has been systematically shown to improve voice in patients with Parkinson hypophonia and is first-line therapy for the condition. Deep brain stimulation is presently not a primary indication to treat Parkinson hypophonia. Answers C and D are not indicated for the evaluation or treatment of Parkinson dysphonia. PAGE 1031

45. **Answer: A.** Any epithelial lesion with demonstrating changes in growth or characteristic may represent transformation to a more aggressive disease, including carcinoma, and requires surgical excision. Leukoplakia has not been proven to have a worse or better prognosis than erythroplakia and vice versa. Keratotic lesion can be benign and observed in some settings. PAGE 989

46. **Answer: C.** *Klebsiella pneumoniae* is not a common pathogen in the larynx. (PAGE 978) Causative bacteria, also similar to those in the pediatric population, include *Haemophilus influenzae*, *Streptococcus* species, and *Staphylococcus* species.

47. **Answer: A.** Indirect voice therapy focuses on decreasing phonotrauma and vocal hygiene. This can typically be done in 1 to 2 sessions. The bulk of the voice therapy program focuses on direct voice therapy, which works on coordinated voice production. PAGE 1048

48. **Answer: A.** Mitomycin is commonly used topically in airway surgery based on its theoretic reduction of fibroblast proliferation. It has not been proven beneficial in prospective trials, and was first used in ophthalmology for scar reduction. PAGE 887

49. **Answer: E.** All of the answers are approaches that allow access to the body of the vocal fold for injection. PAGES 1082–1086

50. **Answer: D.** Each choice given plays a role in formulating a comprehensive plan for this patient with dysphagia. Taking into account family goals, severity of the patient's dysphagia, along with complications that have occurred due to dysphagia, will direct appropriate management. PAGE 866

51. **Answer: A.** The larynx has several different receptors, including negative pressure receptors. These are primarily mediated through the SLN. PAGE 875

52. **Answer: B.** Stimulation of neck musculature, uncoordinated from the precise mechanics of swallowing may actually make patients more at risk for aspiration than the nonstimulated state. PAGE 843

53. **Answer: D.** Answers A–C are all involved with esophageal motility. PAGES 844–845

54. **Answer: D.** The lack of pathologic findings on initial laryngoscopy should prompt the clinician to seek more definitive imaging. (PAGE 954) Stroboscopy is an essential evaluation tool for dysphonia when no gross abnormalities are found on initial laryngoscopy. Answers B and C are treatments that cannot be used until a diagnosis has been established.

55. **Answer: C.** The vocalis muscle, the medial aspect of the thyroarytenoid muscle, is primarily involved with tonic contraction, which typically requires fatigue-resistant slow twitch muscle. PAGE 948

56. **Answer: E.** Pepsin may be detected in some cases of subglottic stenosis. Tracheal resection can usually be accomplished without releasing maneuvers. Though balloon dilation may have some theoretic advantages in endoscopic airway surgery, it has not been proven to be superior to other methods of dilation. PAGE 885

57. **Answer: C.** The mere presence of mast cells in the esophagus is not enough for diagnosis. Biopsy confirms the diagnosis, requiring 15 to 20 eosinophils per HPF. (PAGE 852) Chronic ulceration is not a feature of eosinophilic esophagitis.

58. **Answer: B.** These histologic features are classically seen in schwannomas found throughout the body. PAGE 985

59. **Answer: A.** Mixed voice is the register between head and chest voice. It is often referred to as the middle voice, or vocal passagio. The other answers are incorrect. (Vocal registration is described on PAGE 1066 .)

60. **Answer: D.** The purpose of CPAP is to stent open the airway, which typically collapses during end-expiration in OSA patients. CPAP can stent open the collapsed segment during end-expiration. This may be one mechanism by which CPAP therapy is effective. CPAP causes a decrease in genioglossus muscle activity during wakefulness in patients with sleep apnea, but not in normal persons, suggesting that the increased activity in the waking OSA syndrome patient represents compensation for a mechanically obstructed airway, not defective reflexes. PAGE 869

61. **Answer: B.** As opposed to the other methods of swallow evaluation described, this study does not detect silent aspiration (by definition). A bedside swallow evaluation does not involve specialized equipment and can be done in patients following acute stroke. Although this study does not offer direct information about vocal fold mobility, this is not a weakness particular to this study, as videofluoroscopic swallow study also gives limited information in this regard. PAGES 827–828

62. **Answer: C.** The intermediate layer has numerous elastin fibers and is also the thickest layer of the lamina propria. The vocal ligament is composed of collagen, and Answer A is not a layer within the vocal fold. PAGE 874

63. **Answer: A.** Answer B suggests that eating a large bolus of food will be safer in a patient with pulmonary impairment. Answer C suggests that the patient should eat safely when they are acutely short of breath. Answer D suggests that poor oral hygiene will actually improve swallowing function. PAGE 846

64. **Answer: E.** Initial intervention is to provide the patient alimentation and prevent asipration complications. NPO and NGT placement provide this. Following this, PEG, tracheotomy, and laryngeal stent placement are the next steps in providing the possibility for PO (per oral) intake. Laryngotracheal separation or laryngectomy could be considered after this. PAGE 861

65. **Answer: D.** PPIs do not prevent reflux; they simply raise the pH of gastric secretions and can reduce direct acid irritation of laryngopharyngeal tissues, and reduce the activity of pepsin, a digestive enzyme in refluxate. PAGE 971

66. **Answer: B.** Sulcus vocalis implies loss of lamina propria, leading to vocal fold mucosal defects that can significantly affect healthy vocal production depending on size and location. PAGE 993

67. **Answer: E.** Increased state of inflammation, increasing age, and high complexity stenosis generally lead to poorer outcomes in open airway surgery. PAGES 888–889

68. **Answer: C.** "Head back" positioning places the larynx in a more posterior position, which may lead to more risk of laryngeal penetration and aspiration. PAGE 839

69. **Answer: B.** Hyaluronic acid is a temporary injectable. All of the other mentioned materials are permanent implants. PAGES 1014–1016

70. **Answer: B.** The pharyngeal squeeze maneuver allows for improved assessment of pharyngeal function (PAGE 828). The presence or absence of a gag reflex is not predictive of swallow dysfunction. A laryngeal adductor reflex is tested by the FEESST examination. Intrabolus pressure can only be assessed via manometry.

71. **Answer: C.** The other three issues can be worked around when performing office-based procedures. However, if someone cannot be examined with an endoscope, there is no ability to visualize the field during a procedure. PAGES 1078–1079

72. **Answer: C.** Fundoplication is the only treatment presently available that consistently reduces reflux of gastric contents. Acid reducers do not reduce reflux. Prokinetic agents can theoretically reduce reflux by promoting gastric emptying, but few agents are available that are effective. PAGE 972

73. **Answer: C.** While there are different practice patterns with regard to timing of intervention, the finding of poor prognosis on LEMG strongly argues in favor of permanent treatment. LEMG, especially serial, can be used to shorten the time until permanent treatment can be implemented. None of the other answers describe firm criteria for permanent treatment over waiting or temporary treatment. PAGE 1013

74. **Answer: B.** Upper motor neurons involved in laryngeal control synapse in the nucleii ambiguous, not the spinal trigeminal nucleus or nucleus tractus solitarius. Answer D describes the lower motor neurons. The extrapyramidal system neurons are higher order to the upper motor neurons. PAGE 1026

75. **Answer: E.** The posterior cricoarytenoid muscle is the only abductor of the vocal fold (PAGE 871). Answer B is a strap muscle, Answer C does not exist, and the cricothyroid is traditionally thought to be involved in vocal fold lengthening for pitch elevation.

76. **Answer: A.** This patient likely has multiple system atrophy (MSA) given the vocal fold paralysis. Sleep disorders are common in this disease and warrant further evaluation. Although Lee Silverman Voice Therapy (LSVT) is effective for Parkinson hypophonia, it is not effective for vocal fold paralysis. In this case, Parkinson disease is a confounder and this patient is more likely to have MSA. This warrants intervention first, with LSVT reserved for Parkinson disease. PAGE 1032

77. **Answer: D.** Tendon rupture is not a risk of systemic steroids. However, patients should be counseled on possible mental status changes, sleep disturbance, predisposition to vocal fold hemorrhage, and, rarely, aseptic or avascular necrosis of the hip. (PAGE 1074 has more information on using systemic steroids in professional voice users.) PAGE 1074

78. **Answer: A.** All the other materials listed are temporary injectables. Silicone elastomer (Silastic) is a solid, permanent implant. PAGE 1016

79. **Answer: B.** An exit procedure refers to an *ex utero* intrapartum treatment procedure and is performed when there is a known or suspected serious airway problem anticipated during delivery. The airway is secured while the newborn is still receiving oxygenation through placental circulation. PAGE 898

80. **Answer: C.** The Bullard laryngoscope has a stylet to the right of the viewing lens and is designed to match the shape of the indirect laryngoscope. It was originally designed for use in the difficult pediatric airway and is available in both adult and pediatric sizes. PAGE 900

81. **Answer: A.** Killian dehiscence is located posteriorly between the cricopharyngeus muscle and the inferior constrictor muscle. PAGE 856

82. **Answer: C.** Thyroid surgery carries a higher risk of bilateral vocal fold paralysis, as many of these surgeries include total removal of the gland putting both recurrent laryngeal nerves at risk. PAGE 1017

83. **Answer: B.** During a normal physiologic swallow, static motor unit recruitment to the UES ceases during hyolaryngeal elevation, allowing passive opening of the UES to allow passage of boluses subject to positive oropharyngeal propulsive forces and negative hypopharyngeal suction forces. PAGE 820

84. **Answer D.** Interventional procedures typically require larger working channels and more time to perform. While possible through a TNE, larger endoscopes and sedation are preferred for these types of cases. Complication profile, tolerance, and Barrett esophagus screening are either similar or improved with TNE over traditional EGD PAGES 831–834.

85. **Answer: B.** Answer B is the best choice: suture lateralization provides airway improvement that is reversible should movement of one or both vocal folds recover. Tracheotomy may be simultaneously avoided. Permanent intervention (destructive glottis enlargement procedure) at 2 months following surgery is not indicated due to the possibility of recovery. PAGE 884

86. **Answer: B.** Vocal tremor involves multiple sites, often including the pharynx, tongue base, and palate. Botulinum toxin can mitigate some of the symptoms associated with vocal tremor, particularly glottal stops. Patients should be counseled that tremor symptoms usually will not completely resolve due to more diffuse vocal tract involvement. Medications tend to have limited effectiveness for axial tremor. PAGE 1033

87. **Answer: E.** An LMA is typically inserted blindly and specifically cannot be used in the situations described in choices A, B, and C. PAGE 904 .

88. **Answer: C.** Premature spillage of boluses from the oral cavity to the pharyngeal cavity represents poor oromotor control of food boluses. A variety of conditions may lead to this occurrence. PAGE 819

89. **Answer: E.** Answer A could be considered safe, but, most commonly, patients with impossible direct laryngoscopy can be intubated safely with awake fiberoptic intubation, provided an airway management plan including possible awake tracheotomy is organized to manage intubation failures. PAGE 911

90. **Answer: B.** The conus elasticus originates on the upper border to the cricoid cartilage and rises to the glottic aperture, forming the convergent shape of the subglottis. PAGE 946

91. **Answer: E.** Caseating nodules on histology should lead the clinician to suspect a diagnosis other than granuloma. The most common location of vocal fold granulomas is near the vocal process, often related to intubation, and can be recurrent—particularly in cases with nonintubated etiology. PAGE 995

92. **Answer: E.** The answers describe ideal characteristics for any tool used for laryngeal surgery. PAGE 1086

93. **Answer: D.** Wegener disease has a predilection for the subglottis. Though unproven at this point, monoclonal antibody therapy may prevent long-term airway scarring and stenosis. PAGES 880–881

94. **Answer: E.** Paralysis of the left vocal fold creates asymmetry by decreasing the uptake on the left side, making the right side seem too hot by comparison. In truth, the right side is displaying normal physiologic uptake of FDG. This uptake is in the wrong location for either type of recurrence. There are no CT findings of infection or chondroradionecrosis. PAGE 160

95. **Answer: B.** The calcified matrix within this tumor consists of arcs and circles, which are features seen in chondrosarcoma. Osteosarcoma and SCC would be more aggressive. Hemangiomas and polyps would not calcify in this pattern. PAGE 152

96. **Answer: B.** A smooth posterior indentation at the level of C5/6, measuring 1 cm in vertical dimension, is usually an unrelaxed cricopharyngeus muscle. Mucosal tumors would have an irregular margin. Denervation presents as asymmetric pharyngeal contractility. PAGE 822

97. **Answer: A.** This image shows severe subglottic tracheal stenosis. Goiter usually causes severe stenosis only at the thoracic inlet. There are no erosive changes to suggest cancer. Prior tracheostomy is the most common cause of subglottic tracheomalacia. PAGE 936

98. **Answer: C.** VFSS permits evaluation of hyolaryngeal elevation, which is important in stroke patients. With FEES, this cannot be assessed. Both methods can identify frank aspiration. Answer A is an advantage of FEES. PAGE 830 AND TABLE 57.5

5 Trauma

1. Which of the following is an indication for vascular evaluation in patients with penetrating trauma to the face?

   A. Active bleeding
   B. No exit wound
   C. Signs of neurological compromise
   D. Penetration posterior to the orbital apex
   E. Penetration posterior to the mandibular angle plane

2. When using the coronal flap approach to expose the zygomatic arch, the dissection should:

   A. Remain above the deep temporal fascia throughout
   B. Be superficial to the temporoparietal fascia
   C. Transition deep to the deep temporal fascia onto the temporal fat pad above the arch
   D. Transition deep to the temporalis muscle above the arch

3. A 46-year-old man sustained an assault to the face with a glass bottle and presents with lower lid laceration medial to the punctum on the left. Evaluation is likely to reveal injury to:

   A. Canalicular system
   B. Medial rectus
   C. Orbital septum
   D. Nasal bone
   E. Levator aponeurosis

4. The upper labial sulcus approach is best utilized to repair:

    A. Zygomaticomaxillary complex fractures
    B. Frontal sinus fractures
    C. Orbital floor blowout fractures
    D. Mandibular condyle fractures

5. Medial orbital wall exposure is accomplished by which of these statements?

    A. Best accomplished through a transcutaneous or "Lynch" incision
    B. Optimally done through a transcaruncular, transconjunctival approach
    C. Best approached from the upper labial sulcus
    D. Ideally gained through an eyebrow or "gullwing" incision

6. A 12-year-old boy sustained a blow to the eye from an elbow while jumping on a trampoline. There was no loss of consciousness. He is brought to the emergency department 6 hours after the injury and has had one episode of emesis. Pulse rate is 45 bpm, blood pressure 120/80 mm Hg, and respirations 18/minute. Examination reveals periorbital ecchymosis and restriction of extraocular motion, and CT of the head shows a fracture of the orbital floor. What is the most appropriate approach to management?

    A. Emergent surgical intervention
    B. Surgery in 24 to 72 hours
    C. Surgery in 4 to 7 days
    D. Observation with reassessment in 7 to 10 days

7. Which of the following is the most common midface fracture (other than nasal fracture)?

    A. Nasoorbitoethmoid (NOE) fracture
    B. Le Fort 1 fracture
    C. Le Fort 2 fracture
    D. Le Fort 3 fracture
    E. Zygomaticomaxillary (ZMC) fracture

8. Rounding of the inferior rectus on CT imaging is predictive of:

   A. Permanent diplopia on upgaze
   B. Injury to the lacrimal drainage system
   C. Development of delayed enophthalmos
   D. Permanent injury to the infraorbital nerve

9. A 7-year-old patient sustains a fall and presents with altered mental status and an upper eyelid hematoma. Which is the most likely diagnosis?

   A. Orbital floor blowout fracture
   B. Medial orbital wall fracture
   C. Frontal sinus fracture
   D. Orbital roof fracture

10. A 6-year-old girl is brought to the emergency department after being struck in the nose with a fist while playing with her sisters. She had immediate epistaxis, which is now resolved, but she cannot breath through the right side of her nose. Examination reveals a painful and blue right-sided intranasal mass which is compressible with a Q-tip. What is the next best step in management?

    A. Drainage at the bedside
    B. Operative drainage
    C. Placement of nasal packing
    D. Decongestion with oxymetazoline and follow-up in 7 days when edema has resolved

11. A 23-year-old man was found down after being trapped while mountain climbing. The temperature reached below 0°C and he sustained frostbite involving his nose, cheeks, and ears. What is the most appropriate first step?

    A. Surgical debridement
    B. Antibiotic prophylaxis
    C. Gradual warming beginning at 40°F
    D. Rapid rewarming in baths at 104°F to 108°F
    E. Administration of a vasodilator

12. A 3-year-old child presents to the emergency room with a deep puncture wound to the left cheek. The family reports the child was playing with the family cat when the injury occurred. What is the most common organism isolated from cat bites?

    A. *Moraxella* sp.
    B. *Pasteurella* sp.
    C. *Corynebacterium* sp.
    D. *Streptococcus* sp.
    E. *Staphylococcus* sp.

13. Which type of shock is most common after trauma?

    A. Hypovolemic shock
    B. Neurogenic shock
    C. Septic shock
    D. Cardiogenic shock
    E. Central nervous system shock

14. The appropriate treatment strategy for management of frontal sinus fractures can be made from assessing which of these five anatomic parameters?

    A. Nasoorbitoethmoid (NOE) complex fracture, orbital fracture, frontal recess, anterior table fracture, and posterior table fracture
    B. Anterior table fracture, posterior table fracture, nasofrontal recess injury, dural tear/ cerebrospinal fluid (CSF) leak, and fracture displacement/comminution
    C. Dural tear/CSF leak, NOE complex fracture, nasofrontal recess injury, orbital roof fracture, and posterior table fracture
    D. Through-and-through lacerations, orbital roof injury, frontal recess injury, anterior table fracture, and posterior table fracture

15. Intraoperative mydriasis is noted while repairing an orbital floor fracture. Which of the following is the most likely cause?

    A. Pressure on the ciliary ganglion
    B. Transection of the optic nerve
    C. Occlusion of the ophthalmic artery
    D. Retrobulbar hematoma

16. All of the following are absolute indications for open reduction of condyle fractures *except*:

    A. Displacement into the middle cranial fossa
    B. Foreign body in the joint capsule (e.g., gunshot wound)
    C. Lateral extracapsular deviation of the condyle
    D. Unilateral condylar fracture associated with a single midfacial fracture
    E. Inability to open mouth or achieve occlusion after 1 week
    F. Open fracture with facial nerve injury

17. Which of the following is the most common sequela in patients with a gunshot wound to the mandible zone?

    A. Airway obstruction
    B. Globe injury
    C. Intracranial penetration
    D. Vascular injury
    E. Trismus

18. Which of the following is *correct* concerning immediate facial nerve paralysis after penetrating trauma?

    A. The nerve injury is usually a contusion.
    B. The nerve injury is usually a transection.
    C. With observation alone, most patients will recover some facial nerve function.
    D. Surgical repair almost always requires a 12 to 7 crossover or jump-graft technique.
    E. Functional result after repair is usually a grade 2 on the House–Brackmann scale.

19. Which of the following fractures is most common in childhood?

    A. Frontal sinus
    B. Orbital
    C. Nasal
    D. Le Fort

20. Malunion of a fracture should be interpreted as:

    A. Instability at 8 to 12 weeks after fixation
    B. Bony union in nonanatomic position
    C. Fibrous union of fracture site
    D. Pseudoarthrosis

21. Where are septal fractures most commonly seen?

    A. Above the interface with the maxillary crest
    B. At the caudal septum
    C. At the junction of the cartilage with the perpendicular plate of the ethmoid bone
    D. Right where the cartilage interfaces with the maxillary crest

22. The majority of mandibular angle fractures are horizontally favorable/unfavorable based on which of these statements?

    A. Unfavorable as the masseter, lateral pterygoid, and temporalis muscles contribute to the superior and lateral displacement of the proximal segment.
    B. Favorable as the masseter, medial pterygoid, and temporalis muscles contribute to the superior and medial closure of the proximal segment.
    C. Unfavorable as the masseter, medial pterygoid, and temporalis muscles contribute to the superior and medial displacement of the proximal segment.
    D. Favorable as the masseter, medial pterygoid, and temporalis muscles contribute to the superior and medial closure of the distal segment.

23. What has improved trauma care the most?

    A. Widespread cardiopulmonary resuscitation use
    B. Coordinated prehospital and hospital care
    C. Automatic defibrillator devices
    D. Seatbelts
    E. Bicycle helmets

24. Which of the following is correct regarding the use of lag screws for mandibular fixation?

    A. Comminuted fractures of the symphysis can be readily treated with lag screws.
    B. The screw holes on the proximal and distal sides of the fracture should match the diameter of the screw shaft.
    C. Lag screws are an effective means of fracture compression.
    D. The lag screw should traverse the fracture line at an oblique angle.

25. When a screw is overtightened it may "strip," resulting in microfracture of the drill hole. What is the most appropriate solution?

    A. Redrill at another location
    B. Employ a different plate
    C. Use a different screw of same length and shaft diameter with greater thread diameter
    D. Use a longer screw

26. Which of the following mandible fractures is most appropriately treated with 2.0-mm miniplates?

    A. Comminuted fracture of the mandibular angle
    B. Edentulous mandibular body fracture
    C. Linear fracture of the right angle and left subcondylar region
    D. Mandibular nonunion with bone resorption

27. Regarding nasal fractures in children, which of these statements is correct?

    A. Earlier intervention is required as compared to adults.
    B. Epistaxis occurs more often than with adult nasal fractures.
    C. Imaging is of greater benefit than in adults because the clinical examination can be more challenging.
    D. The incidence is higher than in adults as accidental injury is more common in childhood.

28. A 10-year-old boy is evaluated because of severe pain when opening his mouth. One week ago he fell from his bicycle, striking his chin. Examination reveals deviation of the chin to the right and premature contact in the right molar region. The most likely cause of these findings is a fracture of which segment of the mandible?

    A. Angle
    B. Body
    C. Ramus
    D. Condyle
    E. Parasymphysis

29. Endoscopic repair of anterior table fractures is indicated in which patient population?

    A. Elderly patients with comminuted anterior table fractures
    B. Young patients with anterior table fractures that extend below the orbital rim
    C. Patients with isolated anterior table fractures and thin skin
    D. Patients with mildly displaced anterior table fractures (2 to 6 mm) that do not extend below the inferior orbital rim

30. The primary survey consists of which three areas of assessment?

    A. Airway, mental status, and perfusion
    B. Head, heart, and extremities
    C. Oxygen, pulse, and heart rate
    D. Color, pallor, and skin turgor
    E. Airway, breathing, and circulation

31. Which clinical scenario is the most appropriate for use of a stent in laryngeal trauma?

    A. Extensive lacerations of the anterior commissure
    B. Bilateral vocal fold hematomas
    C. Massive laryngeal cartilage fractures with adequate stabilization
    D. Cricotracheal separation

32. Which of the following tests is the most appropriate diagnosis imaging for a frontal sinus fracture?

    A. Axial CT scan with 3-mm slices
    B. Axial and coronal CT scans with 3-mm slices
    C. Plain radiographs and thin-cut axial, coronal, and sagittal CT scans with three-dimensional reconstructions
    D. Thin-cut (1.0 to 1.5 mm) axial CT scan with coronal, sagittal, and three-dimensional reconstructions

33. The decision to reduce a nasal fracture is based on which of these factors?

    A. A facial bone CT scan
    B. History and clinical examination
    C. Plain radiographs
    D. The age of the patient

34. Which is the single best site at which the accuracy of zygomaticomaxillary (ZMC) fracture reduction may be assessed?

    A. Zygomaticofrontal suture
    B. Zygomaticomaxillary suture
    C. Zygomaticosphenoid suture
    D. Zygomaticotemporal suture
    E. Infraorbital rim

35. A 19-year-old male wrestler presents to your clinic with evidence of a large auricular hematoma. This was treated appropriately with incision and drainage with bolster placement. In follow-up he is without symptoms following resolution of his hematoma. Within what layer(s) did the hematoma form?

    A. Skin
    B. Subcutaneous
    C. Intracartilaginous or subperichondrial
    D. Auricular musculature
    E. Supraperichondrial

36. Class II occlusion is best described as:

    A. The mesiobuccal cusp of the maxillary first molar occludes distal to the buccal groove of the mandibular first molar.
    B. Intercuspation of the mesial buccal cusp of the maxillary first molar with the buccal groove of the mandibular first molar.
    C. The mesiobuccal cusp of the maxillary first molar occludes mesial to the buccal groove of the mandibular first molar.
    D. The mesiobuccal cusp of the mandibular first molar is buccal to the buccal cusp of the maxillary first molar.

37. Which of the following is the most common complication that occurs after a transconjunctival approach?

    A. Symblepharon
    B. Ectropion
    C. Entropion
    D. Epiphora

38. A 26-year-old man suffers laryngeal trauma in a bull riding injury. Physical examination findings include mild anterior cervical ecchymosis, palpable laryngeal landmarks, and quiet breathing. Fiberoptic flexible laryngoscopy shows a small hematoma of the right true vocal fold but with good mobility. CT displays a nondisplaced fracture of the cricoid cartilage. Which of the following is the next best step in management?

    A. Direct laryngoscopy to evaluate for mucosal lacerations and arytenoid mobility
    B. Conservative management with humidified room air, proton pump inhibitors, and voice rest
    C. Fiberoptic intubation with a small-diameter endotracheal tube
    D. Awake tracheostomy under local anesthesia

39. A 58-year-old man suffers laryngeal trauma in a motor vehicle collision. His physical examination findings include anterior cervical ecchymosis, loss of laryngeal landmarks, biphasic stridor, and moderate respiratory distress. The next best step in management would be?

    A. Admission for observation, humidified room air, and intravenous steroids
    B. Awake fiberoptic intubation
    C. Secure airway through awake tracheostomy with local anesthesia
    D. Needle cricothyroidotomy with jet ventilation

40. A 14-year-old boy presents to your office. One day prior he was struck in the forehead with a baseball. Evaluation with CT at an emergency department reveals a nondisplaced fracture of the anterior table of the frontal sinus. Examination reveals central forehead ecchymosis without periorbital ecchymosis or rhinorrhea. There is no restriction of extraocular movement, and intercanthal distance measures 29 mm. What is the next best step in management?

    A. Transnasal wiring of nasoorbitoethmoid region
    B. Frontal sinus obliteration
    C. Observation and reevaluation in 5 days
    D. Neurosurgical referral

41. Which of the following is one of the most important factors in successful frontal sinus obliteration?

    A. Choosing the correct obliteration material
    B. Complete removal of all sinus mucosa
    C. Choosing the appropriate plate size for posterior table reconstruction
    D. Use of atraumatic technique for elevation of the pericranial flap

42. Which of the following is *not* a recommended option in the initial evaluation of a patient with a penetrating injury to Zone 1 of the neck?

    A. Four-vessel angiogram
    B. Contrast esophagram
    C. Esophagoscopy
    D. Surgical exploration
    E. Fiberoptic laryngoscopy

43. Placing which of these incisions offers the least risk of scleral show and ectropion?

    A. Transconjunctival with cantholysis
    B. Lateral brow
    C. Tranconjunctival without cantholysis
    D. Subciliary
    E. Subtarsal

44. A 34-year-old woman presents 1 year after laceration closure of a dog bite injury to her lower lip with a noticeable soft tissue deficiency deep to the cutaneous scar. Inappropriate closure of which anatomical component has likely led to this defect?

    A. Inner mucosal layer
    B. Vermilion border
    C. Orbicularis oris muscle
    D. Facial skin and red lip junction
    E. Mental crease

45. Which of the following nasal bone fractures are most likely to be associated with other facial fractures?

    A. Displaced nasal fractures
    B. Fractures of the caudal aspect of the nasal bones
    C. Fractures of the cephalic end of the nasal bones
    D. Fractures of the nasal sidewall

46. Valid options for fixation at the orbital rim so as to avoid a palpable or visible plate include:

    A. 2.0-mm equivalent midface plate
    B. 1.7-mm equivalent midface plate
    C. 1.5-mm equivalent midface plate
    D. Wire fixation
    E. Lag screw fixation

47. What neuroendocrine response is most commonly seen in trauma?

    A. Release of catecholamines epinephrine and norepinephrine
    B. Release of antidiuretic hormone (ADH)
    C. Increase in thyroid-stimulating hormone
    D. Decrease in testosterone
    E. Adrenal gland shuts down

48. Regardless of whether closed or open techniques are utilized in pediatric mandible fractures, early mobilization:

    A. Reduces the risk of limited mobility due to fibrosis/ankylosis, and should be a tenet of treatment
    B. Increases the risk of limited mobility because of placing a load on the fractured mandible prior to proper healing
    C. Increases the risk of limited mobility of the jaw due to fibrosis and ankylosis from infections
    D. Increases the risk of limited mobility of the jaw by creating a nonunion fracture, thus furthering the risk of complications

49. Initial airway management requires attention to:

    A. The extremities
    B. The brain
    C. The neck
    D. The heart
    E. The lungs

50. Which of the following is *correct* concerning shotgun injuries to the face?

    A. Treatment depends on the entry zone of the injury.
    B. Major vascular injury is common.
    C. Airway compromise is common.
    D. Eye injuries are common.
    E. Soft tissue loss is rare.

51. Which nerve is at greatest risk during transcutaneous exposure of mandibular fractures?

    A. Greater auricular nerve
    B. Marginal branch of the facial nerve
    C. Infraorbital branch of the trigeminal nerve
    D. Frontal branch of the facial nerve

52. Which of the following clinical findings suggests a septal fracture?

    A. A compound fracture
    B. A tear in the septal mucoperichondrium
    C. Bilateral nasal bone fractures
    D. Epistaxis

53. A horizontal distance of 6 mm between the maxillary and mandibular incisors is best described as:

   A. Normal
   B. Overjet
   C. Overbite
   D. Open bite

54. A 12-year-old is struck in the left eye with a baseball and complains of diplopia and severe pain on upward gaze. A CT scan confirms presence of an orbital floor fracture. When should be the treatment performed?

   A. If diplopia does not resolve in 5 to 7 days
   B. Urgently
   C. If enophthalmos develops
   D. Within 2 weeks

55. Shear failure of resorbable screws with open reduction and internal fixation of laryngeal cartilage is best prevented by utilizing:

   A. Tapped, undersized drill bits
   B. Untapped, undersized drill bits
   C. Tapped, same-sized drill bits
   D. Untapped, same-sized drill bits

56. Anatomic locations with an increased propensity for fracture include:

   A. The mandibular angle (especially if the third molar is impacted), the mental foramen region, and the condylar neck
   B. The mandibular angle regardless of the third molar status, the temporomandibular joint, and the symphysis
   C. The mandibular angle (especially if the third molar is impacted), ramus, and the condylar neck
   D. The mandibular angle regardless of the third molar status, the mental foramen, and the coronoid

57. After blunt laryngeal trauma, persistent immobility of the vocal fold may be caused by recurrent laryngeal nerve injury or by cricoarytenoid joint dislocation. Which of the following diagnostic tools is able to distinguish arytenoid dislocation from recurrent laryngeal nerve injury in the setting of an immobile vocal fold?

   A. Fiberoptic flexible laryngoscopy
   B. Strobovideolaryngoscopy
   C. Computed tomography
   D. Laryngeal electromyography (LEMG)

58. Which of the following best describes the transconjunctival lower eyelid approach?

    A. It is potentially less prone to postoperative lower eyelid malposition
    B. Can be dissected anterior or posterior to the orbital septum
    C. May be performed with or without a lateral canthotomy and cantholysis
    D. All of the above

59. Which is not a vertical buttress of the face?

    A. Zygomaticomaxillary
    B. Zygomatic arch
    C. Nasomaxillary
    D. Pterygomaxillary

60. Frontal sinus fractures most commonly involve:

    A. Young men involved in interpersonal altercations
    B. Middle-aged to elderly men involved in motor vehicle accidents
    C. Young men involved in motor vehicle accidents
    D. Both men and women equally

61. A 37-year-old patient with blunt neck trauma. What findings are depicted on this image?

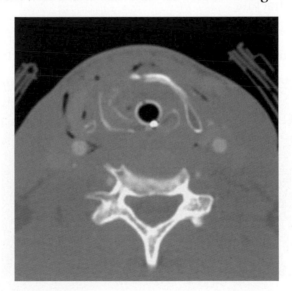

    A. Thyroid cartilage fracture
    B. Cricoid cartilage fracture
    C. Multifocal thyroid and cricoid cartilage fractures
    D. Cricoarytenoid dislocation
    E. Traumatic pseudoaneurysm

62. How is this fracture best classified?

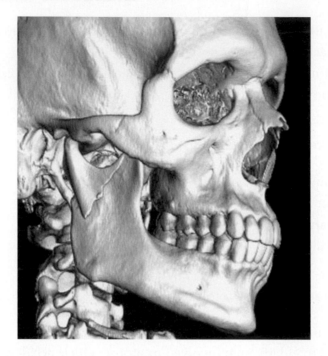

    A. High ramus fracture
    B. Angle fracture
    C. Condylar neck fracture
    D. Subcondylar fracture
    E. Condylar head fracture

63. An 18-year-old trauma patient. Which of the following structures remains intact?

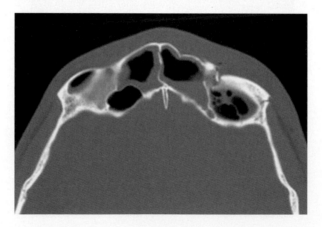

    A. Lateral orbital wall
    B. Orbital roof
    C. Anterior table
    D. Posterior table
    E. Intersinus septum

64. A 19-year-old trauma patient. Which of the following statements is true?

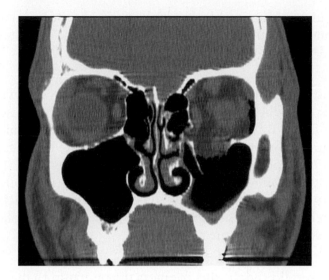

    A. This fracture is classified as Le Fort II.

    B. This fracture should be managed conservatively.

    C. The lamina papyracea requires surgical repair.

    D. This CT was acquired as a direct coronal acquisition.

    E. The inferior rectus muscle has herniated through an orbital floor blowout.

Chapter 5 Answers

1. **Answer E.** Vascular evaluation should be performed when penetrating wounds are in proximity to a major vascular structure or when the wound is posterior to the mandibular angle plane. PAGE 1133

2. **Answer C.** At the level of the zygomatic arch, the facial nerve is vulnerable to injury because the tissues are adherent. Once above the arch, the facial nerve travels within the temporoparietal fascia. By transitioning deep to the deep temporal fascia 2 to 3 cm above the arch and coursing on top of the temporal fat pad, the nerve can be protected as subperiosteal elevation is performed to expose the arch (PAGE 1174). The nerve would likely be injured if the elevation remains above the temporal fascia throughout. While the nerve would be deep to the dissection if the plane chosen were superficial to the temporoparietal fascia, the arch would not be exposed. Likewise, a dissection plane deep to the temporalis muscle would not expose the arch.

3. **Answer A.** The lower lid canaliculus connects the punctum to the lacrimal sac just below the eyelid margin (PAGE 1117). The orbital septum could be injured with lid lacerations but the significance is less than if the canalicular system is involved. The levator aponeurosis is an upper eyelid structure.

4. **Answer A.** The upper labial sulcus provides excellent exposure to the lower midface and to the medial and lateral maxillary buttresses, making it ideally suited for zygomaticomaxillary complex fractures (PAGE 1187). This approach does not provide exposure to the frontal sinus, orbital floor, or mandibular condyle.

5. **Answer B.** The transcaruncular approach provides excellent exposure to the medial orbital wall and can be combined with a lower eyelid transconjunctival incision for fractures or lesions involving both the medial wall and the orbital floor (PAGE 1183). The transcaruncular approach has no external scar and has largely replaced the Lynch incision. The upper labial sulcus incision provides access to the maxillary face and inferior orbital rim, but is not an acceptable approach to the medial orbital wall. The "gullwing" incision should be avoided as the resulting scar is unacceptable. PAGE 1177

6. **Answer A.** The findings in this patient are consistent with a trapdoor or "white-eyed" orbital fracture. The patient has oculocardiac reflex symptoms and should be taken to the operating room on an emergent basis (PAGE 1281). In patients with true entrapment but without the oculocardiac reflex symptoms, surgical exploration should be performed within 24 to 48 hours. Waiting for >48 hours increases the risk of permanent diplopia.

7. **Answer E.** Blunt trauma to the malar eminence, the most prominent feature of the midface, accounts for the high incidence of ZMC fractures (PAGE 1211). Le Fort and NOE fractures are less common and require more energy for disruption.

8. **Answer C.** A 2007 study by Matic et al. suggests that rounding of the inferior rectus on CT imaging may be a predictor of the development of delayed enophthalmos PAGE 1231. (Matic DB, Tse R, Banerjee A, et al. Rounding of the inferior rectus muscle as a predictor of enophthalmos in orbital floor fractures. *J Craniofac Surg* 2007;18(1):127–132.)

9. **Answer D.** Falls are the most common etiology of orbital roof fractures in children and often have associated intracranial findings (PAGE 1229) . Orbital floor and medial orbital wall fractures are unlikely to present with an upper eyelid hematoma, and the frontal sinus is not yet developed in a 7-year-old.

10. **Answer B.** This clinical description is characteristic of a septal hematoma (PAGE 1277) . It should be treated promptly and under general anesthesia. Bedside drainage is poorly tolerated in the pediatric population and may compromise the effectiveness of the treatment. Nasal packing is poorly tolerated in children. Splints and quilting sutures are a good substitute for packing. If treatment is delayed for 7 days, the patient will have irreversible cartilage damage and is more prone to septal abscess or septal perforation.

11. **Answer D.** Rapid rewarming is the first step in treating frostbite. This is performed with warm compresses or immersion of the body part in a warm water bath maintained at 100°F to 108°F (PAGE 1128) . Antibiotic treatment and eventual surgical debridement may be warranted but are not first steps in treatment. Gradual rewarming may lead to further tissue damage and should be avoided. Vasodilation will occur with rewarming, and administration of a vasodilator is not indicated.

12. **Answer B.** Cat bites have a higher rate of infection when compared to dog bites, and *Pasteurella multocida* is responsible for 50% to 75% of infections from cat bites. Cat bites may also be polymicrobial (PAGE 1127) . Dog bite infections are frequently polymicrobial and involve the bacterial species listed in Answers A, C, D, and E.

13. **Answer A.** Hypovolemia (assumed to be related to hemorrhage until proven otherwise) is the most common form of shock in the trauma patient (PAGE 1098) . Neurogenic shock may be found in patients with brainstem dysfunction or spinal cord injury. Cardiogenic shock is associated with tension pneumothorax, cardiac tamponade, and myocardial contusion.

14. **Answer B.** The five parameters listed in Answer B are sufficient to design a treatment plan (PAGE 1257) . Fractures of the NOE complex and orbit may be associated with severe facial trauma including frontal sinus fractures, but they are not necessarily a part of most frontal sinus fractures. Wide exposure of the fracture, usually by a coronal approach, is necessary to adequately treat frontal sinus fractures, and lacerations do not typically provide sufficient access for repair.

15. **Answer A.** Excessive retraction of the globe during orbital fracture repair may transmit pressure to the ciliary ganglion, resulting in mydriasis (PAGE 1238) . Retraction should be released and the pupil should be allowed to recover before proceeding. Transection of the optic nerve would also result in dilation of the pupil but would be difficult while dissecting along the orbital floor with sound surgical technique. Although ophthalmic artery occlusion may present with an afferent pupillary defect and vision loss, this is uncommon in the setting of orbital fracture repair.

16. **Answer D.** Open reduction of condyle fractures is absolutely indicated in all of the listed situations except Answer D (PAGE 1204, TABLE 80.3) . Repair of unilateral condylar fractures associated with a single midfacial fracture may not be necessary if vertical maxillary height is restored with repair of the midface.

17. **Answer A.** Mandibular zone gunshot wounds frequently cause bleeding, edema, and hematoma formation requiring airway intervention. Consideration should be given to elective airway stabilization even without symptoms (PAGE 1134). Globe injury and intracranial penetration occur more commonly with maxillary zone injuries, and vascular injury should be suspected when the entry wound is posterior to the mandibular angle plane.

18. **Answer B.** Immediate facial paralysis after penetrating trauma should be considered a nerve transection and the patient should be surgically explored when the wound is lateral to the lateral canthus (PAGE 1134). A facial nerve contusion is more likely to result in delayed-onset paralysis. Recovery of facial nerve function depends on the site of injury and the presence of arborizing branches. Surgical repair of a transected facial nerve branch is best accomplished with a tension-free primary repair or cable nerve grafting. The best outcome after either primary nerve repair or cable nerve grafting is House–Brackmann 3 to 4.

19. **Answer C.** Nasal fractures are the most frequent facial fracture (PAGE 1272). Frontal sinus fractures are uncommon in childhood since the frontal sinus is not fully developed until after age 15. Orbital fractures are the second most common midfacial fractures after nasal fractures. Midface fractures are uncommon and account for 5% to 10% of pediatric facial fractures.

20. **Answer B.** By definition, bony union in a nonanatomic position is a malunion (PAGE 1153). Instability at 8 to 12 weeks after fixation is a delayed union. Fibrous union occurs when indirect fracture healing does not lead to ossification. Pseudoarthrosis is a fibrous union mobile enough to function as a joint.

21. **Answer: A.** Dislocations are more commonly seen where the quadrangular cartilage is thicker (right at the bony-cartilaginous interfaces), while fractures are more common in areas where the cartilage is thinner—the central portion of the quadrangular cartilage above the maxillary crest. (PAGE 1244)

22. **Answer C.** Mandible fractures are unfavorable when the mandibular musculature tends to displace the fracture fragments (PAGE 1196). Most mandibular angle fracures are horizontally unfavorable and allow displacement of fractures in the vertical plane.

23. **Answer B.** Early trauma deaths account for approximately one-third of all trauma deaths. This statistic emphasizes the importance of coordinated prehospital and hospital care. (PAGE 1093). Answers A and C are helpful in increasing survival in cardiac arrest. Answers D and E are useful in preventing or minimizing trauma.

24. **Answer C.** Lag screws are one of the most effective ways to compress and stabilize a fracture (PAGE 1157). Lag screws are contraindicated in comminuted fractures. The drill hole proximal to the fracture line should be the diameter of the screw threads (gliding hole) and the drill hole distal to the fracture line should be the diameter of the screw shaft. The lag screw should be placed as perpendicular to the fracture line as possible.

25. **Answer C.** The use of an "emergency" or "rescue" screw is a fairly common occurrence. The greater thread diameter allows this screw to engage stable bone (PAGE 1157). If multiple holes are stripped with the use of "rescue" screws, it may be necessary to redrill at another location or to employ a different plate, but this is uncommon. Choosing a longer screw of the same thread diameter will not result in stability if the drill hole is stripped.

26. **Answer C.** This fracture pattern is quite common and because the fractures are linear, the cortical bone edges will interdigitate and load-sharing fixation with 2.0-mm miniplates may be used (PAGE 1200). Comminuted fractures, edentulous fractures, and defect fractures (resorption at site of nonunion) are all challenging fractures and lack intrinsic stability. In these situations, load-bearing stabilization with a 2.4- or 2.7-mm reconstruction plate is necessary.

27. **Answer: A.** Facial and nasal fractures are less common in children than adults. With respect to nasal fractures, both the clinical examination and imaging can be unreliable. Pediatric nasal bone fractures begin to heal and unite much quicker than in adults, so earlier intervention is recommended when necessary. (PAGE 1250–1251)

28. **Answer D.** Statistically, the condyle is the most commonly involved site of pediatric mandible fractures (PAGE 1279). In this case, the clinical findings of chin deviation to the right and premature contact in the right molar region (likely has a left open bite as well), all suggest a right condylar fracture with right-sided vertical shortening of mandibular height. A displaced fracture of the ramus or angle could allow similar findings but are less common. Fractures in the other regions listed would not produce the clinical findings noted. Careful evaluation should be performed to detect associated fractures of the contralateral condylar region or parasymphyseal regions any time a unilateral condylar or subcondylar fracture is identified.

29. **Answer D.** The endoscopic repair of anterior table fractures is a camouflage technique used in a delayed fashion. It is reserved for patients with mildly displaced fractures (PAGE 1261). Comminution of the anterior table, extension below the orbital rim, displacement greater than 6 mm, and thin skin, all make the coronal approach more desirable than the endoscopic technique.

30. **Answer E.** The primary survey should address the "ABC's" of trauma (PAGE 1094–1100). Answer A combines areas addressed during both primary and secondary surveys. Answer B is addressed during the secondary survey. Answer D lists physical examination findings that can assist in patient evaluation but are not specifically related to the primary survey.

31. **Answer A.** Laryngeal stenting should be avoided whenever possible, but lacerations of the anterior commissure and endolarynx may lead to webbing and loss of the normal laryngeal configuration. In these situations, stenting should be considered (PAGE 1145). Vocal fold hematomas typically resolve without intervention. Stabilized laryngeal cartilage fractures do not require stenting unless mucosal lacerations are extensive. Cricotracheal separation should be repaired primarily after stabilization of the airway with tracheotomy.

32. **Answer D.** The thin-cut CT is the diagnostic imaging modality of choice. Axial and sagittal views are helpful to assess the patency of the frontal recess and provide information on frontal contour. Coronal images allow visualization of the frontal sinus floor and orbital roof. Three-dimensional reconstructions provide an excellent overview of the fractures and frontal contour (PAGE 1256). Plain radiographs are not indicated in frontal sinus fracture diagnosis.

33. **Answer: B.** New change in alignment of the nose externally and new-onset nasal airway obstruction are the two most important indications for surgical intervention. Both of these can be determined with an attentive history and physical examination. Although radiographs may corroborate the diagnosis, they are not routinely required to direct the management of isolated nasal bone fractures. (PAGE 1245)

34. **Answer C.** The zygomaticosphenoid articulation is three-dimensionally complex and is the best site to evaluate the accuracy of ZMC fracture reduction (PAGE 1215). The zygomatico-frontal suture is easily accessible and provides a reasonable degree of stability when plated, but does not provide the best alignment. The zygomaticomaxillary suture is easily accessed by a gingivobuccal incision. It provides excellent stability, but is not the best site for verifying alignment. The zygomaticotemporal suture is not typically accessed for routine ZMC fractures and would offer only limited assistance with alignment. The infraorbital rim likewise offers only limited information for the overall alignment of the ZMC complex.

35. **Answer C.** The classical auricular hematoma forms in the subperichondrial plane or among cartilaginous fracture fragments in more severe trauma. (PAGE 1125) The skin is densely adherent to the underlying perichondrium and the auricle does not have significant subcutaneous tissue making Answers A, B, and E incorrect. The auricular musculature likewise plays no role in auricular hematoma formation.

36. **Answer C.** Angle's classification of malocclusion is based on where the buccal groove of the mandibular first molar contacts the mesiobuccal cusp of the maxillary first molar. Answer C defines Angle Class II (PAGE 1161). Answer A defines Angle Class III. Answer B defines Angle Class I. Answer D defines a buccal crossbite and does not correlate to Angle's classification.

37. **Answer C.** Although infrequent, an entropion or lower lid retraction is the most common complication after a transconjunctival approach and can often be attributed to excessive retraction or thermal cautery injury (PAGE 1238). Symblepharon is an adhesion developing between the palpebral and bulbar conjunctiva. Entropion more commonly results from transcutaneous approaches to the lower eyelid. Epiphora has multiple etiologies including injury to the lacrimal system, dry eye, and ectropion with pooling of tears.

38. **Answer B.** This patient is clinically stable with preserved laryngeal landmarks and a small hematoma. Conservative management is indicated (PAGE 1144). Direct laryngoscopy is not indicated given the fiberoptic laryngoscopy findings, and since the airway is stable, intubation and tracheostomy are unnecessary.

39. **Answer C.** This patient has impending airway compromise and awake tracheostomy should be performed without delay (PAGE 1144). Fiberoptic intubation should be avoided to prevent further trauma to his traumatized larynx. Observation does not play a role in this patient and could result in loss of the airway. Jet ventilation is recommended by some authors for children under 12 years of age but is difficult in the patient with loss of laryngeal landmarks.

40. **Answer C.** With the described clinical findings, this patient is unlikely to have a contour deformity requiring surgical intervention (PAGE 1282). Transnasal wiring is not indicated and the patient has a normal intercanthal distance. Frontal sinus obliteration is not indicated without disruption of the frontal recess and outflow tract. Neurosurgical referral is not necessary.

41. **Answer B.** Complete removal of sinus mucosa is essential to reduce the incidence of delayed mucocele formation (PAGE 1268). Many different obliteration materials have been

successfully used. Plates are not typically applied to the posterior table of the frontal sinus. Although atraumatic elevation of a pericranial flap is essential to preserve the flap integrity and blood supply, not all frontal sinus obliteration cases will require a pericranial flap.

42. **Answer D.** Surgical exploration is indicated in symptomatic patients with Zone II penetrating trauma and may be considered in asymptomatic patients with Zone II penetrating trauma. Because of the high risk of injury to the great vessels and the esophagus in Zone I injuries, angiography and esophageal evaluation are indicated (PAGE 1137) . While fiber-optic laryngoscopy is especially useful in diagnosing Zone II airway injuries, it may detect blood in the airway even in Zone I injuries.

43. **Answer B.** Although a transconjunctival incision is thought to have a lower incidence of scleral show and ectropion than a subciliary or subtarsal incision, all three of these incisions are placed in the lower lid and carry some risk of lid complications (PAGE 1216) . The lateral brow incision can be used to access the zygomaticofrontal suture and does not violate the lower lid. There is no risk of ectropion or scleral show with the lateral brow incision.

44. **Answer C.** Soft tissue deficits of the lip result from failure to adequately repair the muscular layer (PAGE 1126) . Failure to properly repair the vermilion border results in readily noticeable lip irregularities, but does not typically result in a deep soft tissue deficiency.

45. **Answer: C.** The cephalic end of the nasal bones is the thicker than the thin caudal end. As a result, more force is required to fracture the nasal bones at their cephalic end, which implies greater risk of facial bone fractures. (PAGE 1242)

46. **Answer D.** Extremely thin plates (typically 1.0 mm) or wire must be used on the inferior orbital rim to avoid visibility or palpability (PAGE 1221) . The plates listed in Answers A, B, and C are all too thick to be used on the inferior rim. Although the use of a lag screw would in theory be possible with an oblique fracture of the inferior rim, it would be technically difficult and is not used in common practice.

47. **Answer A.** Release of catecholamines is the body's most fundamental hormonal reaction to trauma. (PAGE 1094) ADH may be released in response to pain and volume loss. The adrenal gland is activated in trauma.

48. **Answer A.** Ankylosis is one of the most dreaded complications of pediatric condyle fractures (PAGE 1205) . Early mobilization reduces the likelihood of this complication.

49. **Answer C.** The primary risk during early airway management is neck movement in the setting of an occult cervical spine fracture. (PAGE 1095)

50. **Answer D.** In multiple series, globe injuries are common and ophthalmologic evaluation should be obtained (PAGE 1133) . Shotgun wound classification is based on proximity (close range vs. long range) and not on the entry zone used to describe other penetrating injuries (including nonshotgun gunshot wounds). Although airway compromise is possible in close-range injuries involving the mandible or when significant oral cavity bleeding is present, the need for emergency airway establishment is uncommon in shotgun injuries to the face.

51. **Answer B.** The marginal mandibular nerve exits the parotid and courses anteriorly to innervate the lower lip depressor muscles (PAGE 1190). As it travels anterior, it dips below the mandibular border and must be protected during exposure of the mandible by placing the skin incision 1.5 to 2 cm inferior to the mandibular border and by performing subplatysmal dissection to the mandible. The facial artery and vein can be ligated, divided, and retracted superiorly if necessary to protect the nerve and improve exposure.

52. **Answer: B.** In a 2004 Korean study all patients undergoing surgical treatment of isolated nasal bone fractures had the septum explored via a hemitransfixion incision. In that study, mucosal tears, noted either on rhinoscopy or endoscopic examination, were the clinical finding most suggestive of an associated septal fracture. (PAGE 1246)

53. **Answer B.** The normal anterior dental relationship occurs when the maxillary anterior dentition is 1 to 3 mm anterior to the mandibular anterior dentition (PAGE 1161). Increased horizontal distance between the teeth is termed overjet. Increased vertical overlap of the anterior dentition is termed overbite. Insufficient anterior dental overlap results in an open bite.

54. **Answer B.** The associated pain and entrapment in this adolescent patient is concerning for a "white-eyed" fracture that traps periorbital tissues and possibly the inferior rectus muscle (PAGE 1231). Radiographic findings are often minimal. These fractures should be treated urgently to prevent irreversible ischemic damage to the inferior rectus.

55. **Answer B.** Because both resorbable and nonresorbable screws tend to pull out of cartilage, careful surgical technique with an untapped and undersized drill bit is helpful. (PAGES 1146–1147)

56. **Answer A.** An impacted third molar increases the likelihood of fracture at the mandibular angle because of reduced bone stock. Likewise, the mental foramen region is a common site for fracture, often in conjunction with a contralateral mandibular angle or condylar neck fracture (PAGE 1195). Coronoid fractures are relatively uncommon.

57. **Answer D.** Of the answers listed, LEMG is the most useful tool for differentiating recurrent laryngeal nerve injury from arytenoid dislocation and may also offer prognostic information regarding spontaneous recovery in cases of recurrent laryngeal nerve injury (PAGE 1150). The other diagnostic modalities are useful adjuncts in the patient with laryngeal trauma.

58. **Answer D.** The transconjunctival approach is quite versatile and has a lower incidence of ectropion than the subciliary approach. The dissection plane may be either pre- or postseptal (PAGE 1178). If excessive retraction is required for exposure, addition of a lateral canthotomy and inferior cantholysis should be considered.

59. **Answer B.** The zygomatic arch provides anterior facial projection and as such is not a vertical buttress (PAGE 1209). Each of the other options is a vertical buttress that transmits the forces of mastication to the skull base and provides vertical facial height.

60. **Answer C.** The frontal sinus is protected by thick cortical bone, and fractures of this region require high-energy transfer. This most commonly occurs in motor vehicle accidents in young men (PAGE 1255). Although interpersonal altercations can result in frontal sinus fractures, the forces delivered in motor vehicle accidents tend to be greater.

61. **Answer: C.** There are fractures of the anterior midline thyroid cartilage, posterior right cricoid cartilage, and lateral right cricoid cartilage. The arytenoid cartilages are not depicted on this image, and the vessels are normal. PAGE 1143

62. **Answer: D.** Subcondylar fractures extend from the sigmoid notch to the posterior edge of the ramus. PAGE 1203

63. **Answer: D.** Fractures are depicted in the left anterior table, extending across the intersinus septum. The medial orbital roof is involved, and the fracture extends along the superior orbital rim to involve the lateral orbital wall. PAGE 1259

64. **Answer: E.** This CT depicts a large orbital floor blowout fracture that will require surgical repair. The inferior rectus muscle has herniated through the defect into the maxillary antrum. The other elements of a Le Fort II fracture are not present. Most of the lamina papyracea is intact. This CT was originally acquired in axial plane, as the dental artifact demonstrates. PAGES 1227–1229

6

Pediatric Otolaryngology

1. An 11-month-old infant is brought to the emergency room at 22:00 hours by his parents as a result of an increase in drooling following ingestion of a silver object. There is no stridor. A chest X-ray is taken and this demonstrates a radiopaque circular object on anteroposterior view. On lateral view, there is a small irregularity noted in the profile of the object. What is the next most appropriate step?

   A. Emergency endoscopy and removal of the foreign body
   B. Defer esophagoscopy until the following morning as the patient is in no respiratory distress
   C. CT scan of his chest to better characterize the ingested object
   D. Fluoroscopic removal

2. What is the incidence of infant hearing loss per 1,000 births?

   A. 0.02 to 0.04
   B. 0.2 to 0.4
   C. 2 to 4
   D. 20 to 40
   E. 200 to 400

3. The virus most commonly identified as a cause of congenital hearing loss is:

   A. Adenovirus
   B. Respiratory syncytial virus
   C. Cytomegalovirus (CMV)
   D. Rubella

4. Which of the following most predisposes the anterior neuropore to incomplete closure?

   A. Reduced blood supply to anterior neural tube
   B. Relatively late neural tube closure and low concentration of neural crest cells
   C. Lack of extracellular stromal support for neural crest cell migration
   D. Early apoptosis of anterior neuropore cells

5. Congenital recessive genetic hearing loss is most commonly associated with mutations in:

   A. Waardenburg syndrome genes
   B. Usher syndrome genes
   C. Pendred syndrome gene (*SLC26A4*)
   D. *GJB2* (Connexin 26) gene

6. Kasabach–Merritt phenomenon is associated with which vascular anomaly?

   A. Infantile hemangioma
   B. Congenital hemangioma
   C. Kaposiform hemangioendothelioma
   D. Pyogenic granuloma

7. Which of the following surgical techniques is *not* a standard surgical treatment for velopharyngeal insufficiency?

   A. Bardach hard palate flaps
   B. Furlow palatoplasty
   C. Hogan modification of posterior pharyngeal flap
   D. Hynes sphincter pharyngoplasty

8. Which of the following is the best initial surgical procedure for chronic pediatric rhinosinusitis?

   A. Adenoidectomy
   B. Anterior ethmoidectomy
   C. Maxillary antrostomy
   D. Anterior ethmoidectomy with maxillary antrostomy

9. Which of the following is an advantage of tracheotomy compared with prolonged endotracheal intubation?

   A. Tracheotomy requires a surgical procedure.
   B. Tracheostomy tubes are less likely to cause injury to the larynx, including the vocal folds and subglottis.
   C. Tracheotomy can be performed by a variety of health care providers.
   D. Tracheostomy tubes lead to increased airway dead space.

10. The major diagnostic criteria of Apert syndrome include:

    A. Craniosynostosis
    B. Syndactyly of the hands and feet
    C. Prominent forehead
    D. All of the above
    E. None of the above

11. If a pediatric patient with chronic rhinosinusitis continues to be symptomatic after adenoidectomy, which of the following is a reasonable next step?

    A. Workup for allergies
    B. Workup of the immune system for deficiencies
    C. CT image after prolonged course of broad-spectrum antibiotics
    D. All of the above

12. A 4-month-old otherwise healthy infant presents with tachypnea and "washing-machine" breathing that has worsened with upper respiratory tract infections. A high-kilovolt airway radiograph is likely to suggest:

    A. Supraglottic stenosis
    B. Pneumonia
    C. Tracheal stenosis
    D. Tracheomalacia

13. Which of the following is true regarding the diagnostic evaluation of pediatric patients with sensorineural hearing loss (SNHL)?

    A. All patients should undergo a comprehensive diagnostic evaluation, including temporal bone imaging and genetic screening.
    B. If temporal bone imaging is normal, there is no reason to order genetic testing.
    C. Children with bilateral severe-to-profound SNHL should undergo temporal bone imaging as the initial step in the diagnostic workup.
    D. If an enlarged vestibular aqueduct or Mondini deformity is identified on CT scan, testing for *SLC26A4*, or Pendred, should be performed.

14. Which of the following is the best description of neurofibromatosis 2 (NF2)?

    A. Posterior capsular cataracts occur in 80% of patients.
    B. Café-au-lait spots are consistent findings.
    C. Cutaneous neurofibromas are not consistent findings.
    D. A and C.
    E. B and C.

15. Third and fourth branchial cleft anomalies are characterized by all of the following *except*:

    A. May present as recurrent neck abscesses
    B. May be treated with excision
    C. Usually occur on the right side of the neck
    D. Have a sinus opening in the pyriform sinus
    E. May be treated with cautery of the sinus in the pyriform

16. A child with velocardiofacial syndrome (VCFS) has tonsillar and adenoid hypertrophy causing severe obstructive sleep apnea. Which of the following potential associated anomalies most significantly affects operative intervention?

    A. Facial paresis
    B. Carotid artery medialization
    C. Subglottic stenosis
    D. Tracheal stenosis

17. Pediatric sleep-disordered breathing (SDB) has been associated with all of the following behavioral problems in children *except*:

    A. Hyperactivity
    B. Aggression
    C. Somatization
    D. Anxiety
    E. Hyperphagia

18. You provide consultation on a slightly hypotensive 1-day-old infant in whom a pediatrician was unable to pass a 6F catheter into the nose. A CT scan is obtained that demonstrates a solitary maxillary median central incisor and nasal pyriform aperture stenosis. Your next recommendation should be:

    A. Tracheotomy
    B. Transpalatal repair of congenital nasal pyriform aperture stenosis
    C. Endocrine consultation
    D. Sublabial repair of congenital nasal pyriform aperture stenosis

19. A high-quality fetal ultrasound performed at 19 weeks gestational age suggests cystic, dilated lungs, ascites, and no other significant fetal abnormalities. The next most likely step in diagnosis and management is:

    A. Perform chorionic villus sampling
    B. Recommend termination of the pregnancy
    C. Recommend ex-utero intrapartum treatment (EXIT) to secure the airway at Cesarean delivery
    D. Recommend fetal MRI and further evaluation

20. Robin sequence is characterized by:

    A. Micrognathia, cleft palate, and glossoptosis
    B. Micrognathia, cleft palate, and airway obstruction
    C. Cleft palate, airway obstruction, and glossoptosis
    D. Micrognathia, glossoptosis, and airway obstruction

21. A 2-year-old male child accidentally ingests a large quantity of lye. What type of injury will this compound cause?

    A. Liquefaction necrosis
    B. Coagulation necrosis
    C. Ischemic necrosis
    D. Aseptic necrosis

22. Which of the following is the second most commonly occurring type of tracheoesophageal fistula (TEF)?

    A. Proximal TEF with distal esophageal atresia (EA)
    B. Proximal EA with distal TEF
    C. H-type TEF
    D. Proximal and distal TEF with EA

23. The major diagnostic criteria of Robin sequence are:

    A. Micrognathia
    B. Glossoptosis
    C. Inverted U-shaped cleft palate
    D. None of the above
    E. All of the above

24. Which of the following is the most commonly used adjuvant for recurrent respiratory papillomatosis (RRP) among members of American Society of Pediatric Otolaryngology (ASPO)?

    A. Bevacizumab (Avastin)
    B. Intralesional cidofovir (Vistide)
    C. Celecoxib (Celebrex)
    D. Interferon

25. A 2-year-old male child presents with chronic nasal obstruction and slight widening of the nasal dorsum. The patient has been treated conservatively for a presumed nasal polyp without improvement. Endoscopic examination reveals a pulsatile mass medial to the middle turbinate. Which of the following is the most likely diagnosis?

    A. Sincipital nasoethmoidal encephalocele
    B. Nasal glioma
    C. Basal transethmoidal encephalocele
    D. Nasal dermoid

26. What size airway raises concern for subglottic stenosis in a premature infant?

    A. >5.0 mm
    B. <7.0 mm
    C. <5.0 mm
    D. <3.5 mm

27. Which of these is the most likely diagnosis in a neonate with expiratory stridor and a brassy cough?

    A. Congenital subglottic stenosis
    B. Tracheomalacia
    C. Robin sequence
    D. Bilateral vocal fold paralysis

28. Which of the following statements regarding the DFNB1 locus is true?

    A. A mutation at DFNB1 is present in 10% to 15% of patients with hearing loss ≥70 dB.
    B. A mutation at DFNB1 is present in 40% of patients with mild-to-moderate hearing impairment.
    C. The gene at locus DFNB1 is gap junction beta 2 (*GJB2*), which has a carrier frequency of 1 in 40 in the United States.
    D. All patients with DFNB1 have a deletion of a guanine at nucleotide position 35 (35delG).

29. **Segmental facial hemangiomas can be associated with PHACES, which is an acronym standing for:**

    A. Precocious puberty, hemangioma, acromegaly, cardiac anomalies, eye anomalies, and spinal deformities

    B. Posterior cranial fossa malformations, hemangioma, arterial anomalies, cardiac anomalies, eye anomalies, and spinal deformities

    C. Posterior cranial fossa malformations, hemangioma, acromegaly, cardiac anomalies, eye anomalies, and sternal cleft

    D. Posterior cranial fossa malformations, hemangioma, arterial anomalies, cardiac anomalies, eye anomalies, and sternal cleft

30. **Which of the following is an advantage of using speaking valves in children with tracheostomies who can tolerate them?**

    A. The speaking valve allows children with tracheostomy tubes to generate higher subglottic pressures, which lead to improved coughing and laryngeal function during swallowing.

    B. The speaking valve allows for improved communication, even for patients on the ventilator with cuffed tracheostomy tubes.

    C. The speaking valve leads to improved laryngeal elevation during swallowing.

    D. The speaking valve permits children with tracheostomy tubes to talk even if they have severe subglottic stenosis.

31. **Which of the following is a true statement about complications following tonsillectomy?**

    A. Secondary bleeding is more common than primary bleeding.

    B. In a child with submucous cleft palate, tonsillectomy is contraindicated.

    C. Children under 3 years are more likely to have respiratory complications.

    D. Children have more postoperative complications than adults.

    E. A and C

32. **A 2-month-old infant has a history of a patent ductus arteriosus (PDA) ligation at 1 month of age. The infant's cry is very weak and breathy. The infant is choking and gagging with feeds and has been on thickened formula. What would you expect to find on endoscopy/stroboscopy?**

    A. Recurrent respiratory papillomatosis

    B. Large vocal polyp

    C. Unilateral vocal fold paralysis

    D. Muscle tension dysphonia

33. **Imaging for pediatric rhinosinusitis is most accurately accomplished with:**

    A. Plain films
    B. CT scans
    C. MRI
    D. Maxillary sinus transillumination

34. **Which of the following is true regarding Stickler syndrome?**

    A. It is associated with mutations in collagen genes.
    B. Hearing loss is uncommon.
    C. It is inherited in an autosomal recessive fashion.
    D. Ocular abnormalities are present in all patients.

35. **What is the overall 5-year survival of children with salivary gland malignancy?**

    A. <20%
    B. 50%
    C. 75%
    D. >90%

36. **A child with bilateral second branchial cleft anomalies (BCA) may have all of the following *except*:**

    A. Bilateral preauricular pits
    B. Sensorineural hearing loss
    C. Renal disease
    D. Microtia
    E. Autosomal recessive inheritance

37. **A 12-month-old infant is brought to the emergency room after he was seen swallowing a coin. He is drooling more than normal and there is no stridor. Where would the coin be most likely lodged?**

    A. Upper esophageal sphincter
    B. Midesophagus
    C. Lower esophageal sphincter
    D. Laryngeal inlet

38. Recurrent respiratory papillomatosis (RRP) demonstrates a predilection for which of the following sites?

    A. Junction of ciliated and squamous epithelium
    B. The undersurface of the vocal folds
    C. The laryngeal ventricle
    D. All of the above

39. Which of the following bacteria are most likely to result in permanent sensorineural hearing loss after meningitis?

    A. *Streptococcus pneumoniae*
    B. *Haemophilus influenzae* (type B) (Hib)
    C. *Neisseria meningitidis*
    D. *Listeria monocytogenes*

40. Which of the following is the most common inflammatory disorder of the salivary glands in the United States?

    A. Mumps
    B. Juvenile recurrent parotitis (JRP)
    C. Rheumatoid arthritis
    D. Sarcoidosis

41. Which of the following would likely require neurosurgical intervention via craniotomy during resection of a nasal dermoid tract approaching the skull base?

    A. Presence of a fibrous stalk within 1 mm of the skull base
    B. Need for a transglabellar approach if exposure via open rhinoplasty is insufficient
    C. Inability to confirm the point of termination of dermoid tract on physical examination
    D. Histologic evidence of an open epithelial-lined tract at the level of the skull base

42. What structure in the cochlea generates otoacoustic emissions (OAEs)?

    A. Inner hair cells
    B. Outer hair cells
    C. Deiter cells
    D. Stria vascularis
    E. Basement membrane

43. Contraindications to an endoscopic laryngotracheal cleft repair include the following *except*:

    A. Low-birth-weight neonate
    B. Cleft extends into the cervical trachea
    C. Micrognathia
    D. Concomitant subglottic stenosis

44. A patient with choanal atresia, external ear anomalies, congenital heart defects, and an irregular pupil secondary to an iris defect likely has which of the following associated defects?

    A. *CHD7* mutation
    B. VACTERL
    C. *SHH* mutation
    D. Pallister–Hall syndrome

45. Which of the following may place a child "at risk" for developmental delay?

    A. Permanent hearing loss
    B. Learning disability
    C. Language delay
    D. Blindness
    E. All of the above

46. A 3-year-old with congenital hearing loss was found to have abnormal electroretinography. This child most likely has:

    A. Pendred syndrome
    B. Usher syndrome
    C. Jervell and Lange-Nielsen syndrome
    D. Nonsyndromic hearing loss

47. What vaccines are recommended for acute otitis media (AOM) for infants and children?

    A. *Haemophilus influenzae* type B
    B. *Streptococcus pneumoniae*
    C. Influenza
    D. A and B
    E. B and C

48. A mass that splays apart the nasal bones and has an intranasal component in a child may have all of the following characteristics *except*:

    A. Be a dermoid cyst
    B. Be a glioma
    C. Be an encephalocele
    D. It is safe to biopsy at the initial visit
    E. May require surgery that results in significant nasal deformity

49. Which of the following is most suggestive of intracranial involvement of congenital nasal lesions?

    A. Bifid crista galli and enlarged foramen cecum
    B. Widened nasal dorsum and hypertelorism
    C. Lateral displacement of the medial orbital walls
    D. Previous history of meningitis

50. An 18-month-old child presents to the hospital 30 minutes following an accidental ingestion of a small amount of hydrochloric acid. She is hemodynamically stable, and there are no oral mucosal injuries noted on examination. What is the next most appropriate step in the management of this patient?

    A. Diagnostic esophagoscopy 12 to 48 hours following ingestion
    B. Barium swallow while in the emergency room
    C. Discharge home without further investigation
    D. CT scan of her neck and chest

51. The most common anatomic site of stridor in the neonate is:

    A. Larynx
    B. Trachea
    C. Nose
    D. Oral cavity

52. Which are the most commonly isolated bacteria in the acute otitis media (AOM)?

    A. *Haemophilus influenzae*
    B. *Staphylococcus aureus*
    C. *Streptococcus pneumoniae*
    D. *Moraxella catarrhalis*
    E. None of the above

53. Which of the following is *not* part of the summary statement from the 2010 Clinical Practice Guideline on Tonsillectomy?

    A. In children with abnormal polysomnography and hypertrophic tonsils, tonsillectomy can provide a means to improve health.
    B. Children undergoing tonsillectomy do not need perioperative antibiotics.
    C. Children undergoing tonsillectomy will benefit from perioperative antibiotics.
    D. Clinicians should evaluate their rates of primary and secondary postoperative hemorrhage annually.
    E. A single dose of intraoperative intravenous dexamethasone during tonsillectomy can significantly reduce postoperative nausea and vomiting.

54. What is the narrowest portion of the pediatric airway?

    A. Trachea
    B. Supraglottis
    C. Glottis
    D. Subglottis

55. Of those listed below, which is the most common syndrome associated with cleft lip and palate (CL/P)?

    A. Apert syndrome
    B. Velocardiofacial syndrome
    C. Van der Woude syndrome
    D. Turner syndrome

56. Which of the following statements best describes the management of recurrent respiratory papillomatosis (RRP)?

    A. Complete eradication of disease is essential.
    B. The goal of surgical therapy is to maintain a patent airway, improve voice quality, and avoid harm.
    C. Adjuvant therapies such as cidofovir should be used in children with mild RRP that require surgical intervention two times or fewer per year.
    D. Tracheostomy is a mainstay of treatment and should be considered in all infants diagnosed with RRP.

57. The highest rate of success in treating sialorrhea is seen with:

    A. Four duct ligation
    B. Submandibular duct rerouting
    C. Submandibular gland excision and parotid rerouting
    D. Bilateral total parotidectomy

58. Work type 2 first branchial cleft anomalies are characterized by all of the following *except*:

    A. Are frequently misdiagnosed
    B. Present following previous inadequate surgery
    C. May contain tissues derived from ectoderm and mesoderm
    D. May contain tissues derived from ectoderm only
    E. Require facial nerve dissection for safe and complete excision

59. The first step in caring for the neonate in respiratory distress is to:

    A. Obtain a thorough history of the pregnancy and delivery
    B. Perform flexible laryngoscopy
    C. Rapidly assess the patient's clinical condition
    D. Obtain a pulse oximetry reading

60. A 3-month-old infant presents with biphasic stridor. A laryngeal web is identified on endoscopic examination. Which of the following syndromic diagnoses needs to be considered?

    A. Oculoauriculovertebral syndrome
    B. Stickler syndrome
    C. Treacher Collins syndrome
    D. Velocardiofacial syndrome

61. A 6-year-old child presents with complaints of double vision and right periorbital discomfort. Examination shows obvious exopthalmus, strabismus, and a lesion of the right upper eyelid. CT scan shows a lesion involving the right upper eyelid, soft tissue around the right lateral orbital rim, and a small amount of orbital extension. There are no suspicious lesions on CT that would suggest nodal disease or metastases. A biopsy reveals rhabdomyosarcoma. What is the best treatment?

    A. Surgical treatment only with exoneration of the eye and debulking of the soft tissue component of the tumor
    B. Radiation of the affected area and systemic chemotherapy
    C. Radiation of the affected area and lymph node basins of the right parotid region and right cervical neck
    D. Wide local excision of affected skin, complete surgical removal of the affected soft tissue, right lateral orbital wall removal, right parotidectomy, and neck dissection

62. Which two complications are the most common causes of tracheostomy-related morbidity and mortality?

    A. Accidental decannulation and tracheostomy tube occlusion
    B. Pneumothorax and tracheoinnominate artery fistula formation
    C. Tracheitis and airway hemorrhage
    D. Accidental decannulation and tracheoinnominate artery fistula formation

63. A 5-year-old boy presents with 2 years of hoarseness. He has no symptoms of coughing or throat clearing. His mother reports that he is a screamer. He has a breathy raspy voice, and stroboscopy reveals symmetric bilateral lesions in the midmembranous vocal fold. What is the most appropriate step in the initial management of this patient?

    A. Diagnostic/operative endoscopy
    B. Voice therapy
    C. Laser surgery
    D. Proton pump inhibitor

64. A 12-year-old boy presents with bilateral enlarged lymph nodes that have been present for almost 3 months without significant change in size. They are firm, rubbery, and nontender. He has associated nighttime fevers, malaise, and weight loss. A chest X-ray shows mediastinal involvement. What is the best diagnostic procedure?

    A. Fine-needle aspirate biopsy
    B. Small incisional biopsy of single node with frozen sections and cultures
    C. Biopsy with permanent hematoxylin/eosin sections, and immunohistochemistry and cytogenetics studies
    D. Needle aspirate of enlarged node with fungal and atypical mycobacterial cultures

65. The most common inflammatory disorder of the salivary glands worldwide is:

    A. Mumps
    B. Juvenile recurrent parotitis (JRP)
    C. Rheumatoid arthritis
    D. Sarcoidosis

66. Which of the following is the most common cause of stridor in the newborn?

    A. Laryngomalacia
    B. Subglottic stenosis
    C. Tracheomalacia
    D. Vocal fold paresis

67. Sclerotherapy with OK-432 for branchial cleft anomalies is associated with all of the following *except*:

    A. Fever
    B. Highly successful for multilocular lesions
    C. Odynophagia
    D. Approximately a 60% complete response rate
    E. Pain

68. Which of the following is a risk factor for otitis media?

    A. Cleft palate
    B. Family history positive for otitis media
    C. Breastfeeding for less than 6 months
    D. Second-hand tobacco smoke exposure
    E. All of the above

69. Which of the following is the safest way to perform a tracheotomy in a child?

    A. In the operating room but with the patient awake and breathing spontaneously
    B. In the operating room, under general anesthesia, with the airway secured with an endotracheal tube or rigid bronchoscope
    C. In the pediatric intensive care unit with a percutaneous technique
    D. In the operating room with a laryngeal mask airway (LMA) in place

70. Which of these is the most common salivary gland malignancy in children?

    A. Acinic cell carcinoma
    B. Squamous cell carcinoma
    C. Mucoepidermoid carcinoma (MEC)
    D. Warthin tumor

71. A 3-year-old girl presents with a 2-cm right-sided neck mass. According to the mother, the mass initially developed quickly and then had a more gradual increase in size in the past 2 weeks. There are no associated fevers or other constitutional symptoms. The skin overlying the mass is a violaceous red hue and is very thin. A purified protein derivative skin test is positive, and a chest X-ray shows hilar nodular abnormalities. How do you treat this mass?

    A. Surgical excision
    B. Radiation therapy to the neck and systemic chemotherapy for the chest lesions
    C. Multiagent antibiotic therapy for at least 12 months
    D. Observation as the lesion is self-limiting and will resolve on its own

72. Characteristics of congenital hemangiomas include:

    A. Does not stain for glucose transporter 1
    B. Rapidly involutes after birth
    C. Does not involute
    D. All of the above

73. A 2-year-old child presents with a 5-day history of bilateral enlarged lymph nodes. His mother reports that the child had an associated sore throat and low grade fever 1 week ago that has resolved essentially. On examination, there are multiple small (about 1 cm in diameter), bilateral, tender lymph nodes. There are no areas of fluctuance or overlying skin changes. The examination also demonstrates mild posterior oropharyngeal erythema and slightly enlarged tonsils, without exudates. There is also an associated clear rhinorrhea. What is the best treatment option?

    A. Observation with symptomatic treatment of fever and sore throat
    B. One-week course of amoxicillin
    C. Admit to the hospital for IV antibiotics until afebrile for at least 48 hours, and then switch to an oral antibiotic such as amoxicillin and claculanic acid
    D. Excisional lymph node biopsy with systemic chemotherapy

74. Which of the following factors predisposes to a more severe clinical course in children with juvenile-onset recurrent respiratory papillomatosis (RRP)?

    A. Diagnosis of RRP at less than 3 years of age
    B. Human papillomavirus (HPV) subtype 6
    C. Maternal history of condylomata
    D. Family history of RRP

75. A 6-year-old girl presents to your clinic from a family doctor with a 6-month history of wheezing that is refractory to the first-line asthma treatments. There is no history of foreign-body aspiration or choking. You perform a complete history and physical examination. What is the next most appropriate step?

    A. Inspiratory and expiratory views on chest X-ray
    B. Chest CT with contract to rule out vascular compression of the airway
    C. Referral to a pulmonary physician for asthma testing and treatment
    D. Initiate second-line medications for the treatment of asthma

76. In CHARGE syndrome, which of the following is the best description?

    A. Choanal atresia is associated with more than 65% of cases.
    B. It is unilateral in more than two-thirds of the patients.
    C. In unilateral cases, it is more common on the right side.
    D. A only.
    E. B and C only.

77. **A diagnosis of auditory dyssynchrony in a neonate should be considered if there is:**

    A. Presence of otoacoustic emissions (OAEs), presence of cochlear microphonic, absence/abnormal auditory brainstem response (ABR) waveforms
    B. Absence of OAEs, presence of cochlear microphonic, absence/abnormal of ABR waveforms
    C. Absence of OAEs, presence of cochlear microphonic, presence of ABR waveforms
    D. Absence of OAEs, absence of cochlear microphonic, absence/abnormal ABR waveforms

78. **Genetic testing of a child with aminoglycoside-induced hearing loss would most likely reveal:**

    A. A paternally inherited 12S rRNA mutation
    B. A maternally inherited 12S rRNA mutation
    C. A maternally inherited *GjB2* mutation
    D. An X-linked mutation

79. **Which bacteria have been specifically linked to tonsillar hypertrophy?**

    A. *Haemophilus influenzae*
    B. *Staphylococcus aureus*
    C. *Prevotella*
    D. Group C β-hemolytic streptococci
    E. *Acinetobacter*

80. **All neonates with suspected airway obstruction should undergo:**

    A. Flexible airway endoscopy
    B. Airway fluoroscopy
    C. Rapidly assess the patient's clinical condition
    D. Obtain a pulse oximetry reading

81. **A 14-year-old girl presents with a history of exercise-induced asthma. She reports that the symptoms occur during soccer games but do not occur during practice. She initially undergoes therapy with a speech-language pathologist; however, she continues to have symptoms. What would be the appropriate next steps in the management of this child?**

    A. MRI brain scan
    B. Psychiatric or psychological evaluation
    C. Awake flexible endoscopy
    D. All of the above

82. **Reasonable initial medical management of recurrent or chronic pediatric sinusitis includes:**

    A. Prolonged course of oral broad-spectrum antibiotics
    B. Topical nasal steroid sprays
    C. Nasal irrigations
    D. All of the above

83. **Bilateral choanal atresia can cause significant airway distress in the newborn because of which of these statements?**

    A. Infants with choanal atresia usually have concomitant cardiac anomalies.
    B. Infants are initially obligate nasal breathers.
    C. The neonatal larynx is smaller and collapses easily.
    D. Neonates have low oxygen reserves.

84. **Which of the following best characterizes the order of embryogenesis of the anterior neuropore?**

    A. Neural crest migration, neural grove formation, neural tube closure
    B. Neural crest migration, neural tube closure, neural groove formation
    C. Neural groove formation, neural tube closure, neural crest migration
    D. Neural groove formation, neural crest migration, neural tube closure

85. **The current national goals for hearing screening were developed by the federal Early Hearing Detection and Intervention (EHDI) program. What are they called?**

    A. 1-2-3 plan
    B. 3-6-9 plan
    C. 1-3-6 plan
    D. 2-4-8 plan

86. **All of the following pairings between cough quality and etiology are correct** *except*:

    A. Barking cough → Croup
    B. Staccato cough →Psychogenic
    C. Paroxysmal cough →Parapertussis
    D. Cough productive of casts →Plastic bronchitis
    E. Cough with a whoop → Pertussis

87. Which group of patients has the lowest chance for successful decannulation?

    A. Children with airway obstruction from subglottic stenosis
    B. Children with bronchopulmonary dysplasia from prematurity
    C. Children with neurologic impairment
    D. Children with craniofacial abnormalities

88. Which statement about visual reinforcement audiometry (VRA) is *false*?

    A. It may be used on infant as early as 5 to 6 months of age.
    B. It does not provide information about response thresholds.
    C. Speech and pure tone stimuli may be used.
    D. Ear specific and sound field testing is possible.
    E. It requires cooperation of the infant to participate in the tasks.

89. If your patient has failed an adenoidectomy and there is a normal immune system without allergies, your next step would be to proceed with:

    A. Anterior and posterior ethmoidectomy
    B. Anterior and posterior ethmoidectomy and maxillary antrostomy
    C. CT of the sinuses after a prolonged course (20 days) of oral antibiotics
    D. Prolonged course of IV antibiotics

90. Which of the following is currently the most common indication for tracheotomy in the pediatric population?

    A. Providing access for pulmonary toilet
    B. Airway obstruction from subglottic stenosis
    C. Airway obstruction from craniofacial abnormalities
    D. Respiratory failure and ventilator dependence

91. A 2-year old boy with a tracheotomy is evaluated for decannulation. He has a history of eosinophilic esophagitis and has undergone previous endoscopic attempts at repair. Endoscopy reveals firm grade III subglottic stenosis that does not include the vocal folds. What surgical intervention would be the least likely to succeed?

    A. Single-stage laryngotracheal reconstruction with anteroposterior costal cartilage graft
    B. Endoscopic laser resection
    C. Cricotracheal resection
    D. Two-stage laryngotracheal reconstruction with anteroposterior costal cartilage graft

92. Which of the following is true regarding the treatment of cough in children?

    A. A 10-day course of antibiotics reduces persistence of short- to medium-term cough.

    B. In children whose cough responds to antibiotics, the nasopharynx is most commonly colonized by *Streptococcus pneumoniae.*

    C. Antihistamine decongestant combinations are not effective in treating acute cough in children.

    D. Both A and C.

    E. All of the above.

93. Incidence of the cleft lip deformity is highest in which of the following ethnic subgroups?

    A. African Americans

    B. Caucasians

    C. Native Americans

    D. Asians

94. A 2-year-old patient presents with mild aspiration with liquids. All diagnostic examinations were unremarkable. Direct laryngoscopy and palpation of larynx revealed a dehiscence above the level of cricoid through the arytenoid musculature. What grade laryngeal cleft does the child have?

    A. Grade I

    B. Grade II

    C. Grade III

    D. Grade IV

95. A prenatal ultrasonogram revealed a large cervicofacial mass that had both cystic and solid components. A fetal MRI performed at 35 weeks of gestation demonstrated a heterogeneous, sharply circumscribed mass with solid and variable signal characteristics of the solid component consistent with teratoma. Radiology report did not indicate direct complete airway obstruction, but expressed concern due to the large mass in the neck. What is your next step?

    A. Wait for natural birth

    B. Induce birth immediately, to avoid further growth that could compromise natural vaginal delivery

    C. Have airway management team available at Cesarean delivery

    D. Plan for the ex-utero intrapartum treatment (EXIT) procedure

96. All of the following are appropriate associations on radiologic evaluations *except*:

    A. Steeple sign–laryngotracheitis
    B. Thumbprint sign–epiglottitis
    C. Air trapping on chest radiograph–vocal cord immobility
    D. Thickened soft tissue overlying C-spine–retropharyngeal abscess/phlegmon

97. The optimal timing for alveolar bone grafting is described best for which situation below?

    A. In the skeletally mature adolescent patient
    B. In the patient with primary dentition, prior to eruption of the permanent dentition
    C. At any time during the patient's lifetime
    D. In the patient with mixed dentition, prior to eruption of the cleft-side canine

98. What is the most common type of laryngeal stenosis in children?

    A. Acquired subglottic stenosis
    B. Congenital subglottic stenosis
    C. Congenital laryngeal web
    D. Complete tracheal rings

99. Which of the following is completely developed at the time of birth?

    A. Eustachian tube
    B. Mastoid antrum
    C. Mastoid tip
    D. Ossicular chain

100. A 10-year-old boy presents with long-standing "hoarseness." He presents with chronic coughing and throat clearing. Endoscopy reveals thickened vocal folds, small nodules, and vocal fold erythema. He has been on a proton pump inhibitor (PPI) for 3 months. What would be the appropriate next step in therapy?

    A. Referral to a gastroenterologist for esophagogastroduodenoscopy (EGD), biopsy, and impedance probe testing
    B. Increase the dose of the PPI
    C. Add ranitidine (Zantac)
    D. Pulsed steroid therapy

101. A 3-month-old, who was a former 26-week premature infant with a 2-month history of intubation, presents with biphasic stridor. What test or procedure would be the most useful in establishing a diagnosis?

    A. Flexible nasopharyngoscopy
    B. Microlaryngoscopy and bronchoscopy
    C. High kilovolt radiograph
    D. CT scan of the trachea/airway

102. When is "watchful-waiting" not indicated in the treatment of acute otitis media (AOM)?

    A. <6 months of age
    B. Temp ≥ 39°C
    C. Bilateral AOM
    D. Otorrhea
    E. All of the above

103. Which statement about otoacoustic emissions (OAEs) is *false*?

    A. It is an objective measure.
    B. The middle and external ear status influences the results of the emission.
    C. Accurate measurement of hearing levels may be predicted.
    D. In young infants, the low-frequency emission may be reduced.
    E. The presence of emissions does not assure normal hearing.

104. In patients with a complete cleft of the palate (CP), the three abnormal attachments of the levator veli palatini (LVP) are:

    A. The muscularis uvulae, palatopharyngeus, and superior pharyngeal constrictor muscles
    B. The posterior edge of the hard palate, tensor aponeurosis, and superior pharyngeal constrictor muscle
    C. The stylopharyngeus muscle, palatoglossus muscle, and vomer
    D. The tensor veli palatini muscle, lateral nasal mucosa, and lateral pharyngeal constrictor muscle

105. Screening based only on high-risk indicators identifies what percent of infants with significant hearing loss?

    A. 5%
    B. 10%
    C. 25%
    D. 50%
    E. 75%

106. Y-linked genes are best described by which of these phrases?

    A. Occur only in males.
    B. They are transmitted to all the sons and none of the daughters.
    C. There are very few genes known to be definitely on the Y chromosome.
    D. None of the above.
    E. All of the above.

107. Which of the following is the most common cause of dysphonia in school-aged children?

    A. Vocal fold nodules
    B. Vocal fold papilloma
    C. Vocal fold paresis
    D. Vocal fold web

108. Universal screening guidelines for hearing loss in newborns recommend that if an infant fails the initial screening test, the confirmatory testing should be carried out no later than:

    A. 3 months
    B. 6 months
    C. 12 months
    D. 18 months

109. Sturge–Weber syndrome is associated with:

    A. Capillary malformations
    B. Venous malformations
    C. Congenital hemangiomas
    D. Arteriovenous malformations

110. What is the most common cause of pediatric dysphonia?

    A. Airway reconstruction
    B. Unilateral vocal fold paralysis
    C. Paradoxical vocal fold dysfunction
    D. Vocal fold nodules

111. **Infantile hemangiomas in a bearded distribution can be problematic because:**

    A. They can be associated with airway hemangiomas.
    B. They can cause nasal airway obstruction.
    C. They do not involute like other infantile hemangiomas.
    D. They do not respond to medical management.

112. **Which of the following bacteria have not been discovered in appreciable quantity in diseased adenoidal/tonsillar tissue?**

    A. *Haemophilus influenzae*
    B. *Staphylococcus aureus*
    C. *Prevotella*
    D. Group C β-hemolytic streptococci
    E. *Acinetobacter*

113. **The most common presenting symptoms in children with recurrent respiratory papillomatosis (RRP) are:**

    A. Dysphagia and poor weight gain
    B. Dyspnea with exertion
    C. Progressive hoarseness and stridor
    D. Odynophagia

114. A 3-year-old boy with rapidly enlarging neck mass. Which category of disease is most likely diagnosed?

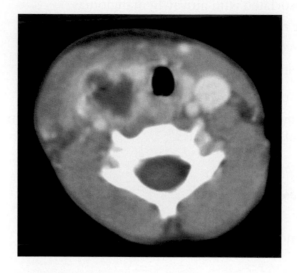

    A. Superinfection of congenital malformation

    B. Suppurative adenopathy

    C. Malignancy

    D. Benign neoplasm

    E. Trauma

115. A 3-year-old girl with neck mass. What is the most likely diagnosis?

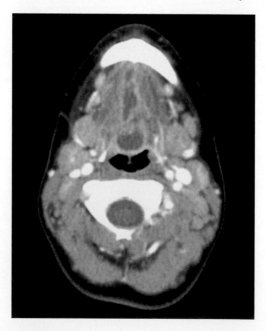

    A. Thyroglossal duct cyst

    B. Branchial cleft anomaly

    C. Suppurative lymphadenopathy

    D. Hemangioma of infancy

    E. Lymphatic malformation

Chapter 6 Answers

1. **Answer: A.** In patients who are asymptomatic, endoscopy can be postponed for 12 to 24 hours. There are two important exceptions to this principle. The first is a foreign body that appears to be a disc battery. The second is if the foreign object is sharp and/or has the potential to perforate the esophagus, such as an open safety pin. PAGE 1406

2. **Answer: C.** Data from newborn hearing screening programs show that the incidence of hearing loss is twice as high as all other diseases screened at birth, occurring in about 2 to 4 per 1,000 births. PAGE 1507

3. **Answer: C.** Prenatal exposure to CMV, a β-herpes virus, is the most common congenital viral infection and currently the most common viral cause of congenital sensorineural hearing loss. PAGE 1527

4. **Answer: B.** The anterior neuropore is the most distal point of the neural crest cell migration; the lack of neural crest cells and the relatively late tube closure predispose this region to developmental defects. PAGE 1445

5. **Answer: D.** Genetic etiology to hearing loss. Mutations in the Pendrin gene (PDS, *SLC26A4*) cause Pendred syndrome but are also responsible for a nonsyndromic form of recessive sensorineural hearing loss, DFNB4. PAGE 1535

6. **Answer: C.** This process is a rare, life-threatening condition associated with two specific subtypes of vascular tumors, tufted angioma and kaposiform hemangioendothelioma. It is not associated with infantile hemangiomas. In point of fact, the tumor traps and destroys platelets and is associated with other coagulopathies. PAGE 1579

7. **Answer: A.** Answers B (Furlow palatoplasty), C (Hogan modification), and D (Hynes pharyngoplasty) are the recommended procedures. PAGE 1568

8. **Answer: A.** Most pediatric otolaryngologists would recommend adenoidectomy as the first step. Whether the adenoid pad is large and obstructing or small in size, adenoidectomy should improve symptoms. PAGES 1459–1460

9. **Answer: B.** The advantages of tracheotomy as opposed to prolonged endotracheal intubation include the following: shorter, larger tube can be placed, decreased airway dead space, less damage to larynx, more comfortable for the patient, may allow the child to be discharged from the hospital, even on a ventilator, and care for a tracheotomy can be performed by trained caregivers/family members who are not health care professionals. PAGE 1385

10. **Answer: D.** Acrocephalosyndactyly type 1. Features of this autosomal dominant syndrome include craniosynostosis of the coronal suture. PAGES 1622–1623

11. **Answer: D.** If maximum medical therapy and adenoidectomy failed, a complete workup for allergy and/or immune problems should be done, in addition to obtaining a CT scan to assess the need for sinus surgery. PAGE 1459

12. **Answer: C.** Children with tracheal stenosis generally exhibit a biphasic wet-sounding breathing pattern referred to as "washing-machine" breathing. This pattern transiently clears with coughing. PAGE 1361

13. **Answer: D.** The gene that causes Pendred syndrome has been identified and is named *SLC26A4* (or PDS). The hearing impairment in Pendred syndrome is associated with abnormal iodine metabolism, which typically results in a euthyroid goiter. PAGE 1546

14. **Answer: D.** Café-au-lait spots and cutaneous neurofibromas are not consistent findings of NF2. Axillary freckling is uncommon. Other neurogenic tumors are common, such as schwannomas, intracranial or spinal meningiomas, or astrocytomas. Lisch nodules are absent in NF2. Posterior cataracts are common (80%). PAGE 1630

15. **Answer: C.** More than 90% of both third and fourth branchial cleft anomalies occur on the left side. PAGES 1609–1610

16. **Answer B.** Prior to performing an adenotonsillectomy, one should always palpate the palate to check for a submucous cleft and evaluate the oropharynx for abnormal pulsatile vessels. This is especially important in syndromic children so that surgery can be modified appropriately. PAGE 1301

17. **Answer: E.** SDB is known to increase the risk for hyperactivity and symptoms of attention deficit hyperactivity disorder (ADHD). The children may have enuresis, behavior problems, poor school performance, reduced quality of life, and growth problems. PAGE 1436

18. **Answer: C.** In addition to nasal obstruction, pituitary disorders along with dental and facial anomalies are seen with congenital nasal pyriform aperture stenosis. PAGE 1316

19. **Answer D.** Ultrasound is currently the most important and commonly used means to diagnose aerodigestive disease because it is anatomic, physiologic, and noninvasive. However, the use of MRI is widening, and reports exist that document the utility of this modality in the diagnosis of aerodigestive tract abnormalities that may predict respiratory embarrassment at delivery. PAGE 1309

20. **Answer: D.** The findings of micrognathia and glossoptosis in the neonate with airway obstruction are pathognomonic for Robin sequence. Cleft palate is seen in approximately 50% of these patients. PAGE 1331

21. **Answer: A.** Alkaline agents cause liquefaction necrosis, wherein the mucosa disintegrates, allowing the agent to penetrate into the surrounding tissues. PAGE 1399

22. **Answer: C.** Five anatomic configurations typically are described with TEF: EA with distal TEF (85%), EA alone (8%), TEF alone (H-type TEF) (4%), EA with proximal and distal TEF (3%), and EA with proximal TEF (1%). PAGE 1322

23. **Answer: E.** The major diagnostic criteria of Robin sequence are micrognathia, glossoptosis, and inverted U-shaped cleft palate. It is very heterogeneous, with a birth prevalence of 1 in 8,500 births. PAGE 1631

24. **Answer: B.** Specific recommendations have been made by the Task Force on RRP from ASPO in regard to the use of cidofovir. Informed consent must be obtained from the patient's parents because this drug is being used in an off-label setting. PAGE 1421

25. **Answer: A.** Sincipital encephaloceles, also known as frontoethmoidal encephaloceles, constitute 15% of the encephaloceles (three types). They occur between the frontal and ethmoid bones at the foramen cecum immediately anterior to the cribriform plate. These lesions are usually pulsatile and classically show expansion with crying, or jugular vein compression (Furstenberg sign). PAGE 1449

26. **Answer: D.** The narrowest part of an infant's airway is the subglottis and it normally measures 4 to 7 mm. Less than 4 mm in size in a newborn or 3.5 mm in a premature infant is diagnostic of subglottic stenosis. PAGE 1343

27. **Answer: B.** Patients with tracheobronchial obstruction, including tracheomalacia, usually present with a normal cry, expiratory stridor, brassy cough, and sometimes wheezing. With severe obstruction, the stridor may become biphasic. PAGE 1334

28. **Answer: C.** The gene at the DFNB1 locus is gap junction beta 2 (*GJB2*), which produces a protein called connexin 26. DFNB1 was the earliest autosomal recessive gene locus to be mapped and characterized. PAGE 1544

29. **Answer: D.** This association of findings is far more common in females. More than 50% of patients are affected by neurologic sequelae, including seizures, stroke, developmental delay, and migraines. PAGE 1577

30. **Answer: A.** In children who can tolerate them, speaking valves can help with both verbal communication and swallowing. Contraindications to speaking valves include significant laryngeal stenosis or other forms of airway obstruction that would prevent adequate exhalation and severe neurologic dysfunction. PAGE 1396

31. **Answer: E.** Hemorrhage can be primary (within 24 hours of surgery) and secondary (more than 24 hours after surgery). The incidence of primary hemorrhage ranges from 0.2% to 2.2%, while secondary hemorrhages range from 0.1% to 3%. PAGE 1439

32. **Answer: C.** Unilateral vocal fold paralysis is more common than bilateral paralysis, and because of the longer course of the left recurrent nerve, left-sided paralysis is more common than right-sided. PAGE 1377

33. **Answer: B.** CT scan has become the gold standard for the evaluation of chronic sinusitis in children. There are increased concerns that children are receiving significant doses of radiation from CT scans. Pediatric radiologists are now practicing ALARA (as low as reasonably achievable). PAGES 1456–1457

34. **Answer: A.** Stickler syndrome type 1 (STL1) is the classic phenotype. It is associated with mutation in the *COL2A1* gene, which encodes a fibrillar collagen that is arrayed in quarter-staggered fashion to form fibers. Stickler syndrome type 2 (STL2) is caused by a mutation in the *COL11A1* gene. PAGE 1549

35. **Answer: D.** The prognosis of malignant salivary neoplasms in the pediatric population is dependent on the type and grade. A recent study showed that for salivary gland malignancy the overall 5-year survival was 93%, and 26% developed a recurrence. PAGE 1474

36. **Answer: E.** Patients with a combination of bilateral preauricular sinuses, bilateral second or third BCA in the neck, and renal disease most likely have branchiootorenal syndrome. This is an autosomal dominant syndrome with variable penetrance. The hearing loss can be conductive or sensorineural. PAGE 1611

37. **Answer: A.** Children with foreign bodies lodged at the upper esophageal sphincter frequently present with early symptoms of dysphagia and drooling. As a result of this, earlier surgical intervention is typically is recommended. PAGE 1405

38. **Answer: D.** RRP lesions occur most often at anatomic sites in which ciliated and squamous epithelium are juxtaposed. The most common sites for RRP are the limen vestibuli, the nasopharyngeal surface of the soft palate, the midline of the laryngeal surface of the epiglottis, the upper and lower margins of the ventricle, the undersurface of the vocal folds, the carina, and at bronchial spurs. PAGE 1410

39. **Answer: A.** In a 2010 systematic review and meta-analysis, although Hib meningitis was the most common, hearing loss occurred most commonly after pneumococcal meningitis. PAGE 1530

40. **Answer: B.** JRP is the most common inflammatory salivary gland disorder in children in the United States and is second only to mumps worldwide. PAGE 1469

41. **Answer: D.** On approaching the skull base, the lesion should come free or terminate in a fibrous stalk. If there is any question about the stalk representing an epithelial-lined tract penetrating the skull base, a frozen section may be taken of its most superior, extracranial extent. PAGE 1453

42. **Answer: B.** The sensory or outer hair cells, within the organ of Corti, are thought to be responsible for the generation of OAEs, specifically the electromotility of the outer hair cells. The presence of an emission provides a reasonable assurance that hearing thresholds are 30 to 40 dB or better in the frequency range where the emission is present. PAGE 1512

43. **Answer: B.** Endoscopic repair of laryngeal clefts may be attempted if the patient does not have concomitant subglottic stenosis or other airway limitations. This would include low-birth-weight newborns, individuals with craniofacial anomalies, especially micrognathia, and clefts that extend beyond the second tracheal ring. PAGE 1321

44. **Answer: A.** The anomalies described are seen with CHARGE syndrome. Mutations in the *CHD7* gene (*8q12.2*) cause more than half of CHARGE cases. PAGE 1317

45. **Answer: E.** Risk factors for developmental difficulties include permanent hearing loss independent of otitis media with effusion, suspected or diagnosed speech and language delay or disorder, autism spectrum disorder and other pervasive developmental disorders, craniofacial disorders that include cognitive and linguistic delays, blindness or uncorrectable visual impairment, and cleft palate with or without a syndrome. PAGE 1494

46. **Answer: B.** An ophthalmologic evaluation is integral to the diagnosis of Usher syndrome. Results of electroretinographic studies have been reported to be subnormal in patients 2 to 3 years of age, before functional or fundoscopic abnormalities can be detected. Early diagnosis of Usher syndrome can have important implications on the rehabilitation of an affected child and on educational planning. PAGE 1547

47. **Answer: E.** Presently, the *Streptococcus pneumoniae* vaccines (Pneumovax, Prevnar, and Prevnar 13) are the only bacterial vaccines available in the United States for otitis media. Other respiratory viruses, such as respiratory syncytial virus, influenza, adenovirus, parainfluenza, and rhinovirus, have been isolated in middle ear effusions using polymerase chain reaction (PCR). Influenza vaccine is the only available recommended viral vaccine today that may impact otitis media. PAGE 1488

48. **Answer: D.** When a cyst-appearing mass occurs in the dorsum of the nose or in the intranasal region deformity in a child the differential diagnosis includes dermoid, glioma, and encephalocele. Since the mass may have an intracranial extension, biopsy or excision of the mass without a prior CT scan and possibly MRI is to be condemned as it may cause cerebrospinal fluid leak and meningitis. PAGE 1614

49. **Answer: A.** The presence of a bifid crista galli and enlarged foramen cecum is highly suggestive of intracranial involvement and implore the need for neurosurgical consultation. PAGE 1451

50. **Answer: A.** The timing of endoscopy is crucial. If the examination is performed earlier than 12 hours following ingestion, adequate time may not have passed for injury to fully manifest. As a result, the examination may underestimate the extent of injury. However, examination during the period of structural weakness of the esophageal wall will increase the risk of iatrogenic injury during the examination. As a result, endoscopy should be performed between 12 and 48 hours following ingestion to achieve the highest degree of patient safety while providing the most information. PAGE 1401

51. **Answer: A.** The larynx is the most common anatomic site of stridor in the neonate. Noisy breathing **resulting from** nasal **airway** obstruction is typically described as **stertor**. PAGE 1332

52. **Answer: C.** Though there has been some change in the relative frequency of organisms recovered from ears with AOM, *Streptococcus pneumoniae* remains the most frequent organism recovered. However, there has been a relative increase in the frequency of *H. influenzae*. PAGE 1486

53. **Answer: C.** Children undergoing tonsillectomy do *not* benefit from perioperative antibiotic treatment based on clinical studies. PAGE 1441, TABLE 95.4

54. **Answer: D.** The subglottis is the narrowest part of the airway because of the complete ring structure of the cricoid cartilage. PAGE 1356

55. **Answer: C.** The most common syndrome with CL/P is Van der Woude syndrome, an autosomal dominant syndrome characterized by blind lower lip pits in addition to CL/P. PAGE 1557

56. **Answer: B.** No single modality has been consistently effective in eradicating RRP. As a result, the current standard of surgical therapy is to maintain an airway with voice improvement while avoiding complications. Overzealous surgical therapy may result in significant scar which can lead to airway and voice problems even after disease remission. PAGE 1415

57. **Answer: C.** A recent meta-analysis found overall surgical success to be 81.6% across all studies. The highest rate of success was with bilateral submandibular gland excision and parotid rerouting. PAGE 1476

58. **Answer: D.** A work type 2 first branchial cleft lesion will contain derivates of two germ cell layers, ectoderm and mesoderm. PAGE 1608

59. **Answer: C.** When presented with a neonate in respiratory distress, the physician must decide initially whether the airway needs to be managed emergently or is it safe to proceed with a detailed history and physical examination. PAGE 1328

60. **Answer: D.** Of the various syndromes considered, laryngeal abnormalities are typically found only in children with the velocardiofacial syndrome. is it PAGE 1295

61. **Answer: B.** In large or extensive rhabdomyosarcomas of the head and neck in which the morbidity of surgical resection is excessive or complete resection is unobtainable, or both, treatment with combination chemotherapy and radiotherapy is indicated. In some limited orbital tumors, surgical removal can be utilized. Radiation therapy is avoided in certain circumstances as well. PAGE 1602

62. **Answer: A.** The rates of accidental decannulation are probably higher than reported in the literature, as many episodes are not documented unless there is significant morbidity or requirement to return to the operating room for a stomal revision as a result. Tracheostomy tube obstruction/plugging tends to occur more frequently in premature infants and newborns compared with children older than one year of age and is likely related to the smaller diameter of the tracheostomy tubes used in this population. PAGES 1386, 1387, 1392

63. **Answer: B.** The initial management of children with vocal fold nodules, cysts, and polyps often involves a course of voice therapy with a speech-language pathologist with expertise in voice disorder. Most children who are 4 years or older and developmentally normal can actively participate in voice therapy. PAGE 1376

64. **Answer: C.** Over half of pediatric neck malignancies are lymphomas. They present in two distinct histopathologic and clinical types, Hodgkin disease and non-Hodgkin disease. The long-term outcome is dependent on the stage of the disease at the time of diagnosis. PAGE 1601

65. **Answer: A.** Mumps is the most common inflammatory gland disorder worldwide; JRP is the most common inflammatory salivary gland disorder in children in the United States. PAGE 1469

66. **Answer: A.** The most common laryngeal anomaly is laryngomalacia, which in some respects is considered normal neonatal supraglottic development. Though the etiology is debated, most recent research suggests that immature sensorimotor integration and tone may be the factor most responsible. PAGE 1296

67. **Answer: B.** Unilocular lesions have a higher success rate than multilocular lesions, which have only partial or no response to OK-432. PAGE 1607

68. **Answer: E.** Risk factors can be host-related (young age, male sex, Caucasian, prematurity, allergy, immunocompetence, cleft palate and craniofacial abnormalities, genetic predisposition) as well as environmental (upper respiratory tract infections, breastfeeding, lower socioeconomic status, pacifier use, and obesity), and are considered important in the occurrence, recurrence, and persistence of middle ear disease. PAGE 1482

69. **Answer: B.** An LMA can be used if intubation is not possible or a rigid bronchoscope cannot be passed or is unavailable. PAGE 1386

70. **Answer: C.** MEC is the most common malignant salivary gland in the pediatric population (46% to 55%). It has been reported that the majority of MECs appear in major salivary glands. PAGE 1474

71. **Answer: C.** The clinical picture is most consistent with *Mycobacterium tuberculosis*. Multiagent antituberculous antibiotic therapy for 12 to 18 months is the standard treatment. PAGE 1595

72. **Answer: D.** Congenital hemangiomas are an uncommon variant of infantile hemangiomas. They differ from infantile hemangiomas in clinical behavior, appearance, and histopathology and are occasionally present in utero. They present as fully grown lesions and do not undergo additional postnatal growth. Some of them demonstrate rapid involution and others do not involute. PAGE 1575

73. **Answer: A.** The clinical scenario is most consistent with a viral upper respiratory tract infection. Symptomatic care is all that is necessary. PAGE 1594

74. **Answer: A.** Children whose RRP has been diagnosed at younger ages (less than 3 years have been found to be 3.6 times more likely to have more than four surgeries per year and almost 2 times more likely to have two or more anatomic sites affected than were children whose RRP was diagnosed at later ages (greater than 3 years). PAGE 1409

75. **Answer: A.** The most important noninvasive study to evaluate for foreign bodies is the chest radiograph. However, up to 25% of plain films in children with known foreign bodies are interpreted as normal. This may be due to the fact that the hallmark radiographic signs associated with foreign-body aspiration, mediastinal shift, and air tracking are most readily demonstrated only on expiratory films or fluoroscopy instead of a single inspiratory view. As a result, inspiratory and expiratory views on the chest film often are recommended. PAGE 1403

76. **Answer: D.** The components of the CHARGE are: *C* (coloboma of the eye), *H* (heart disease), *A* (atresia of the choanae), *R* (retarded development and growth), *G* (genital anomalies), and *E* (ear anomalies, deafness, or both). Choanal atresia is associated with more than 65% of the cases. It is bilateral in more than two-thirds of the patients. In unilateral cases, it is more common on the left side. PAGE 1624

77. **Answer: A.** Auditory dyssynchrony spectrum disorders comprise of up to 10% of hearing loss in infants. In an infant with auditory dysscynchrony, robust OAEs may be present, but on ABR tracings only a cochlear microphonics, followed by indistinct or absent ABR waveforms, will be seen. Therefore, no matter which test is used for screening, follow-up diagnostic testing should utilize both modalities. PAGE 1525

78. **Answer: B.** Mitochondrial inheritance is distinctly matrilineal and affects both male and female offspring equally. Mitochondrial mutations have been associated with nonsyndromic hearing loss and ototoxicity. Patients with 12SrRNA mutation have been found to have a genetic predisposition to aminoglycoside-induced hearing loss. PAGE 1551

79. **Answer: A.** Studies support a bacterial etiology for tonsillar hypertrophy. Some authors have argued for an etiologic role of *H. influenzae* in the pathogenesis of tonsillar hypertrophy in children. PAGE 1433

80. **Answer A.** A standard part of the physical examination in any neonate with suspected airway obstruction should be flexible endoscopy with a pediatric flexible laryngoscope. PAGE 1329

81. **Answer: D.** The management involves the expertise of both a speech-language pathologist and a psychologist to help the patient gain insight into what trigger the condition. For recalcitrant cases, further workup and treatment are warranted and may include a MRI brain scan, Botox injection, and testing for myasthenia gravis. PAGE 1379

82. **Answer: D.** The cornerstones for the medical management of chronic sinusitis continue to be prolonged broad-spectrum antibiotic therapy, irrigation with normal saline, and topical nasal steroid spray. PAGE 1458

83. **Answer: B.** With complete nasal airway obstruction in the newborn, cyanotic episodes are frequent and may be alleviated during crying, a phenomenon known as cyclical cyanosis. PAGE 1330

84. **Answer: A.** As neural tube closure progresses, neural crest cells in the lateral portions of the neural tube migrate between the tube and the surface ectoderm into the mesenchyme that will eventually form bone and cartilage. The anterior neuropore is the most distal point of neural crest cell migration; the lack of neural crest cells and the relatively late tube closure predispose this region to developmental defects. PAGE 1445

85. **Answer: C.** The 1-3-6 plan involves the following: (1) all newborns will be screened for hearing loss by 1 month of age, preferably prior to discharge; (2) all newborns who screen positive will have a diagnostic audiologic evaluation before the age of 3 months; and (3) all infants with an identified hearing loss will receive appropriate early intervention services by the age of 6 months. PAGE 1525

86. **Answer: B.** A barking/brassy cough often is found with tracheomalacia, croup, or a habit cough. A honking type of cough is seen most often from psychogenic causes. A paroxysmal cough which may contain a whoop is seen most often with pertussis, parapertussis, or with a psychogenic cough. A staccato cough is most commonly associated with *Chlamydia* in infants. PAGE 1349

87. **Answer: C.** The underlying indication for a tracheotomy influences the chance for successful decannulation. As a result, children with neurologic impairment in whom their underlying disease process frequently progresses have a lower rate of successful decannulation and a higher mortality rate than those without neurologic impairment. PAGE 1395

88. **Answer: B.** In children developmentally at 5 to 6 months of age, it is possible to measure hearing threshold levels using VRA. PAGES 1513–1514

89. **Answer: C.** If maximum medical therapy and adenoidectomy failed, a complete workup for allergy and/or immune problems should be done, in addition to obtaining a CT scan to assess the need for sinus surgery. PAGE 1459

90. **Answer: D.** The three main indications for tracheotomy in the pediatric population are respiratory failure and anticipated need for prolonged ventilation, upper airway obstruction, and providing access for pulmonary toilet. PAGE 1383

91. **Answer: B.** Factors predisposing to failure in treating subglottic stenosis with a CO_2 laser include failure of previous endoscopic procedures, significant loss of cartilaginous framework, combined laryngotracheal stenosis, circumferential cicatricial scarring, fibrotic scar tissue in the interarytenoid area of the posterior commissure, abundant scar tissue >1 cm in vertical dimension, severe bacterial infection of the trachea after tracheotomy, exposure of perichondrium or cartilage during CO_2 laser excision predisposing to perichondritis and chondritis, and concomitant tracheal disease. PAGE 1363

92. **Answer: D.** A Cochrane review has concluded that a 10-day course of antibiotics reduces the duration of short- to medium-term cough. There is no data that the use of antihistamine/decongestant therapy is any more effective than placebo. PAGE 1353–1354

93. **Answer: C.** For cleft lip and/or palate (CL/P) the prevalence varies between ethnic subgroups: 3.6 per 1,000 in Native Americans, 2.1 per 1,000 in Asians, 1 per 1,000 in Caucasians, and 0.41 per 1,000 in African Americans. PAGE 1556

94. **Answer: A.** Laryngeal clefts are graded as Grade I involving only the interarytenoid muscle, Grade II involving part of the cricoid, Grade III involving the entire cricoid, and Grade IV extending into the trachea. PAGE 1345

95. **Answer: D.** With the prenatal diagnosis of a large mass, which is expected to cause life-threatening airway obstruction, an EXIT procedure is planned in order to secure the airway via a Cesarean delivery during ongoing placental perfusion. PAGE 1600

96. **Answer: C.** Children with vocal cord immobility most often will have a normal radiographic examination. Biphasic radiographs may reveal hyperinflation from obstructing lesions or lower airway disease such as infiltrates or pneumonia. PAGE 1339

97. **Answer: D.** Bone grafting of the maxillary and alveolar bone defects should be performed during the period of mixed dentition prior to the eruption of the permanent lateral incisor and canine. The patients benefit from presurgical orthodontic treatment to expand the maxillary dental arch and optimize the position of the teeth bordering the cleft. PAGE 1568

98. **Answer: A.** With the advent of long-term nasotracheal intubation in the management of the unstable neonatal airway, acquired subglottic stenosis resulting from this process is now more common than congenital stenosis in the pediatric age group. PAGE 1359

99. **Answer D.** In addition to the ossicular chain, the tympanic membrane is adult-sized at birth. However, due to incomplete ossification of the external auditory canal, it lies in a nearly horizontal position, thus impairing its visualization on routine otoscopic examination. PAGE 1292

100. **Answer A.** When the dysphonia and related symptoms persist, the patient should be referred to a gastroenterologist for an EGD, impedance probe testing, and biopsies. These diagnostic procedures will distinguish between laryngopharyngeal reflux, eosinophilic esophagitis, and other disorders. PAGE 1374

101. **Answer: B.** Flexible fiberoptic laryngoscopy provides information on dynamic vocal cord function. However, rigid endoscopy with Hopkins rod-lens telescopes provides the best possible examination in establishing a diagnosis of subglottic stenosis. PAGE 1358

102. **Answer: E.** Absolute contraindications for observation in children with AOM include age <6 months, immune deficiency or disorder, severe illness or treatment failure or inability to insure follow-up and rescue antibiotic. Relative contraindications include a relapse within 30 days of treatment, otorrhea, bilateral disease if <2 years of age, or a craniofacial malformation. PAGE 1491

103. **Answer: C.** Prediction of hearing levels is not possible by measuring OAEs. The absence of OAE can be associated with hearing loss of mild to moderate degree, and presence does not ensure normal hearing. PAGE 1512

104. **Answer: B.** In patients with CP, the LVP has three abnormal attachments: the superior pharyngeal constrictor, the tensor aponeurosis, and the posterior edge of the hard palate. PAGE 1560, FIGURE 103.2

105. **Answer: D.** Risk indicator screening identifies only 50% of infants with significant hearing loss. PAGE 1508

106. **Answer: E.** Y-linked genes occur only in males and are transmitted to all sons and none of the daughters. There are very few genes identified on the Y chromosome. PAGE 1619

107. **Answer: A.** Vocal fold nodules are the most common cause of hoarseness in preschool and school-aged children, but a laryngeal examination is justified to rule out other more serious etiologies such as recurrent respiratory papillomas. PAGE 1301

108. **Answer A.** The earlier institution of amplification, ideally between 6 weeks and 3 months of age, is the goal of universal newborn hearing screening programs. PAGE 1298

109. **Answer: A.** Sturge–Weber syndrome typically presents with a facial port-wine stain in the ophthalmic distribution of the trigeminal nerve, glaucoma, and vascular eye abnormalities and in ipsilateral intracranial vascular malformations. These patients often develop progressive neurologic symptoms, including seizures, migraines, stroke-like episodes, learning difficulties or mental retardation, visual field impairment, or hemiparesis. PAGE 1584

110. **Answer: D.** Vocal fold nodules are the most common cause of pediatric dysphonia (5% to 40%). Patients generally present with a harsh breathy voice, and they often have limited pitch range. These children may be either heavy voice users or vocal abusers who frequently scream and yell. PAGE 1375

111. **Answer: A.** Sixty-five percent of patients with hemangiomas that occur in a beard distribution (i.e., the chin, jawline, and preauricular areas) have associated airway involvement, and most airway hemangiomas are localized in the supraglottic or subglottic region. PAGE 1578

112. **Answer: E. Acinetobacter** has not been identified in adenoidal/tonsillar tissue obtained from postoperative specimens. PAGE 1433

113. **Answer: C.** Besides hoarseness and stridor, children with severe RRP may present with progressive dyspnea. PAGE 1414

114. **Answer A.** The key to this case is recognizing that the inflammatory mass is within the thyroid gland. Abscess within the thyroid gland is usually attributable to a lower branchial cleft anomaly. Superinfection causing abscess and cellulitis brings the anomaly to medical attention. Thyroid gland fracture would be more linear. PAGE 1610

115. **Answer E.** The key to this case is recognizing that the cystic mass is not isolated to the tongue base but also extends into the floor of mouth. A trans-spatial mass should suggest venolymphatic malformation. PAGES 1584–86

7

Head and Neck Surgery

1. The optimal treatment of advanced-stage nasopharyngeal (NP) carcinoma is:

   A. Surgery and postoperative radiotherapy
   B. Induction chemotherapy and radiotherapy (CRT)
   C. Concomitant CRT
   D. Adjuvant CRT
   E. Radiotherapy and brachytherapy

2. A 62-year-old man presents with a mass extending from the right true vocal cord superiorly into the ventricle and false vocal cord, which is biopsy-proven squamous cell carcinoma. The true vocal cord is fixed. There is only unilateral disease. What is the best treatment option?

   A. Chemoradiation therapy
   B. Laser resection
   C. Supraglottic laryngectomy
   D. Supracricoid laryngectomy

3. Radiographic imaging for cN0 patients results in a significant false-positive rate and the potential for some patients' necks to be overtreated. True or false?

   A. True
   B. False

4. What is *not* part of MEN IIa syndrome?

   A. Medullary thyroid carcinoma
   B. Pheochromocytoma
   C. Primary hyperparathyroidism
   D. Marfanoid habitus

5. A 48-year-old has surgery for a T2N0 squamous cancer of the lateral tongue. Pathology reveals the margins are negative. There is no perineural tumor and 5 of 24 nodes are involved with extracapsular extension. Best evidence suggests that the patient needs:

   A. No further therapy
   B. Conventional radiation
   C. Hyperfractionated radiation
   D. Chemoradiation therapy

6. Which laryngeal site is the most at risk of developing radionecrosis?

   A. Cricoid
   B. Thyroid lamina
   C. Arytenoid
   D. Epiglottis

7. The utility of sentinel node biopsy is higher in patients with tumors in:

   A. Floor of the mouth
   B. Oral tongue
   C. Lower gum
   D. Base of the tongue
   E. Larynx

8. What is the most common cause for failed tracheoesophageal (TE) voice?

   A. Microstomia
   B. Valve failure
   C. Hypopharyngeal bar
   D. Granuloma

9. Which of the following is the first priority in selecting reconstructive options for any size full-thickness lip defect?

   A. Preserve or restore the dynamic function of the lip
   B. Restore competence of the oral sphincter
   C. Optimize the cosmetic result
   D. Retain ability to use dentures
   E. Single-stage reconstruction

10. A 47-year-old presents with a firm submucosal mass adjacent to the maxillary first molar. What is the most likely diagnosis?

    A. Squamous cancer
    B. Minor salivary gland tumor
    C. Odontogenic tumor
    D. Pseudoepitheliomatous hyperplasia

11. What structures does the head and neck surgeon have to include when resecting a tumor of the posterior pharyngeal wall that can lead to significant dysphagia?

    A. Prevertebral fascia
    B. Pharyngeal constrictors
    C. Pharyngeal plexus
    D. Cricoarytenoid muscles

12. The development of a cutaneous malignancy is associated with chronic exposure to:

    A. Ammonia
    B. Arsenic
    C. Chromium
    D. Benzene

13. Successful parathyroidectomy is usually best predicted by:

    A. Localization with ultrasound
    B. Frozen section
    C. Intra operative parathyroid hormone (PTH) reduction to normal
    D. Ionized serum calcium

14. A 15-year-old boy presents with epistaxis and right orbital proptosis with diplopia. Radiographic studies, including a CT scan with and without contrast, and an MRI with contrast are consistent with an advanced juvenile nasopharyngeal angiofibroma extending intracranially on the right with inferior orbital fissure invasion and middle cranial fossa invasion. Your proposed surgical management should include:

    A. Endoscopic resection
    B. Endoscopic resection following angiographic embolization
    C. Combined endoscopic and open resection
    D. Transfacial resection following angiographic embolization with follow-up potential transcranial resection

15. Which of the following is true regarding organ preservation therapy for a T4aN1 squamous cell carcinoma of the larynx?

    A. Is associated with reduced survival due to distant metastatic disease
    B. Is more likely when cetuximab is added to radiation
    C. Is more likely to require salvage laryngectomy
    D. Is more likely using induction chemotherapy, followed by radiation

16. Which of the following salivary cancers is most associated with pain and perineural spread of tumor?

    A. Acinic cell cancer
    B. Adenoid cystic cancer
    C. High-grade mucoepidermoid cancer
    D. Squamous cell cancer

17. In a patient with elevated serum calcium, elevated parathyroid hormone, and elevated urine calcium, the most common diagnosis is:

    A. A single parathyroid adenoma
    B. Parathyroid hyperplasia
    C. Hypocalciuric hypercalcemia
    D. Secondary hyperparathyroidism

18. What is the advantage of intensity-modulated radiation therapy (IMRT) over 3D?

    A. Reduced dose to the parotid glands and other normal tissues
    B. Increased dose to the tumor
    C. Shorter treatment time
    D. All of the above

19. Which diagnostic procedure is the gold standard in the diagnosis of lymphoma in patients presenting with enlarged cervical lymph node?

    A. Excisional biopsy
    B. Fine-needle aspiration (FNA) biopsy
    C. Core needle biopsy (CNB)
    D. Contrast-enhanced CT scan

20. Which melanoma subtype demonstrates neurotropism, a low rate of lymph node metastases and is often treated with postoperative radiation therapy?

    A. Superficial spreading
    B. Nodular
    C. Lentigo maligna
    D. Desmoplastic

21. Which of the following represents indications for the use of radiation therapy in patients with tracheal malignancy?

    A. Positive surgical margins
    B. Resected tumors that are high grade
    C. Resected tumors that demonstrate perineural invasion
    D. Regional nodal metastasis
    E. All the above

22. Patients with Sjogren disease have which relative risk of developing lymphoma within the involved parotid gland compared to age-matched controls?

    A. 10 times
    B. 20 times
    C. 30 times
    D. 40 times

23. Neck dissection for a T3N0 well-differentiated left lower lip cancer patient for whom XRT is not indicated should involve:

    A. Right level I and left I–III selective neck dissection
    B. Left parotid and left I–III selective neck dissection
    C. Left modified radical (I–V) neck dissection
    D. Left I–III selective neck dissection
    E. No neck dissection as the risk of cervical metastasis is low

24. What is the most important predictor of better functional outcomes in conservation surgery for supraglottic tumors?

    A. Pulmonary function status
    B. Age
    C. Type of surgical approach
    D. Extent of resection

25. Which of the following is a major constraint to the application of transoral laser microsurgical (TLM) approach for resection of early supraglottic cancer?

    A. Advanced age
    B. Inadequate access
    C. Recurrent tumor
    D. Questionable preepiglottic space involvement

26. Indications for adjuvant chemoradiation include:

    A. Extracapsular spread
    B. Three or more lymph nodes involved by tumor
    C. Stage IV disease
    D. Perineural invasion

27. Permanent parotid salivary dysfunction can be expected after what total dose of radiation (mean dose to parotid)?

    A. 10 Gy
    B. 25 Gy
    C. 55 Gy
    D. 70 Gy

28. A chylous fistula develops following a neck dissection. Upon exploration of the neck to control it, the surgeon would anticipate the thoracic duct to be located:

    A. Anterior to the carotid and posterior to the jugular vein
    B. Anterior to the carotid and the jugular vein
    C. Posterior to the thyrocervical trunk
    D. Posterior to the carotid artery
    E. In between the subclavian artery and vein

29. Which of these statements best describes lymphoscintigraphy?

    A. Radiation treatment of the lymph node basin
    B. Use of radioactive colloid to map the lymphatic pathway
    C. A type of positron emission tomography scanning to visualize the lymph nodes
    D. Use of external beam radiation to identify sentinel lymph nodes

30. For cutaneous squamous cell carcinoma, which of the following locations is considered a high-risk feature for staging purposes?

    A. Junction of the ala and nasolabial fold
    B. Chin
    C. Ear
    D. Medial canthal area

31. What is the most reliable method to prevent pharyngeal spasm at the time of primary tracheoesophageal (TE) puncture?

    A. Single layer pharyngeal closure
    B. Botox injection
    C. Pharyngeal constrictor myotomy
    D. Pharyngeal neurectomy

32. Which of these melanoma subtypes is also referred to as melanoma in situ?

    A. Superficial spreading
    B. Nodular
    C. Lentigo maligna
    D. Desmoplastic

33. Patients who have undergone chemoradiation are more likely to:

    A. Develop wound problems after salvage surgery
    B. Develop deep vein thrombosis after salvage surgery
    C. Develop local recurrence than if treated by radiation alone
    D. Suffer free flap loss after salvage surgery
    E. Maintain their body weight during treatment

34. Which of the following statements is true?

    A. Osteogenic sarcomas, the most common arising from the jaw in the head and neck, are primarily treated with wide-field surgical excision with reconstruction followed by adjuvant radiation for improved outcomes.
    B. Chondrosarcomas, arising from cartilaginous structures, are treated with wide-field excision and postoperative radiation if vital structures are involved.
    C. Rhabomyosarcomas of the paranasal sinuses are treated with triple intrathecal chemotherapy, whole brain radiation, and spinal radiation in both the pediatric and adult populations.
    D. Fibrosarcomas, arising from fibroblasts, are treated with induction chemoradiation, followed by wide-field radiation.

35. Which of the following arteries can be a source of secondary hemorrhage or major bleeding during transoral laser resection of a supraglottic tumor?

    A. Inferior laryngeal artery
    B. Superior laryngeal artery
    C. Ascending pharyngeal artery
    D. Superior thyroid artery

36. A 40-year-old male smoker presents with hoarseness for 4 months. Office fiberoptic laryngoscopy reveals a superficial hyperkeratotic lesion on the right anterior vocal cord. Cord mobility is normal. What would be the next logical step in management?

    A. MRI
    B. Administration of antireflux agents and speech therapy
    C. Direct laryngoscopy with transoral laser microsurgery (TLM) excisional biopsy
    D. Fiberoptic laryngoscopy after 1 month

37. A 45-year-old presents with a left level II neck mass. It measures 28 mm with a cystic center and thick wall. Needle aspiration demonstrates fluid with no cells. What is the likely diagnosis?

    A. Branchial cleft cyst, previously infected
    B. Warthin tumor
    C. Lymphangioma
    D. Metastasis from the oropharynx

38. The ophthalmic artery branches off the internal carotid artery medially just after it exits the cavernous sinus and dural rings and runs in which of these directions to the optic nerve inside the optic canal?

    A. Inferolateral
    B. Supralateral
    C. Inferomedial
    D. Supralateral

39. Merkel cell carcinoma is highly specific for which of the following immunostains?

    A. S100
    B. Synaptophysin
    C. CK-20
    D. Neuron-specific enolase

40. Which of the following salivary gland tumors is associated with the highest rate of cervical metastases?

    A. Adenoid cystic cancer
    B. High-grade mucoepidermoid cancer
    C. Salivary duct cancer
    D. Squamous cell cancer

41. The most common cause of false-positive intraoperative parathyroid hormone (IOPTH) is:

    A. Double adenoma
    B. Multigland hyperplasia
    C. Poor PTH clearance
    D. Renal compromise

42. In patients undergoing chemotherapy and radiation as definitive therapy for hypopharyngeal carcinoma, how should the patient be counseled to minimize significant dysphagia?

    A. Referral to speech pathology with administration and performance of therapeutic exercises
    B. Maintaining a minimal level of PO intake to avoid long-term dysphagia
    C. Both A and B
    D. Neither A nor B

43. The following ultrasound features of a thyroid nodule are associated with high probability of malignancy *except*:

    A. Hyperechogenicity
    B. Hypoechogenicity
    C. Increased intranodular vascularity
    D. Microcalcification

44. Which statement is most accurate?

    A. Patients with orbital invasion rapidly develop ocular symptoms, such as proptosis, diplopia, decreased visual acuity, diminished motility, chemosis, lid edema, and epiphora.
    B. Bone erosion of the lamina papyracea is an absolute indication for orbital invasion.
    C. Resection of the inferior orbital wall, but not the medial wall, produces enophthalmos and hypophthalmos.
    D. To better restore the orbital anatomy and to prevent lagophthalmos, due to ectropion, the lateral canthus should be reattached 1 cm superior to the corresponding anatomical site of insertion.

45. Which of the following patients is most likely to benefit from elective neck dissection of levels I to IV?

    A. T1N0 left true vocal fold
    B. T2N0 right true vocal fold
    C. T2N0 nasopharynx
    D. T2N0 right lateral tongue

46. Which of the following treatments is the most appropriate therapy for a patient with a T2N1 human papillomavirus-positive oropharyngeal cancer?

    A. Induction chemotherapy with docetaxel, cisplatin, and 5-FU followed by radiotherapy
    B. Concurrent chemoradiation with cisplatin and cetuximab
    C. Radiation therapy only
    D. Concurrent chemoradiation with cisplatin and 5-FU

47. What is the most commonly encountered cause for squamous cancer of the tongue base?

    A. Tobacco exposure
    B. Human papillomavirus (HPV) type 16 infection
    C. Second-hand smoke
    D. Chronic alcohol use

48. After completion of chemotherapy and radiotherapy for T2N2B HPV squamous cell carcinoma of the left tonsil, what initial follow-up would you recommend?

    A. CT of neck 2 to 3 months after treatment
    B. Staging tonsillectomy 2 to 3 months after treatment
    C. Modified left neck dissection 2 to 3 months after treatment
    D. Positron emission tomography (PET)/CT 3 months after treatment

49. Which of the following is *not* an indication for radioactive iodine treatment?

    A. T1N0M0 thyroid papillary carcinoma, 30-year-old women
    B. Pulmonary metastasis from papillary thyroid carcinoma
    C. 4-cm papillary thyroid carcinoma with extrathyroidal extension
    D. 70-year-old man with 2-cm papillary thyroid carcinoma treated with total thyroidectomy

50. What is the principal difference in oncological resection technique between transoral laser resection and classic oncological surgery?

    A. Smaller enbloc tumor margins
    B. Inability to visualize the deep margins
    C. Transtumoral cut and multibloc resection
    D. Frozen section analysis of resection margins

51. According to 2009 The Bethesda System for Reporting Thyroid Cytopathology, what is the risk of malignancy of follicular lesion of undetermined significance (FLUS)?

    A. 5% to 15%
    B. <5%
    C. 20% to 30%
    D. >50%

52. Which statement best describes reconstructive and rehabilitation goals?

    A. Although functional rehabilitation is important following surgical removal of parana-sal sinus tumors, aesthetic results take precedence.
    B. It is essential to obliterate the maxillary sinus space following a total maxillectomy for optimal functional and cosmetic outcome.
    C. Often, a staged free-tissue transfer procedure to separate the intracranial cavity from the aerodigestive tract is preferred to primary closure with local flaps to allow recognition of postoperative complications in the first 24 hours after surgery.
    D. Rehabilitation after surgical resection of paranasal sinus tumors may be achieved with a dental prosthesis or reconstructive flaps, such as temporalis muscle flaps with and without the inclusion of cranial bone, pedicled or microvascular free myocutaneous flaps (e.g., pectoralis major, latissimus dorsi, trapezius), and cutaneous flaps (e.g., fore-head, scalp, deltopectoral).

53. Cervical lymph nodes involved by lymphomas have which two appearances on CT scan with contrast?

    A. Enlarged lymph nodes with homogenous appearance and poor contrast enhancement
    B. Lymph nodes less than 1 cm in diameter with poor contrast enhancement
    C. Enlarged lymph nodes with heterogeneous contrast enhancement
    D. Enlarged lymph nodes with frequent central necrosis

54. Patients who have failed primary chemoradiation of the larynx are best treated by salvage:

    A. Radiation
    B. Chemotherapy
    C. Chemoradiation
    D. Surgery
    E. Photodynamic therapy

55. Laboratory evaluation of patients with hypopharyngeal and cervical esophageal carcinoma should include:

    A. Iron levels
    B. Vitamin levels
    C. Nutrition parameters (prealbumin, transferrin)
    D. Blood counts
    E. All of the above

56. Overexpression of *BcL-2* and *BcL-X* results in which of these situations?

    A. Reduced cell apoptosis (death)
    B. Over expression of *p53*
    C. Vascular proliferation
    D. Increased cancer stem cells

57. A 3-year-old child presents with hypoglobus and a lesion on examination in the superior orbital rim. A fine-needle aspiration in clinic reveals dendritic histiocytes consistent with Langerhans cell histiocytosis. What is the next step in management?

    A. Surgery with conservative removal
    B. Surgery with radical removal
    C. Bone survey
    D. Radiation therapy

58. Treatment of a dentigerous cyst requires:

    A. Enucleation
    B. Removal of impacted tooth and enucleation
    C. Segmental mandibulectomy
    D. Postoperative radiation

59. **Which one of the following statements is correct with regard to the common type, site, and gender distribution of lip tumors?**

    A. Basal cell carcinoma typically affects the lower lip and is more common in women.

    B. Basal cell carcinoma typically affects the lower lip and is more common in men.

    C. Squamous cell carcinoma (SCCA) typically affects the upper lip and is more common in women.

    D. SCCA typically affects the lower lip and is more common in men.

    E. Pleomorphic adenoma typically affects the lower lip and is more common in men.

60. **During an anterolateral approach with orbitozygomatic osteotomy, all of the following anatomical regions should be addressed for the osteotomies, *except*:**

    A. Capsule of the temporomandibular joint

    B. Superior orbital rim

    C. Inferior orbital fissure

    D. Superior orbital fissure

    E. All of the above-mentioned areas

61. **A 45-year-old woman presents with pulsatile tinnitus and occasional instability. An audiogram demonstrates mixed hearing loss, and further radiographic investigations are consistent with a paraganglioma of the temporal bone extending into the otic capsule and replacing the jugular bulb with erosion of the jugulotympanic spine. Your surgical management recommendation should include a discussion of:**

    A. Conductive hearing loss and facial paralysis

    B. Sensorineural hearing loss (SNHL), temporary facial paralysis, possible risk for stroke

    C. Conductive hearing loss, SNHL, temporary facial paralysis, lower cranial nerve paralysis, and risk for stroke

    D. SNHL, temporary facial paralysis, lower cranial nerve paralysis including aspiration, and risk for stroke

62. **Which of the following patients presents a higher risk for malignant paraganglioma?**

    A. A 28-year-old woman recently diagnosed with bilateral carotid body tumors

    B. A 40-year-old man with an ipsilateral carotid body tumor and a contralateral vagal paraganglioma

    C. A 34-year-old woman with a pheochromocytoma and a carotid body tumor

    D. A patient with a familial history of a pheochromocytoma and a known PGL-4 mutation.

63. What is the most frequently mutated gene in head and neck cancer?

    A. *p53*
    B. *p16*
    C. *p13kca*
    D. *MET*

64. What is the most common odontogenic cyst?

    A. Radicular
    B. Dentigerous
    C. Calcifying odontogenic
    D. Glandular odontogenic

65. What is a potential contraindication for transoral resection of a T2N0 tonsil cancer?

    A. Severe trismus
    B. Human papillomavirus (HPV) positive
    C. HPV negative
    D. Age less than 40

66. A torus is considered:

    A. A developmental over growth
    B. Tumor
    C. Hamartoma
    D. Low-grade sarcoid

67. Fibrous dysplasia is commonly treated with:

    A. Observation
    B. Recontouring and esthetic surgery
    C. Wide local excision
    D. Chemotherapy

68. Which of the following is a disadvantage of elective neck dissection (END) versus elective neck irradiation (ENI)?

    A. The inability to adequately treat retropharyngeal and parapharyngeal lymph nodes
    B. Significantly poorer survival outcomes for patients undergoing END
    C. Regional recurrence is more easily detected in patients who undergo ENI
    D. ENI results in significantly less treatment and posttreatment patient morbidity

69. The highest incidence of nasopharyngeal (NP) carcinoma is among:

    A. North Africans
    B. Caucasians
    C. Southern Chinese
    D. Inuits
    E. Japanese

70. A 70-year-old man presents with a 2-week history of a rapidly enlarging otherwise asymptomatic mass on the right upper lip. Physical examination reveals a 2-cm ulcerated circumscribed lesion with elevated or rolled margins, a keratinized central region, and an indurated base. The initial biopsy report provided by the referring physician was read as "suspicious for squamous cell carcinoma." The next best step in management is:

    A. Perform a second incisional biopsy at the margin of the lesion
    B. Observation for 3 months and excisional biopsy if the lesion persists
    C. Wedge resection with 3-mm margins and primary closure
    D. Definitive radiation therapy to the primary site
    E. Refer for Mohs resection

71. What is the appropriate margin of resection for a 2.2-mm-thick melanoma of the scalp?

    A. 0.5 cm
    B. 1 cm
    C. 2 cm
    D. 4 cm

72. A 44-year-old has a pleomorphic adenoma in the tail of the right parotid gland. What is the best intervention?

    A. Radiation therapy
    B. Enucleation
    C. Partial parotidectomy
    D. Complete superficial parotidectomy

73. The most important indication for surgery in primary hyperparathyroidism is:

    A. Elevated renal calcium
    B. Age less than 50
    C. Osteopenia
    D. Relief of symptoms

74. Which of the following statements is true for osteoradionecrosis?

    A. It is a result of infection of the mandible
    B. It is best treated with hyperbaric oxygen (HBO)
    C. It occurs more commonly in the maxilla than in the mandible
    D. It requires free tissue transfer when advanced
    E. It can be treated with local therapy only

75. Which of these is the most common presenting symptom(s) for tracheal squamous cell carcinoma (SCCA)?

    A. Neck mass
    B. Fever
    C. Dyspnea
    D. Dysphagia
    E. Cough with hemoptysis

76. Which of the following statements best describes the disadvantage of elective neck irradiation (ENI) versus elective neck dissection (END)?

    A. Significantly poorer survival outcomes for patients undergoing ENI
    B. Significantly poorer functional outcomes for patients undergoing radiation to the primary site and ENI than those undergoing surgical treatment
    C. Prognostic information from histopathology is not known
    D. ENI is not able to treat all of the levels of the neck that can be addressed with END

77. What is the most common complication of tracheoesophageal (TE) voice restoration?

    A. TE puncture granulation
    B. Sternoclavicular arthritis
    C. Necrosis of posterior wall of trachea
    D. Failure to learn TE speech

78. Eight hours after an uneventful lateral orbitotomy for biopsy of an orbital tumor, your patient notes progressive unrelenting pain and chemosis. What must be considered as a cause for this pain?

    A. Retrobulbar hematoma
    B. Intraoperative traction on the inferior orbital nerve
    C. Transection of the superior orbital nerve
    D. Infection at the site of miniplate repair

79. **Which statement best describes sinonasal melanomas?**

    A. Postoperative radiation therapy may be beneficial for sinonasal mucosal melanoma, although its impact on survival and local control has not been addressed in scientific trials.
    B. Due to the obstructive nature of the tumor, sinonasal mucosal melanoma is often found early and completely excised.
    C. The most common cause of failure of mucosal melanoma in the nasal cavity and paranasal sinuses is distant metastasis.
    D. Early vascular and lymphatic invasion is infrequently encountered with mucosal melanomas of the nasal cavity and paranasal sinuses.

80. **A 70-year-old man presents with a Mohs resection of a lesion of the vertex of the scalp that has produced a 4-cm defect. The pathologic diagnosis is angiosarcoma, and the pathologic margins are questionable. On examination, there are vascular lesions beyond the resection margin stopping at 2 cm distal to the margin. Your surgical management of this should be:**

    A. No additional treatment, and patient should be treated with adjuvant chemotherapy and radiation
    B. Additional resection to 1 cm beyond the current margin
    C. Additional resection to 2 cm beyond the current margin with frozen section control
    D. Additional resection to at least 4 cm beyond the margin regardless of frozen section control

81. **The most commonly used particle for radiation therapy is:**

    A. Photon
    B. Proton
    C. Electron
    D. Neutron

82. **Which is the most common type of basal cell carcinoma (BCC)?**

    A. Nodular
    B. Morpheaform
    C. Pigmented
    D. Sclerosing

83. The optimal treatment for a small recurrent nasopharyngeal (NP) carcinoma in the nasopharynx after radiotherapy is:

    A. Second course of radiation
    B. Chemotherapy and radiation
    C. Radical surgical resection
    D. Targeted therapy
    E. Local excision and postoperative radiotherapy

84. In the course of a neck dissection, profuse venous bleeding occurs in the area below the posterior belly of the digastrics and anterior to the jugular vein. As multiple clamps are applied to control the bleeding, which of the following nerves is at highest risk of injury?

    A. The spinal accessory
    B. The glossopharyngeal
    C. The hypoglossal
    D. The vagus
    E. The superior laryngeal nerve

85. A 48-year-old patient presents with a 1.5-cm biopsy-proven, poorly differentiated squamous cell carcinoma of the left ear. Which of the following is the most appropriate stage of the primary tumor (T)?

    A. T1
    B. T2
    C. T3
    D. T4

86. Reirradiation as a single treatment modality is a well-defined treatment for recurrent:

    A. Larynx cancer
    B. Tongue base cancer
    C. Nasopharyngeal cancer
    D. Skull base cancer
    E. Skin cancer

87. The most common acute toxicity observed after oral radiation therapy are:

    A. Mucositis, osteonecrosis, and xerostomia
    B. Mucositis, carotid endarteritis, and xerostomia
    C. Mucositis, dysphagia, and xerostomia
    D. Mucositis, fibrosis, and xerostomia

88. Which artery is at greatest risk of injury during endoscopic endonasal anterior cranial base resection?

    A. Frontopolar artery
    B. Frontoorbital artery
    C. Anterior cerebral artery
    D. Anterior communicating artery
    E. Anterior ethmoidal artery

89. What is characteristic of paratracheal and paraesophageal lymphatic metastases from a hypopharyngeal carcinoma?

    A. Lateral pyriform sinus involvement
    B. Retropharyngeal involvement
    C. Vocal cord paralysis
    D. Postcricoid tumor involvement

90. Which is the most common site involved by lymphoma within Waldeyer ring?

    A. Tonsils
    B. Base of tongue
    C. Nasopharynx
    D. Oral tongue

91. How many base pairs are in the human diploid genome?

    A. 6,000,000
    B. 60,000,000
    C. 600,000,000
    D. 6,000,000,000

92. Laryngeal preservation in a patient with a T3N2C hypopharyngeal cancer is most likely to be successful with which of these chemotherapy treatments?

    A. Concurrent chemoradiation with cisplatin and 5-FU
    B. Concurrent chemoradiation with cisplatin and cetuximab
    C. Induction chemotherapy using cisplatin and 5-FU followed by radiotherapy
    D. Induction chemotherapy with docetaxel, cisplatin, and 5-FU followed by radiotherapy

93. What is the 5-year overall survival of laryngeal cancer?

    A. 48%
    B. 63%
    C. 75%
    D. 92%

94. A patient with a T3N0 squamous cell carcinoma of the lateral floor of the mouth is to undergo surgical treatment. Which of the following is an appropriate neck dissection in this case?

    A. Selective neck dissection of levels I and II (suprahyoid dissection)
    B. Selective neck dissection of levels I, II, and III (supraomohyoid dissection)
    C. Selective neck dissection of levels II, III, and IV (lateral dissection)
    D. Modified radical neck dissection preserving the jugular vein and the spinal accessory nerve
    E. Modified radical preserving the spinal accessory nerve

95. Which of the following statements is correct with regard to chemotherapy?

    A. The addition of chemotherapy to radiation improves survival of patients with stage IIa nasopharyngeal cancer.
    B. Combination chemotherapy significantly improves the survival of patients with recurrent disease over single agent chemotherapy alone.
    C. Induction chemotherapy followed by radiation therapy is the standard of care for unresectable disease.
    D. Current standards of care are based on phase III data.

96. Free tissue transfer after ablation for recurrent oropharyngeal cancer will result in:

    A. An improvement of preoperative functional status
    B. A lower recurrence rate than if a pedicled flap was used
    C. Lower hospital costs
    D. Decreased metastatic disease
    E. A lower requirement for further surgery

97. A 65-year-old man being treated for T3N2c squamous cell carcinoma of the larynx with adjuvant chemoradiation has significant pain during the fifth week of radiation, requiring hospitalization for fluids and pain control. What should be done with the patient's treatment during the hospitalization?

    A. Discontinue radiation and do not resume
    B. Defer radiation until patient is discharged
    C. Continue radiation while patient admitted
    D. Stop chemotherapy

98. What is the main advantage of the gastric transposition flap over jejunal flap in reconstruction of the esophagus?

    A. Improved voice outcomes
    B. Less morbidity
    C. Single anastomosis
    D. Larger vessels for microvascular anastomosis

99. After an endoscopic endonasal resection of a craniopharyngioma, the patient presented with serum sodium of 155 mEq/L, high urine output, and a urine-specific gravity of 1.001. What is the diagnosis and the best treatment option?

    A. Inappropriate secretion of antidiuretic hormone/1-deamino-8-d-arginine vasopressin (DDAVP)
    B. Inappropriate secretion of antidiuretic hormone/fluid restriction
    C. Diabetes insipidus/DDAVP
    D. Diabetes insipidus/fluid restriction

100. The goal of surgery in secondary hyperparathyroidism is:

    A. Normal serum calcium
    B. Improve renal function
    C. Control of parathyroid hormone (PTH)
    D. Reduction of cardiovascular events

101. The optimal treatment of recurrent cervical lymph node metastasis in nasopharyngeal carcinoma is:

    A. Second course of radiotherapy
    B. Modified neck dissection
    C. Radical neck dissection
    D. Radical neck dissection followed by radiotherapy
    E. Chemotherapy and radiotherapy

102. **Which of these orbital bones contributes to the orbital rims?**

    A. Sphenoid
    B. Zygomatic
    C. Palatine
    D. Lacrimal

103. **Which of these is the most accurate predictor of disease-related survival for patients with head and neck squamous cell carcinoma?**

    A. T stage
    B. Current use of alcohol and/or tobacco
    C. Presence of cervical lymph node metastasis
    D. Presence of significant comorbid cardiopulmonary disease

104. **Sentinel lymph node biopsy should be offered when a patient has:**

    A. A 0.75-mm-thick melanoma of the scalp without ulceration and no clinical evidence of lymph node metastases
    B. A 3.5-mm-thick melanoma of the scalp without ulceration and no clinical evidence of lymph node metastases
    C. A 3.5-mm-thick melanoma of the scalp without ulceration and with lymph node metastases in two cervical lymph nodes
    D. A 3.5-mm-thick melanoma of the scalp without ulceration, with no clinical evidence of lymph node metastases, and with distant metastases in the spine

105. **The most accurate radiologic method to stage the N0 neck in oral cancer is with:**

    A. CT
    B. MRI
    C. Positron emission tomography (PET)/CT
    D. Palpation

106. **Rituximab is which kind of drug used in the treatment of certain lymphomas?**

    A. Small-molecule tyrosine kinase inhibitor
    B. Monoclonal antibody against CD20
    C. Protease inhibitor
    D. Proteosome inhibitor

107. A 72-year-old man presents with a 25-mm mass in the tail of the parotid on the left. CT show a second 20-mm mass on the right. What is the most likely diagnosis?

    A. Bilateral Warthin tumor
    B. Multifocal pleomorphic adenoma
    C. Adenopathy
    D. Metastases for an unknown primary

108. A 28-year-old undergoes partial parotidectomy with facial nerve dissection for a 22-mm tumor. Pathology shows a low-grade mucoepidermoid carcinoma. Margins are negative. The neck is radiologically negative. What therapy do you recommend?

    A. No further therapy, observation
    B. Completion of total parotidectomy
    C. Total parotidectomy, adjuvant radiation
    D. Total parotidectomy, neck dissection

109. The primary treatment for intrabony ameloblastoma requires:

    A. Dental extraction
    B. Enucleation
    C. Enucleation and curettage
    D. Resection with 1.0 to 1.5 cm bony margin

110. The commonest presenting symptom of nasopharyngeal (NP) carcinoma is

    A. Epistaxis
    B. Hearing loss due to serous otitis media
    C. Enlarged cervical lymph node
    D. Nasal obstruction
    E. Abducent nerve palsy

111. A 35-year-old woman presents with a 3-month history of progressing double vision. On examination you note normal acuity, but there is a left cranial nerve 6 palsy. What is the next step?

    A. Obtain an MRI and CT
    B. Electromyography of lateral rectus
    C. Serial clinical examination in 2 weeks
    D. Begin high-dose steroids

112. A 55-year-old man presents with a 3-cm right-sided neck mass. Flexible laryngoscopy shows a mass originating on the right aryepiglottic fold extending superiorly onto the epiglottis. Both true vocal cords are mobile. CT scan shows paraglottic space invasion and multiple right-sided lymph nodes none larger than 3 cm. What is the TNM stage?

    A. T2N2aM0
    B. T2N2bM0
    C. T3N2aM0
    D. T3N2bM0

113. What is the gold standard/preferred method for alaryngeal speech?

    A. Electrolarynx use
    B. Esophageal speech
    C. Tracheoesophageal (TE) speech
    D. Soft tissue shunting

114. Indications for elective treatment of the neck include all of the following *except*:

    A. T3-T4 primary lip SSCa
    B. Recurrent lip SSCa
    C. Locally advanced basal cell carcinoma (BCC)
    D. If free flap reconstruction is necessary
    E. Histology showing poorly differentiated SSCa

115. During a lateral infratemporal approach to the cranial base, exposure of the petrous carotid artery segment requires:

    A. Lateralization of the mandibular nerve and the middle meningeal artery
    B. Sacrifice of the mandibular nerve and the middle meningeal artery
    C. Sacrifice of the maxillary nerve and the middle meningeal artery
    D. Lateralization of the ophthalmic nerve and sacrifice of the middle meningeal artery
    E. Sacrifice of the vidian nerve and sphenopalatine artery

116. Which of the following statements regarding tracheal cancers is true?

    A. The duration of symptoms prior to presentation is longer for squamous cell carcinoma (SCCA) than for adenoid cystic carcinoma.
    B. The duration of symptoms prior to presentation is longer for adenoid cystic carcinoma than for SCCA.
    C. SCCA is more likely than adenoid cystic carcinoma to present with wheezing.
    D. Adenoid cystic carcinoma is more likely than SCCA to present with hemoptysis.
    E. Prolonged use of corticosteroids is uncommon in tracheal cancers prior to diagnosis.

117. **Which of the following statements about nerve sheath tumors is not accurate?**

    A. The majority of peripheral nerve sheath tumors arise in the nasal cavity and paranasal sinuses.
    B. Peripheral nerve sheath tumors arising in the paranasal sinuses, compared to the neck or internal auditory canal, are fast growing, and symptomatic at an early stage.
    C. Peripheral nerve sheath tumors in the nasal cavity and paranasal sinuses lack encapsulation with neoplastic cells undermining adjacent respiratory mucosa.
    D. Treatment of nerve sheath tumors in the nasal cavity and paranasal sinuses is radiation followed by surgical excision.

118. **What is the main lower eyelid retractor?**

    A. Whitnall ligament
    B. Capsulopalpebral fascia
    C. Inferior oblique muscle
    D. Orbicularis oculi

119. **The preferred management of adenoid cystic carcinoma limited to the trachea, with no evidence of distant metastatic disease, and involving 3 cm of trachea is:**

    A. Bronchoscopy with neodymium YAG laser resection
    B. Tracheal resection with free tissue transfer reconstruction
    C. Bronchoscopy with cryoablation
    D. Tracheal resection with primary repair

120. **Which oral site is most commonly afflicted by cancer?**

    A. Tongue
    B. Floor of mouth
    C. Alveolus
    D. Tongue base

121. **Which of these is the most common presenting symptom(s) for tracheal adenoid cystic carcinoma?**

    A. Hemoptysis
    B. Dyspnea
    C. Fever
    D. Dysphagia
    E. Neck mass

122. **Which of the following is an indication for concomitant chemoradiation after a neck dissection?**

    A. Multiple histologically positive nodes
    B. Positive nodes at multiple levels
    C. One positive node beyond the first echelon of drainage
    D. Extracapsular spread of tumor
    E. Close margins of resection

123. **A patient has a T2 N2A human papillomavirus-positive squamous cancer of the left tonsil. What treatment would you recommend?**

    A. Radical tonsillectomy with left neck dissection (ND)
    B. Transoral tonsillectomy with left ND
    C. Chemoradiation therapy (CRT)
    D. Transoral tonsillectomy with left ND and CRT

124. **A 52-year-old has resection of a buccal cancer with ipsilateral neck dissection. Final pathology reports a 19-mm primary with perineural tumor and 2 of 21 nodes involved with microscopic deposits of tumor, and no extracapsular spread. What is the pathologic stage?**

    A. T1No
    B. T2N1
    C. T1N2a
    D. T1N2b

125. **What is the most frequent genetic alteration found in differentiated thyroid cancer?**

    A. BRAF
    B. FLUS
    C. Thyroglobulin
    D. CEA

126. **What is the only absolute contraindication to primary tracheoesophageal puncture?**

    A. Obesity
    B. Prior radiation
    C. Partial pharyngectomy
    D. Separation of trachea and esophageal party wall

127. A 53-year-old woman with hyperparathyroidism. Where is the adenoma?

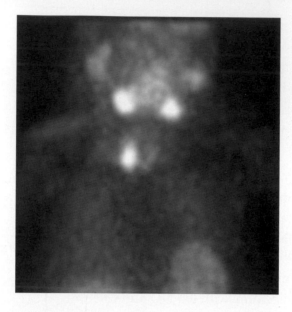

A. Right neck near thyroid gland
B. Left neck near thyroid gland
C. Right side of superior mediastinum
D. Left side of superior mediastinum
E. No adenoma is demonstrated

128. A 23-year-old man with neck mass. What kind of paraganglioma is this?

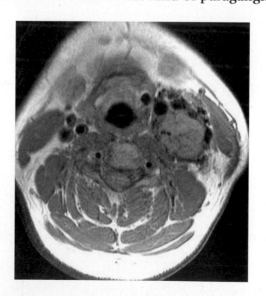

A. Carotid body tumor
B. Glomus tympanicum
C. Glomus jugulare
D. Glomus vagale
E. Laryngeal paraganglioma

129. A 43-year-old man with familial paragangliomas. What is the Shamblin classification of these tumors?

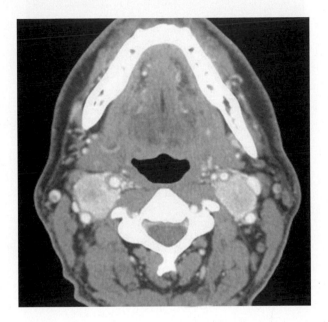

A. Bilateral Shamblin 1
B. Bilateral Shamblin 2
C. Bilateral Shamblin 3
D. Left 1; right 2
E. Left 2; right 3

130. A 28-year-old woman with thyroid enlargement. Based on this transverse ultrasound image, what is the most likely diagnosis?

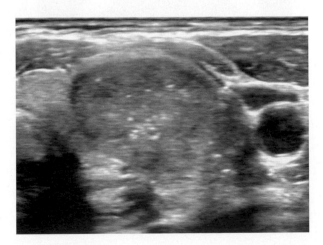

A. Papillary thyroid carcinoma
B. Follicular thyroid carcinoma
C. Medullary thyroid carcinoma
D. Anaplastic thyroid carcinoma
E. Multinodular goiter

131. A 40-year-old man with jaw swelling. What is the most likely diagnosis?

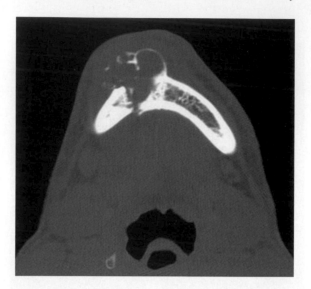

    A. Dentigerous cyst

    B. Apical abscess

    C. Keratocystic odontogenic tumor

    D. Squamous cell carcinoma (SCC)

    E. Ameloblastoma

132. A 48-year-old man with a nasal mass. What is the most likely diagnosis?

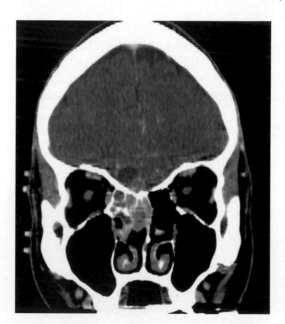

    A. Intranasal melanoma

    B. Squamous cell carcinoma

    C. Minor salivary tumor

    D. Esthesioneuroblastoma

    E. Sinonasal undifferentiated carcinoma

133. A 39-year-old man with neck mass. Fine-needle aspiration reveals squamous cell carcinoma, but endoscopy is negative and no primary lesion is evident clinically. What is the most likely site of primary?

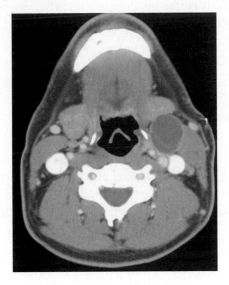

   A. Oral tongue
   B. Nasopharynx
   C. Oropharynx
   D. Hypopharynx
   E. Larynx

134. A 39-year-old man with neck mass. Fine-needle aspiration reveals squamous cell carcinoma (SCC), but endoscopy is negative and no primary lesion is evident clinically. What is the most likely site of primary?

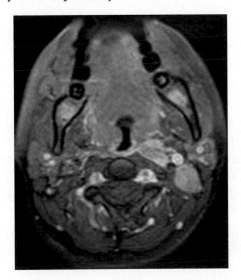

   A. Oral tongue
   B. Nasopharynx
   C. Oropharynx
   D. Hypopharynx
   E. Larynx

Chapter 7 Answers

1. **Answer: C.** Advanced NP carcinoma is technically inoperable. Multiple studies have shown concomitant CRT has the best outcomes when compared to neoadjuvant CRT or surgery followed by adjuvant CRT. PAGES 1887–1888

2. **Answer: A.** Retrospective studies have suggested that voice conserving surgeries can equal or exceed Chemoradiation (CRT) in the setting of stage III laryngeal cancer. At this time, however, the best evidence (level I) is for CRT in terms of disease control. Comparison studies of functional outcomes are pending. PAGE 1695

3. **Answer: A.** Radiologic criteria for suspicious nodes are based on size, shape, and fluorodeoxyglucose (FDG)-uptake criteria and do not distinguish between benign reactive lymph nodes and metastatic nodes, and are associated with a significant false-positive rate. Imaging is not as accurate as elective neck dissection in staging the cN0 neck. PAGES 1840–1841

4. **Answer: D.** The most common type of MENII is MEN IIA, which is characterized by the triad of MTC, pheochromocytoma, and primary hyperparathyroidism. PAGE 2127

5. **Answer: D.** Clinical trial data have shown that patients with the high-risk features of microscopically involved margins or extracapsular spread in lymph nodes in surgical specimens benefited from the addition of platinum-based chemotherapy to postoperative radiation. PAGES 1864, 1701

6. **Answer: C.** Chondroradionecrosis occurs in approximately 5% of patients with laryngeal cancer, and the most common cartilage affected is the arytenoid cartilage. PAGE 1968

7. **Answer: B.** Sentinel node biopsy has been shown to be useful in oral tongue cancer. It is not as useful for floor of mouth or gum tumors because of the proximity of the primary site to the neck which can obscure identification of nodes in level I because of residual radioactivity at the primary site, and is less useful for oropharyngeal and laryngeal cancers because of greater difficulty accessing the primary site for injection and a higher incidence of bilateral nodal drainage. PAGES 1814

8. **Answer: C.** In order for fluent TE speech to occur, there must be sufficient relaxation of the pharynx. Failure to maintain fluent speech is typically due to spasm of the cricopharyngeus and inferior and middle constrictor muscles when speech was attempted. A hypopharyngeal bar corresponding to these muscles can be seen using barium swallow. A column of air distends the esophagus proximal to the bar when phonation is attempted. PAGE 1980

9. **Answer: B.** The oral sphincter is crucial for maintaining oral competence, which is important for eating, speech, and aesthetics. Reconstructive options should attempt to maintain or reconstruct a competent sphincter, without sacrificing tumor extirpation. PAGE 1794

10. **Answer: B.** Minor salivary gland tumors can occur anywhere in the oral cavity, but most commonly arise from the hard palate. These typically present as submucosal masses and may account for 50% of hard palate tumors. PAGE 1868

11. **Answer: C.** Resection of the tumor should include prevertebral musculature if the prevertebral fascia is involved, and a retropharyngeal nodal dissection should be performed with tumors involving the posterior pharyngeal wall. Surgical dissection in this area leads to denervation of the pharyngeal plexus, which can result in significant dysphagia and aspiration. PAGE 1927

12. **Answer: B.** Chronic exposure to arsenic (as seen in Fowlers solution) has been associated with the development of multiple squamous and basal cell carcinomas. PAGE 1723

13. **Answer: C.** A drop in intraoperative PTH levels to normal levels is predictive of surgical success. There is a high false-positive rate when a reduction of intraoperative PTH to 50% of preoperative levels rather than the normal level is used, which can be associated with double adenomas or parathyroid hyperplasia. Ionized calcium levels, intraoperative ultrasound, and frozen sections do not predict biochemical success of surgery. PAGES 2138–2139

14. **Answer: D.** The lateral preauricular approaches are largely reserved for intracranial extension and can be combined with an anterior approach in the same setting or as a separate procedure. The lateral preauricular infratemporal approach provides contiguous access along the middle cranial fossa up to the cavernous sinus. PAGE 2027, TABLE 127.8

15. **Answer: C.** Both the Veterans Affairs Laryngeal Cancer Study and Radiation Therapy Oncology Group 91-11 demonstrated that patients with T4 disease have a higher salvage laryngectomy rate and poorer survival when organ preservation is employed. PAGES 1695–1696

16. **Answer: B.** Adenoid cystic cancer has a proclivity for perineural invasion, which is a hallmark of this disease and traditionally causes pain. PAGE 1765

17. **Answer: A.** A solitary parathyroid adenoma is the most common cause of primary hyperparathyroidism and more common than hyperplasia or double adenomas. Hypercalcemia is not associated with secondary hyperparathyroidism, and the presence of an elevated urine calcium rules out familial hypocalciuric hypercalcemia. PAGE 2132

18. **Answer: A.** The use of IMRT employs multiple beams to allow effective tumor dose while reducing dose to uninvolved tissues. PAGE 1687

19. **Answer: A.** The gold standard for diagnosis of lymphoma in the head and neck is open excisional biopsy because it provides adequate tissue for both diagnosis and definitive subclassification. Due to the new classification schemes (Revised European-American Lymphoma and WHO classifications) which put emphasis on immunophenotypic and cytogenetic characteristics rather than on architectural features in the categorization of these tumors, both FNA and CNB have been investigated as diagnostic tools. FNA is not useful in subclassification of disease or in treatment planning due to insufficient tissue; however, CNB has shown promising results and is accepted as the initial procedure in patients with deep-seated lymph nodes, particularly in the mediastinum or abdomen. PAGES 2034–2035

20. **Answer: D.** Desmoplastic melanoma accounts for less than 1% of melanoma cases, but as many as 75% of these tumors occur in the head and neck region. The predisposition for perineural invasion accounts for the high local recurrence rate despite negative margins. Wider resection margins and adjuvant radiation therapy are recommended. The National Comprehensive Cancer Network guidelines also recommend adjuvant radiation for patients with recurrent disease, extensive neurotropism, gross nodal extracapsular extension, ≥2 lymph nodes, ≥2 cm of tumor in a lymph node, or unresectable nodal, satellite, or in-transit disease. Additionally, radiotherapy should be considered after excision of mucosal melanomas. PAGES 1741–1742, 1751

21. **Answer: E.** Indications for radiation therapy in patients with tracheal malignancies include those who are not considered to be good surgical candidates (primary radiation) and in those requiring adjuvant radiation therapy for positive surgical margins, high-grade histopathology, lymphatic involvement, perineural invasion, and invasion that extends outside of the airway. Hypofractionated tomotherapy allows for three-dimensional coverage of at-risk areas following surgical resection and may limit dose to the esophagus and surrounding trachea, lung, and mediastinum, and therefore, lessen the side effects of radiation. PAGE 1995

22. **Answer: D.** Patients with Sjogren disease have more than 40 times greater relative risk of developing non-Hodgkin lymphoma (NHL) within the affected parotid glands compared to normal age-matched cohorts. These patients also have an overall 4% prevalence of NHL. PAGE 2038

23. **Answer: A.** In patients without clinical evidence of nodal disease, elective neck dissection is indicated for advanced-stage lesions. Because the lower lip lymphatics drain to both ipsilateral and contralateral submental and submandibular lymph nodes, these nodes must be addressed at surgery and comprehensive selective neck dissection of ipsilateral levels I–III is indicated. PAGES 1793–1794

24. **Answer: A.** It is clear that the extent of surgery will impact functional recovery after larynx sparing surgical procedures. At the heart of it all is the fact that all horizontal partial laryngectomy procedures, including endoscopic resections, cause aspiration and patients without the functional reserve to survive will suffer the consequences. PAGE 1949

25. **Answer: B.** The major contraindication to TLM for early supraglottic cancers is inadequate transoral access to the entire tumor. Adequate laryngeal exposure is the basic technical requirement for TLM. Age, recurrent tumor, and preepiglottic space involvement are not contraindications to TLM. PAGES 1943, 1951

26. **Answer: A.** Clinical trial data have shown that only patients with high-risk features of microscopically involved margins or extracapsular spread in lymph nodes in pathologic specimens from surgery benefited from the addition of platinum-based chemotherapy to postoperative radiation. PAGE 1701

27. **Answer: B.** Different tissues have different radiation toxicity levels. The lens of the eye is affected by 10 Gy and the optic chiasm at 55 Gy. PAGE 1685

28. **Answer: D.** The thoracic duct is located at the base of the neck, medial and deep to the carotid artery and vagus nerve. It may have multiple branching tributaries. PAGE 1810

29. **Answer: B.** Localization and mapping of sentinel lymph nodes typically involves preoperative and intraoperative use of technetium-99m-labeled sulfur colloid, which is injected intradermally into the lesion. Single photon emission computed tomography (SPECT) obtained preoperatively can help to identify the nodal basins at risk and, perhaps, the number and location of the sentinel nodes. Intraoperatively, a handheld gamma probe is used to locate sentinel lymph nodes. PAGE 1746

30. **Answer: C.** Primary tumor sites of the ear and non–hair-bearing lip are high-risk features for staging purposes. PAGE 1728, TABLE 113.2

31. **Answer: C.** Management of the pharyngeal constrictor muscles to prevent pharyngeal spasm is key to successful TE speech. The most reliable method for preventing spasm is a pharyngeal constrictor myotomy. PAGE 1983

32. **Answer: C.** Lentigo maligna, also known as melanoma in situ, is a premalignant lesion that frequently develops in the head and neck regions of elderly patients. PAGE 1740

33. **Answer: A.** The history of prior chemoradiation is often associated with worse performance, and poor nutritional status, fibrosis, and small vessel thrombosis result in poor wound healing. PAGES 1708–1709

34. **Answer: B.** The primary therapy of chondrosarcoma is wide local excision. Osteogenic sarcoma may respond best to chemoradiation. Adult rhabomyosarcoma is treated with wide excision when possible. PAGES 2047–2048

35. **Answer: B.** The blood supply to the supraglottic larynx is derived from the superior laryngeal artery, a branch of the superior thyroid artery. The superior laryngeal artery may be encountered while making tumor cuts in the area of the lateral pharyngoepiglottic fold. Transecting this artery without prior ligation can lead to retraction of the cut edge into the lateral soft tissues, causing bleeding. PAGES 1941, 1948

36. **Answer: C.** Direct laryngoscopy with TLM excision of the lesion gives a better estimation of the depth of the lesion, improving diagnostic yield, and has the option of removing the entire gross lesion in the same setting. Watchful waiting and/or conservative treatment often leads to progression of disease. MRI is not indicated in evaluation of a superficial supraglottic lesion. PAGE 1950

37. **Answer: D.** The surgeon must be alert to those asymptomatic patients presenting with a cystic mass in the neck because it may be a cystic metastasis. Positron emission tomography–CT may be helpful in detecting the occult primary in the oropharynx. A branchial cleft cyst is less likely in this age group. Also, the prevalence of human papillomavirus-related cancers has changed the risk profile. PAGE 1902

38. **Answer: A.** The ophthalmic artery is inferolateral to the optic nerve. PAGE 2085

39. **Answer: C.** Merkel cells are of neural crest origin and are highly specific for cytokeratins to include CK-20. PAGE 1736

40. **Answer: C.** Salivary duct cancer is a highly aggressive malignancy with a high rate of nodal metastases, present in more than 50% of patients at diagnosis. This tumor has a poor prognosis due to a high rate of distant metastatic disease. PAGE 1767

41. **Answer: A.** Double adenomas are the most common cause of false-positive intraoperative PTH levels. The second adenoma may not be biologically hypersecretory, and thus, excision of one adenoma may result in a drop in IOPTH to 50% or less, but PTH levels will elevate postoperatively. PAGES 2138–2139

42. **Answer: C.** A study of patients at MD Anderson Cancer Center (2012) revealed a 7% gastrostomy-tube rate 2 years after organ preservation treatment for hypopharyngeal primaries. It was found that those patients who were evaluated and treated by a team of speech pathologists, performed therapeutic exercises, and maintained some oral intake through chemoradiation were less likely to be PEG (percutaneous endoscopic gastrostomy) tube-dependent. PAGE 1936

43. **Answer: A.** Features of benign nodules include coarse calcification, regular margins, and pure cysts (hyperechogenicity). PAGE 2118

44. **Answer: A.** Both CT and MRI may be required to quantify the extent of orbital invasion, but bone erosion does not constitute an absolute indication for exenteration. PAGE 2057

45. **Answer: D.** More than 20% of early stage oral tongue cancers harbor occult nodal metastasis. The likelihood of occult nodal metastases is higher for a T2 oral tongue cancer than for early stage glottic cancer, and nasopharyngeal cancer is rarely treated surgically. PAGES 1840–1842

46. **Answer: C.** The subset of patients with T1 or T2 oropharyngeal cancer and N1 disease, while considered stage III disease, do not appear to benefit from the addition of chemotherapy to radiation therapy. These patients may be treated with radiation alone. PAGE 1698

47. **Answer: B.** Studies have found that oral HPV infection is strongly associated with squamous cell carcinoma (SCCA) of the oropharynx in those patients with and without risk factors of alcohol and tobacco use. In addition, it was found that there is a 14-fold increase in risk of developing SCCA of the oropharynx in those patients who are seropositive for HPV 16. The incidence of tobacco-related tongue base cancer has decreased, while the incidence of HPV-associated tongue base cancer is rising. PAGE 1900

48. **Answer: D.** PET-CT is recommended at 12 weeks posttreatment to evaluate for residual disease. The primary tumor and/or neck are treated accordingly. Staging tonsillectomy and/or neck dissection 2 to 3 months posttreatment are not indicated unless there is clinical (physical examination, PET-CT) evidence of disease. PAGE 1904

49. **Answer: A.** Low risk is characterized by age less than 45, absence of cervical metastasis, absence of local invasion, and low-grade histology. PAGE 2125

50. **Answer: C.** Transoral laser microsurgery (TLM) utilizes *transtumoral* cuts to assess the depth of the tumor and *multibloc* resection as opposed to an *enbloc* tumor resection which

is utilized in open techniques where there is wide exposure of the tumor. The transoral approach allows histologic clearing of tumor margins while the anatomy and functional integrity of the noninvolved tissue is spared. PAGE 1943

51. **Answer: A.** The Bethesda System has three intermediate categories. FLUS has 5% to 15% risk. Follicular neoplasm has 15% to 30% risk, while suspicious category has 60% to 75% risk of malignancy. Individual pathologists should study and report their own accuracy. PAGE 2118

52. **Answer: D.** Sinonasal reconstruction and rehabilitation after surgery often requires a team approach employing both complex flaps and prosthetic devices. PAGE 2050

53. **Answer: A.** Contrast-enhanced CT scans of the head, neck, chest, abdomen, and pelvis are routinely performed for evaluation of both nodal and nonnodal lymphoma involvement. Findings suggestive of lymphoma include large, nonenhancing, homogeneous lymph nodes, particularly in unusual nodal chains such as the retropharyngeal, occipital, and parotid nodes. Because central necrosis is typically seen in large nodes (>3 cm) involved with squamous cell carcinoma, the absence of necrosis in large nodes is suggestive of lymphoma. Pretreatment nodal necrosis, when present, usually implies a high-grade lymphoma. PAGE 2033

54. **Answer: D.** In the setting of salvage after failed initial chemotherapy and radiotherapy, patients with early laryngeal cancer fare better after laryngectomy. PAGE 1710

55. **Answer: E.** Standard laboratory test should be performed on all patients presenting with hypopharyngeal tumors, including complete blood count, electrolytes, thyroid stimulating hormone, iron, prealbumin, albumin, and transferrin levels. PAGE 1921

56. **Answer: A.** Resistance to apoptosin in head and neck squamous cell carcinoma is conferred in part by *BcL-2* overexpression. Disequilibrium between cell proliferation and cell death is characteristic of cancer. These proteins are currently being studied as targets for cancer therapy. PAGE 1661

57. **Answer: C.** Langerhans cell histiocytosis is a disease of mononuclear phagocyte dysregulation and may involve any bone of the body. Prognosis is related to the extent of disease, and a bone survey to rule out disseminated disease is the next step in workup of this disease. PAGE 2068

58. **Answer: B.** These relatively common benign cysts are usually associated with an impacted mandibular third molar. The cyst is unilocular, and well-circumscribed enucleation after tooth removal is usually curative. PAGE 2098

59. **Answer: D.** SCCA is the most common cancer of the lower lip, accounting for 90% of lower lip malignancies. It is seen more commonly in men, in contrast to cancers of the upper lip, which most commonly are basal cell cancers and more common in this location in women. PAGE 1790

60. **Answer: D.** The anterolateral approach does not require osteotomy of the superior orbital fissure. PAGE 2090

61. **Answer: C.** The jugulotympanic paraganglia are distributed within the temporal bone in close association with the tympanic branch of the glossopharyngeal nerve (Jacobson nerve) and the auricular branch of the vagus nerve (Arnold nerve). (PAGES 1999, 2002, SEE FIG 127.3) In the early stages, the jugular paragangliomas and tympanic paragangliomas present differently, but in their later stages, both types produce similar symptoms including cranial nerve deficits. When the jugular bulb is involved, a combined temporal/cervical approach is required. Following an extended mastoidectomy and facial recess approach, the sigmoid sinus is skeletonized and the jugular bulb is exposed. The internal carotid artery is dissected as are the lower cranial nerves 9, 10, and 11, putting all these structures at risk of injury. (PAGE 2013) The stroke rate for paraganglioma is 0% to 2%. (PAGE 2014) In jugulotympanic paragangliomas, the most common nerve deficit is vagal (27%), followed by the glossopharyngeal (18%) and the accessory and hypoglossal (8%). PAGE 2016

62. **Answer: D.** The PGL-4 mutation is associated with 54% malignancy rate. The rate of malignancy is site-specific and is listed in decreasing order: orbital and laryngeal paragangliomas (25%), vagal paragangliomas (10%), jugulotympanic paragangliomas (5%), and carotid body tumors (3% to 6%). Malignancy is confirmed by tumor present in lymph nodes or distant sites, not histologic criteria. Sporadic paragangliomas have a higher rate of malignancy than familial-type paragangliomas. PAGE 2001

63. **Answer: A.** Tobacco smoke preferentially mutates *p53*. High tobacco consumption increases cancer risk 5.8 times. Concurrent alcohol use synergizes to increase risk. PAGE 1646

64. **Answer: A.** The radicular cyst develops at the apex of an erupted tooth in response to pulpal necroses. PAGE 2097

65. **Answer: A.** Trismus, height of mandible, and presence of teeth may hinder visualization of tumor making adequate resection impossible. Visualization of the entire tumor and a 1- to 2-cm resection margin on all sides, including the deep margin, is necessary to successfully resect the tumor. Age and HPV status are not contraindications to transoral resection, only factors that will hinder visualization/exposure of the tumor. PAGES 1905–1906

66. **Answer: A.** Torus is seen in about 20% of individuals. It seems to be a response to stress. PAGE 2106

67. **Answer: A.** Most patients with fibrous dysplasia can be observed. When lesions are disfiguring or create functional impairment, recontouring is appropriate. Recurrence is more likely if treated during a period of active growth. PAGE 2109

68. **Answer: A.** END removes nodes from levels most at risk for harboring occult metastases. It does not address nodes in the retropharyngeal or parapharyngeal space, which are at risk of harboring occult metastases in tumors of the oropharynx, hypopharynx, nasopharynx, and nasal cavity. PAGE 1843

69. **Answer: C.** The highest incidence of NP cancer is observed in Southern China. An intermediate rate is seen in North Africans and Inuits of Alaska. PAGE 1875

70. **Answer: A.** The histologic description of an ulcerated, circumscribed lesion with elevated or rolled margins and a keratinized central region is characteristic of keratoacanthoma, which is a benign self-limiting lesion that often regresses without intervention. Repeat biopsy of the margin is indicated to rule out carcinoma. PAGE 1791

71. **Answer: C.** According to the National Comprehensive Cancer Network guidelines, adequate resection margin for tumors between 2.01 and 4.0 mm in size is 2.0 cm. Excisions are often limited in the head and neck if the lesion is in close proximity with the eyes, nose, ears, and circumoral anatomy. (PAGE 1749)

    Other margins include:
    In situ: 0.5 cm
    ≤1 mm (T1): 1.0 cm
    1.01 to 2.0 mm (T2): 1 to 2 cm
    2.01 to 4.0 mm (T3): 2 cm
    >4 mm (T4): 2 cm

72. **Answer: C.** Partial parotidectomy, removing the tumor and preserving the facial nerve, is standard of care. Higher complication rates are seen with removal of all superficial lobe tissue without benefit for a lesion localized to the tail of the gland. PAGE 1761

73. **Answer: D.** Symptomatic patients with primary hyperparathyroidism are the most likely to benefit immediately from surgery. Guidelines for parathyroidectomy in asymptomatic patients include surgery for patients younger than 50 years, with osteopenia, and poor renal function. PAGE 2136

74. **Answer: D.** Advanced radionecrosis is attributable to small vessel fibrosis and occlusion, which results in bone necrosis. It is more common in the mandible and results in pathologic fracture. This does not respond to HBO or antibiotics, and requires surgical resection and free tissue transfer to achieve wound healing. PAGE 1718

75. **Answer: E.** The most common presenting symptom in SCCA of the trachea is hemoptysis. PAGES 1990–1991, TABLE 126.2

76. **Answer: C.** One advantage of END is the ability to obtain histologic information from the specimen that provides prognostic information and can be used to guide decisions regarding the need for adjuvant treatment. The presence of occult metastases is associated with poorer survival, and when present, can be used to select patients who will benefit from postoperative radiation, or chemoradiation when extracapsular spread is present. PAGES 1840, 1701

77. **Answer: A.** The most common complications encountered following primary and secondary TE puncture include loss of the puncture site by dislodgment of the catheter placed at the time of puncture or partial or complete extrusion of the prosthesis, migration of the puncture site, formation of granulation tissue, aspiration of the prosthesis, cellulitis, stomal stenosis, and pharyngoesophageal stenosis. Less common complications are sternoclavicular arthritis and manual pressure necrosis. Complications unique to secondary TE puncture include violation of the posterior esophageal wall, passage of the catheter through a false passage, and esophageal perforation which can result in deep neck space infections, epidural abscess, vertebral osteomyelitis, and mediastinitis. PAGE 1984

78. **Answer: A.** Postoperative pain after surgery on or near the orbit, particularly when associated with chemosis, should be considered suspicious for a retrobulbar hematoma until proven otherwise, and is a surgical emergency. If untreated, elevated intraocular pressures can result in permanent ischemic injury to the optic nerve. PAGE 2077

79. **Answer: A.** The 5-year survival for sinonasal melanoma is about 20%. Surgery plus radiation helps local control. PAGE 2047

80. **Answer: D.** Radical surgery with negative margins is the treatment of choice for angiosarcomas. However, this is difficult to achieve, particularly in the scalp, due to extensive microscopic spread of tumor. To further complicate this issue, intraoperative frozen section margins are inaccurate at evaluating the presence of microscopically positive margins. (PAGE 2021) Chemotherapy is the primary treatment option for metastatic angiosarcoma. An argument can also be made for the use of adjuvant chemotherapy to prevent distant metastasis in the setting of local failure. PAGE 2022

81. **Answer: A.** Photons are the most commonly used particle. Electrons are widely available, while protons and neutrons require very special and expensive equipment. PAGE 1683

82. **Answer: A.** The most common type of BCC is nodular (noduloulcerative). This lesion typically presents as a discrete, raised circular lesion that often has a central ulceration and rolled borders. The lesion is pink and waxy with a network of capillaries. Morpheaform (also known as sclerosing) is the most aggressive form of BCC. Pigmented BCC is characterized by its brown pigment and differs from nodular BCC by the brown pigmentation only. PAGE 1724

83. **Answer: C.** Most patients with persistent or recurrent NP cancer are inoperable. Those with small tumors may benefit from surgery. One study reports 2-year disease control over 70%. PAGES 1889–1890

84. **Answer: C.** The hypoglossal nerve lies in level II of the neck immediately below and deep to the posterior belly of the digastric tendon. Attempts to control bleeding in this area without nerve identification place the nerve at risk. PAGE 1824

85. **Answer: B.** T2: tumor >2 cm or tumor of any size with two or more high-risk features, which include depth of invasion >2 mm, Clark level IV or greater, perineural invasion, location on ear or non–hair-bearing lip and poorly differentiated or undifferentiated. PAGE 1728, TABLES 13.1, 13.2

86. **Answer: C.** Multiple studies have shown a 5-year local control after reirradiation of nasopharyngeal cancer to be 50% to 60%. PAGE 1712

87. **Answer: C.** Painful mucositis leading to dysphagia and dry mouth are the most common acute toxicities observed. Radionecrosis, fibrosis, and major vessel inflammation manifest as late toxicities. PAGE 1689

88. **Answer: B.** The frontoorbital artery, a branch of the anterior cerebral artery, runs along the inferior surface of the frontal lobe, and so presents an increased risk of injury. PAGE 2082

89. **Answer: D.** Invasion of the pyriform apex (20%), postcricoid mucosa (57%), and subglottis is associated with metastasis in the paratracheal and paraesophageal nodes. `PAGE 1921`

90. **Answer: A.** About 50% of all Waldeyer ring non-Hodgkin lymphomas arise in the palatine tonsil, 20% of which are bilateral. In decreasing order, lymphomas in this region also arise from the pharyngeal tonsil, base of tongue, or lingual tonsil, or involve multiple primary sites. Symptoms correspond with the location of disease and tumors are typically submucosal, not ulcerative. `PAGE 2037`

91. **Answer: D.** In head and neck cancer, on average, 1 to 15 base pairs are mutated for each exome. There may be 6,000 to 90,000 mutations for the 6.4 billion base pairs in the human genome. `PAGE 1647`

92. **Answer: D.** The GORETEC study compared induction chemotherapy with cisplatin and 5-FU to docetaxel, cisplatin, and 5-FU. Laryngeal preservation was higher with the three-drug regimen. `PAGE 1697`

93. **Answer: B.** In between 1999 and 2005, the 5-year survival of laryngeal cancer has statistically decreased to 63%. `PAGES 1961–1962`

94. **Answer: B.** Selective neck dissection for oral cavity cancer of levels I to III is appropriate for oral cavity tumors, with the exception of oral tongue cancer which can spread to level IV and requires dissection of levels I to IV. `PAGES 1821–1822`

95. **Answer: D.** Phase III trials compare the response of a new drug to standard treatment. Phase III clinical trial data provide level I evidence, which is the best evidence to support the use of chemotherapeutic regimens. `PAGE 1694`

96. **Answer: E.** The use of previously unirradiated tissue improves healing and reduces the need for further surgery. It does not increase cancer control. It may indirectly reduce hospital costs through better healing. `PAGES 1710–1711`

97. **Answer: C.** Every effort should be made to continue treatment while treating toxicity. Extended treatment time is associated with reduced tumor control. `PAGE 1684`

98. **Answer: C.** Gastric transposition has the advantage of a robust blood supply and creation of a single pharyngeal anastomosis. Morbidity with gastric pull-up is greater than that associated with jejunal free flaps, and voice outcomes are typically "hollow," whereas voice with jejunal free flap is "wet." `PAGE 1932`

99. **Answer: C.** High urine output of low specific gravity (over 250 mL in 2 hours) with high serum sodium characterizes diabetes insipidus. `PAGE 2094`

100. **Answer: D.** The increased mortality associated with untreated secondary hyperparathyroidism is primarily related to cardiovascular complications induced by ectopic calcifications. The goal of surgery is to reduce PTH secretion when medical management has failed, which is associated with a lower incidence of major cardiovascular events and overall lower mortality. `PAGE 2136`

101. **Answer: C.** Reirradiation results in only a 20% 5-year survival rate. Radical neck dissection reportedly achieved tumor control in over 65% of patients. PAGE 1888

102. **Answer: B.** The orbital rim is comprised of the nasal bone, maxillary bone, zygomatic bone, and frontal bone. The sphenoid and lacrimal bones are part of posterior and medial walls of the orbital vault, while the palatine bone is not part of the orbital vault. PAGE 2065

103. **Answer: C.** While all of the above variables contribute to survival, cervical metastases are the primary determinant of disease-specific survival. Many series report a 50% reduction in survival when nodal metastases are present. PAGE 1840

104. **Answer: B.** A sentinel lymph node biopsy is not offered to patients with lesions measuring 0.75 mm or smaller and to those with clinical nodal or distant metastasis. PAGE 1746, FIGURE 114.4

105. **Answer: A.** High-resolution CT scanning is the imaging modality of choice to stage the cN0 neck in oral cavity cancer and is superior to MRI or PET-CT in evaluation of the neck. Evidence of clinically suspicious lymph node metastases includes size >1 cm, central necrosis, round rather than ovoid shape, and poorly defined borders suspicious for extra-capsular spread. PAGE 1860

106. **Answer: B.** Rituximab is an anti-CD20 monoclonal antibody. In symptomatic patients, combination chemotherapy and immunotherapy is considered to be standard therapy. The addition of rituximab with the standard CHOP (cyclophosphamide, doxorubicin, vincristine, and prednisone) regimen (R-CHOP) has shown significant improvement in outcomes without additional major toxicity and is well tolerated in symptomatic elderly patients with relevant comorbidities. PAGE 2036

107. **Answer: A.** Warthin tumors can be multifocal in up to 50% of cases, and bilateral Warthin tumors are seen in over 10% of patients. These are commonly associated with smoking and have a classic appearance on fine-needle aspiration biopsy. PAGE 1762

108. **Answer: A.** Complete surgical excision of low-grade mucoepidermoid cancer is curative, and with clear margins, adjuvant therapy is not recommended. These tumors have a low incidence of nodal involvement, and if the neck is radiologically negative, elective neck dissection is not recommended for these tumors. PAGE 1764

109. **Answer: D.** When margins are negative, most patients with ameloblastoma can be cured. Incomplete removal is associated with an unacceptable recurrence rate. PAGE 2104

110. **Answer: C.** The presenting symptoms of NP cancer reflect the size and location of the primary tumor. The most common symptom is a neck mass. Cranial nerve involvement reflects intracranial spread. PAGE: 1877

111. **Answer: A.** Cranial nerve deficits should always raise the suspicion of malignancy. Imaging is the next step to identify whether an orbital, skull base, or intracranial tumor is responsible for nerve deficits. PAGES 2064–2065

112. **Answer: D.** PAGE 1964, TABLE 124.2

113. **Answer: C.** TE speech has been rated the most desirable form of alaryngeal speech by both speech pathologists and patients, and is the preferred method of alaryngeal speech by naive listeners. PAGE 1987

114. **Answer: C.** BCC rarely metastasizes to cervical lymph nodes. In the absence of clinical nodal disease, elective neck dissection is not indicated. PAGE 1791

115. **Answer: B.** Exposure of the petrous carotid requires sacrifice of the mandibular nerve, middle meningeal artery, and the eustachian tube. PAGE 2090

116. **Answer: B.** Tracheal tumors are slow-growing, often causing diagnosis to be delayed. The mean duration of symptoms for patients with SCCA and adenoid cystic carcinoma was 12.2 months. The duration of symptoms was longer in adenoid cystic carcinoma than SCCA (18.3 months vs. 4.5 months) and in tumors that were deemed to be unresectable (unresectable adenoid cystic carcinoma 23.7 months; unresectable SCCA 7.58 months). PAGE 1990

117. **Answer: C.** Ninety percent of nerve sheath tumors are benign, the majority being schwannoma or neurofibroma. In the sinonasal tract, they present as a submucosal mass. PAGE 2048

118. **Answer: B.** The capsulopalpebral fascia is the main retractor of the lower lid, while the levator palpebrae is the main retractor of the upper lid. Whitnall ligament is part of the upper lid anatomy, while the orbicularis oculi is responsible for eyelid closure, and the inferior oblique muscle contributes to globe movement. PAGES 2065–2066

119. **Answer: D.** Tracheal resection and primary reanastamosis is the preferred treatment for the majority of both benign and malignant tracheal neoplasms. (PAGES 1992–1993) There are patient and tumor factors that determine if tracheal resection with end to end anastomosis can be performed safely. Important patient factors include body mass index, body habitus, and medical comorbidities such as diabetes mellitus and chronic obstructive pulmonary disease. Tumor factors include the length of the resection needed to remove the tumor with margins. A segmental resection greater than 4 cm or six tracheal rings may put tension on the anastomosis. Tumors with extension into the mediastinum, esophagus, and bronchial tree may require combined cervicothoracic procedures or nonsurgical treatment. Prior radiation therapy and previous tracheotomy with resulting scar tissue (and potential seeding of the anterior neck with tumor) make resection with primary anastomosis more challenging. For those patients in whom resection is contraindicated, tracheotomy, endoscopic tumor ablation, and stent placement are options. PAGES 1992–1993

120. **Answer: A.** The oral tongue is the most common subsite of the oral cavity to develop cancer, occurring in 32% of cases, followed by the floor of mouth. Oral cavity cancer is the most common site for head and neck cancer in the United States. PAGE 1854

121. **Answer: B.** The symptoms of wheezing and dyspnea are more commonly seen in patients with adenoid cystic carcinoma of the trachea. Wheezing is often misdiagnosed as asthma that does not respond to bronchodilator therapy. PAGES 1990–1991, TABLE 126.2

122. **Answer: D.** Microscopically positive margins and extracapsular spread in lymph nodes are the two accepted indications for adjuvant chemoradiation. Outcome analysis of the European Organization for Research and Treatment of Cancer and Radiation Therapy Oncology Group trials examining adjuvant chemoradiation demonstrated a survival benefit for chemoradiation when used in the setting of microscopically positive margins or extracapsular spread, but not for multiple lymph node involvement, angioinvasion, or perineural invasion. PAGE 1827

123. **Answer: C.** Over the past several years, the treatment of oropharyngeal tumors has shifted away from primary surgery to treatment using CRT ("organ preservation"). Although there has been a high rate of complications/morbidity from nonsurgical treatment, it remains the main stay of treatment at this time, particularly for large tumors. (PAGE 1903) . Evidence suggests that CRT offers similar tumor control when compared to surgery and radiation. (PAGE 1905) Nonsurgical management consists of radiotherapy with or without concurrent chemotherapy. Radiation is delivered via intensity-modulated radiation therapy (60 to 70 Gy) and most chemotherapy regimens are platinum based. PAGE 1905

124. **Answer: D.** Staging of oral cavity tumors is based on size and extent of disease in staging the primary tumor, and size and number of nodes to stage the neck. A tumor less than 2 cm is stage T1, while the presence of multiple ispilateral nodes less than 6 cm is stage N2b neck disease. Extracapsular spread is not included in staging algorithms. PAGE 1862

125. **Answer: A.** BRAF mutations are reportedly identified in 40% to 45% of papillary thyroid carcinoma and BRAF B600E mutation is found in 70% to 80% of tall-cell variant. PAGE 2116

126. **Answer: D.** The only absolute contraindication to primary voice restoration is separation of the party wall at the puncture site. This occurs if the surgeon inadvertently separates the party wall or when a patient undergoes a total laryngopharyngoesophagectomy with gastric pull-up. If a puncture is performed following separation of the party wall, abscess formation, sloughing of the posterior tracheal wall, and possibly mediastinitis can occur. PAGE 1981

127. **Answer: A.** This is a sestamibi scan in frontal projection. The increased uptake is on the patient's right side. (To reassure yourself that the patient is oriented correctly, look for uptake in the heart.) The left thyroid lobe is dimly visible, confirming the lower neck location. The uptake in the salivary glands is expected. PAGES 2134–2135

128. **Answer: D.** Both the common carotid artery and the internal jugular vein are displaced forward. Thus, the tumor arose from the back of the carotid sheath, where the vagus nerve normally runs. There is no splaying of the carotid arteries as expected with carotid body tumors. PAGE 1999

129. **Answer: A.** Both carotid body tumors are adjacent to the internal carotid arteries (ICAs), but do not abut 180 degrees of the artery circumference. This meets criteria for Shamblin 1. On the right, the external carotid artery has >180 degrees of involvement, but only the ICA is used for classification. PAGES 2003–2004

130. **Answer: A.** The small bright dots in the middle of the mass are microcalcifications, which are specific for papillary thyroid carcinoma. The well-defined nature of the mass does not exclude malignancy. `PAGE 2116`

131. **Answer: E.** A lucent mass expanding the jaw with areas of cortical remodeling and thinning is most suggestive of ameloblastoma; the "bubbly" appearance of multiple loculations is classic. Keratocystic odontogenic tumors are usually unilocular and are less common. SCC would not erode bone, not remodel. A dentigerous cyst would encompass the crown of a tooth. `PAGE 2012`

132. **Answer: D.** The key finding on this image is the spread of tumor intracranially, above the right cribriform plate. The tumor is cystic on its superior surface. These findings are strongly suggestive of esthesioneuroblastoma. The other tumors can present as aggressive nasal masses, and will occasionally cross the anterior skull base, but this appearance is much more suggestive of esthesioneuroblastoma. `PAGES 2047–2048`

133. **Answer: C.** This is a young patient with a predominantly cystic lymph node in level II. That constellation of findings strongly suggests human papillomavirus-positive oropharyngeal carcinoma, either from the palatine tonsils or from the tongue base. `PAGE 1900`

134. **Answer: B.** The key finding in this case is the left-sided retropharyngeal adenopathy (in addition to the level II node). Nasopharyngeal carcinoma spreads to retropharyngeal nodes far more frequently than SCC arising from other mucosal sites. `PAGES 1885 and 1887`

8

Sleep Medicine

1. Accurate diagnosis of obstructive sleep apnea (OSA) can best be made by:

    A. A careful history with a complete review of systems
    B. Bed partner history
    C. Physical examination of the upper airway
    D. A home sleep study or an in-lab polysomnogram

2. Approximately what percentage of patients with obstructive sleep apnea (OSA) have another coexisting sleep medicine disorder that may be contributing to their symptoms?

    A. 2%
    B. 10%
    C. 20%
    D. 33%
    E. 67%

3. What is the estimated prevalence of snoring in middle-aged men?

    A. 10%
    B. 20%
    C. 30%
    D. 50%

4. In patients with obstructive sleep apnea who have a deviated nasal septum and symptomatic nasal obstruction, nasal surgery has been shown to consistently improve all of the following *except*:

   A. Subjective sleep quality
   B. Daytime sleepiness
   C. Snoring
   D. Apnea–hypopnea index (AHI)
   E. Disease-specific and general health quality-of-life measures

5. In obstructive sleep apnea patients, the most effective method of assessing and following adherence to positive pressure therapy is:

   A. Patient self-report
   B. Asking the bed partner
   C. Data card monitoring software
   D. Epworth Sleepiness scale (ESS)
   E. Sleep diary

6. In patients with poor continuous positive airway pressure (CPAP) compliance and nasal obstruction, lowering nasal resistance with surgical therapy has been shown to:

   A. Improve CPAP compliance
   B. Lower the apnea–hypopnea index
   C. Lower CPAP pressure requirements
   D. Both A and C
   E. All of the above

7. A 56-year-old man with excessive daytime sleepiness and loud snoring is diagnosed with severe obstructive sleep apnea (OSA) (respiratory disturbance index = 65) by polysomnography. Best first-line treatment is:

   A. Positional therapy
   B. Positive airway pressure treatment
   C. Surgical intervention
   D. Oral appliance therapy

8. Which of the following is true of continuous positive airway pressure (CPAP) therapy for pediatric patients?

   A. It is primarily used as adjunct therapy for patients with failed adenotonsillectomy.
   B. The delivery system in children is usually an oral mask.
   C. Many children discontinue CPAP because it is ineffective.
   D. Titration of the CPAP should not be performed during polysomnography.

19. For most patients, the preferred and most effective oral appliance currently used in the management of obstructive sleep apnea is a:

    A. Mandibular repositioning appliance
    B. Tongue-retaining device
    C. Soft palate advancement device
    D. Palatal expander
    E. Prefabricated thermoplastic splint

20. In the population of patients with obstructive sleep apnea (OSA), what is the most common site of obstruction?

    A. Nasals
    B. Retropalatal
    C. Retrolingual
    D. Multilevel

21. Which of the following most accurately describes cine MRI?

    A. It provides a high-resolution view of the static airway.
    B. It produces only a small amount of radiation exposure.
    C. It is particularly helpful for multiple sites of obstruction.
    D. It is routinely performed on children without sedation.

22. In the majority of obstructive sleep apnea patients who fail to improve after traditional uvulopalatopharyngoplasty (UPPP), which is the primary anatomical location of the persistent obstruction?

    A. Nose
    B. Palate
    C. Tonsils
    D. Tongue
    E. Epiglottis

23. Which of the following is the best predictor of the presence of obstructive sleep apnea (OSA) in an adult?

    A. An Epworth sleepiness score > 10
    B. Neck circumference > 17 inches
    C. A history of snoring
    D. A history of frequent nighttime awakening

24. The American Academy of Pediatrics recommends postoperative admission for patients in the "at-risk" group. Which of the following patients should be admitted overnight postoperatively?

    A. Children who had a previous postpartum neonatal intensive care unit stay for jaundice
    B. Children with moderate obstructive sleep apnea on polysomnography
    C. Children with medication-controlled asthma
    D. Children under the age of 3 years

25. The mechanisms by which increased body weight plays an important role in hypopharyngeal obstruction include:

    A. Increase in soft tissue mass
    B. Enlargement of lingual tonsils
    C. Enlargement of palatine tonsils
    D. Change in mandible position

26. What factors correlate with relief of obstructive sleep apnea (OSA) after uvulopalatopharyngoplasty (UPPP)?

    A. Small tonsils, small tongue
    B. Small tonsils, large tongue
    C. Large tonsils, large tongue
    D. Large tonsils, small tongue

27. The most common cause of excessive daytime sleepiness in the United States is:

    A. Obstructive sleep apnea
    B. Restless leg syndrome
    C. Insomnia
    D. Insufficient sleep

28. Which type of palatal surgery is uniquely suited to address an obliquely oriented palate with a large lateral wall component and a circumferential pattern of obstruction?

    A. Traditional uvulopalatopharyngoplasty (UPPP)
    B. Uvulopalatal flap modification
    C. Expansion sphincter pharyngoplasty
    D. Anterior palatoplasty
    E. Transpalatal advancement

29. Portable or home sleep testing for the diagnosis of obstructive sleep apnea is most appropriate for which of the following adult patients?

    A. Patient with a recent cardiovascular accident
    B. Patient with a history of snoring and hypertension
    C. Patient with severe congestive heart failure
    D. Patient with severe chronic obstructive pulmonary disease

30. The first-line treatment for obstructive sleep apnea (OSA) in the pediatric patient with moderate OSA should be?

    A. Weight loss
    B. Continuous positive airway pressure
    C. Adenotonsillectomy
    D. Medical therapy

Chapter 8 Answers

1. **Answer: D.** The physician's subjective impression of the presence or absence of a sleep disorder is inaccurate. The gold standard test for OSA is a sleep study. `PAGE 2152`

2. **Answer: D.** Restless leg syndrome and insomnia are commonly associated with OSA; about one-third of patients may have one of these sleep disorders. These and other sleep pathologies may contribute to symptoms. `PAGE 2186`

3. **Answer: D.** The Wisconsin Sleep Cohort Study reported 51% of middle-aged men snore. For middle-aged women, it is 31%. `PAGE 2191`

4. **Answer: D.** Improved nasal airway reportedly results in objective improvement in all parameters except a statistically significant reduction in the AHI. `PAGE 2193`

5. **Answer: C.** Data card monitoring with the use of smart cards or Web-based technology provides the most accurate information on compliance. `PAGE 2178` The ESS is diagnostic and does not provide information about compliance. Answers A, B, and E are not reliable information compared to the information from continuous positive airway pressure machine usage report.

6. **Answer: D.** Multiple studies demonstrate the potential of nasal airway surgery to improve comfort and reduce required pressure for CPAP users. `PAGE 2194`

7. **Answer: B.** Positive airway pressure such as continuous positive airway pressure is the first-line therapy in the care of severe OSA. `PAGES 2170–2171`

8. **Answer: A.** The treatment of choice for most children with obstructive sleep apnea (OSA) is adenotonsillectomy. CPAP is used adjunctively with persistent OSA. `PAGE 2224`

9. **Answer: B.** OSA is a chronic disease and is rarely "cured." Obviously, continuous positive airway pressure relieves, but does not cure, OSA. Resolution of symptoms after surgery is the most important outcome. `PAGE 2210`

10. **Answer: B.** Surgery has been considered an alternative for patients unable or unwilling to use positive pressure. `PAGE 2192`

11. **Answer: B.** Treatment of nasal obstruction may result in reduced pressure requirements and more comfortable use of CPAP. Answers A, D, and E are incorrect since they denote negative results from nasal obstruction treatment in OSA patients. `PAGES 2179, 2183`

12. **Answer: A.** Complications are largely attributable to excessive soft tissue removal. When circumferential soft tissue is removed, stenosis due to contraction may ensue. `PAGE 2197`

13. **Answer: E.** Chronic nasal obstruction impacts sleep in many ways. `PAGES 2193–2194`

14. **Answer: D.** All evaluations may contribute to the surgeon's ability to identify the site of obstruction during apneic events. Fiberoptic endoscopy is essential. The other testing may also help plan treatment; however, the flexible endoscopy allows three-dimensional evaluation. The value of sleep endoscopy and MRI remains controversial. PAGE 2207

15. **Answer: B.** Skeletal advancement can improve the airway. Greater advancement is associated with better results. Studies suggest results are maintained unless there is weight gain. PAGE 2216

16. **Answer: C.** Glossectomy results in tongue reduction. The other procedures reposition without reducing the soft tissue. PAGES 2210–2214

17. **Answer: D.** An individual's acceptance and adherence to therapy may be established shortly after initiating treatment. Therefore, provision of education with knowledgeable staff is a key to success. PAGE 2179

18. **Answer: B.** Physical examination may alert the physician to the possibility of OSA. PSG remains the traditional and gold standard for diagnosis. PAGES 2221–2222

19. **Answer: A.** The mandibular repositioning appliance is by far the most commonly employed. Data suggest these appliances to be most effective. PAGES 2180–2181

20. **Answer: D.** Multilevel obstruction, including retropalatal and retrolingual, is present in 70% to 80% of patients with OSA. PAGE 2191

21. **Answer: C.** The cine MRI displays the airway like a "real-time movie," allowing for evaluation of obstruction. It requires sedation and, of course, has no radiation exposure. PAGE 2227

22. **Answer: B.** Studies have reported that residual retropalatal obstruction was observed in over 80% following traditional UPPP. PAGES 2195–2196

23. **Answer: B.** The diagnosis of OSA is best made with a polysomnogram (PSG). Neck circumference >17 inches (or 14.5 inches in women) is the best prediction in this question. Other problems such as insufficient sleep may influence the Epworth score. PAGES 2151–2152

24. **Answer: D.** The guidelines call for monitoring in hospital of high-risk groups, such as morbidly obese children and those with craniofacial disorders, including those under age 3. PAGE 2226

25. **Answer: A.** There is good evidence that weight gain results in fat deposits in the tongue and pharynx. This appears to exacerbate the problem of soft tissue collapse. PAGE 2206

26. **Answer: D.** The Mallampati and Friedman systems emphasize how removal of large tonsils in the setting of a normal (small) tongue is a highly reliable predictor of UPPP success. The presence of a large tongue or OSA in a patient with small tonsils suggests a retrolingual site of obstruction. PAGE 2196

27. **Answer: D.** There are over 80 specific sleep disorders currently classified. The most common cause of daytime sleepiness remains basic sleep deprivation. PAGE 2152

28. **Answer: C.** Expansion pharyngoplasty is specifically tailored to patients with an obliquely oriented palate who may fail UPPP. PAGE 2199

29. **Answer: B.** A monitored sleep study measures more parameters and allows for intervention during the study. Portable evaluation is best suited to assessment in the nonacute setting. PAGE 2170

30. **Answer: C.** Adenotonsillectomy is the treatment of choice for most children. Morbid obesity and craniofacial anomaly represent a more difficult-to-treat population. PAGE 2225

9 Otology

1. A 1.5-year-old child with bilateral aural atresia should be offered:

   A. Atresia surgery on at least one ear by age 3 years
   B. Bone-anchored hearing aid (BAHA) soft band
   C. BAHA implant by age 2 years
   D. Aural–oral rehabilitation

2. A 55-year-old man presents with intermittent frontal headaches. History and physical examination are unremarkable, and he has no history of neurotologic disease. A CT of the temporal bone reveals smooth bony expansion. A contrasted MRI of the brain is performed, which reveals a nonenhancing lesion in the right petrous apex which is hypointense on T1 and hyperintense on T2. Which imaging technique would provide the most helpful information in distinguishing it from other lesions that occur in this region?

   A. Fat-suppressed T1-weighted MRI sequence
   B. Digital subtraction cerebral angiogram
   C. Fluid-attenuated inversion recovery (FLAIR) MRI sequence
   D. Fast-spin echo T2-weighted MRI sequence

3. Which of the following is true regarding calyx endings in the vestibular neuroepithelium?

   A. Innervate type I and type II hair cells
   B. Are equally distributed throughout the epithelium
   C. Are seen only on calyx afferent neurons
   D. Do not express calretinin
   E. Receive postsynaptic afferent input

4. **When making a post auricular incision for mastoid surgery in an infant, the incision should be made more posteriorly than in an adult for which of these reasons?**

    A. The mastoid antrum is located more posteriorly.

    B. The mastoid is small and the facial nerve may exit directly from the cortex.

    C. In infants, the emissary vein exits directly out of the mastoid.

    D. In infants, the blood supply to the pinna may be compromised if the incision is too far anterior.

5. **Which consideration in tympanic-membrane reconstruction is unique to the canal-wall-down scenario?**

    A. Careful planning of ear canal incisions

    B. Need to palpate and inspect the ossicular chain to assess mobility

    C. Application of the principles of ossicular and acoustic coupling

    D. Requirement to directly seal off the anterior epitympanic wall from the supratubal recess and middle ear

6. **Which of the following is true with regard to cerebrospinal fluid (CSF) leak after temporal bone fracture?**

    A. High-resolution CT shows potential sites of CSF leak in less than half of cases.

    B. CSF leak after temporal bone trauma rarely closes with conservative management.

    C. Prophylactic antibiotics should be administered in all patients who have temporal bone fractures.

    D. The most significant risk factor for meningitis after temporal bone fracture is duration of CSF leak.

7. **Hearing conservation programs are required by Occupational Safety and Health Administration for workers whose time-weighted average TWA(s) exposures are at least which dBA level?**

    A. 80

    B. 82

    C. 85

    D. 87

    E. 90

8. In a patient with prior history of chronic otorrhea unresponsive to topical antibiotics, the new onset of headache, lethargy, and high fever, without meningeal symptoms, is most worrisome for which of the following pathologic processes?

    A. Epidural abscess
    B. Sigmoid sinus thrombophlebitis
    C. Subdural empyema
    D. Gradenigo syndrome
    E. Meningitis

9. Lead toxicity results in hearing loss from which of the following mechanisms?

    A. Outer hair cell damage
    B. Injury to the stria vascularis
    C. Impairment of neural transmission in auditory pathways
    D. Formation of reactive oxygen species
    E. All of the above

10. Which of the following is the current recommendation for the primary treatment of autoimmune inner-ear disease?

    A. Cyclophosphamide at an initial dose of 1 mg/kg/day orally for 4 to 6 weeks
    B. Intratympanic corticosteroid therapy with systemic methotrexate
    C. Systemic corticosteroid therapy tapered according to patient response
    D. Systemic etanercept for 4 weeks

11. Modalities to monitor ototoxicity include:

    A. Standard pure-tone audiometry
    B. High-frequency audiometry
    C. Distortion-produced otoacoustic emissions (OAEs)
    D. All of the above
    E. A and C

12. Which measure is not used in the calculation of hearing handicap according to the AMA Guidelines?

    A. Better ear
    B. 3,000 Hz
    C. 2,000 Hz
    D. 500 Hz
    E. Speech discrimination score

13. Most cases of sudden sensorineural hearing loss (SSNHL) are caused by:

    A. Temporal bone trauma
    B. Genetic predisposition
    C. Neurologic disease
    D. No identifiable source

14. Which of following factors is the *least likely* to affect functional outcome of a person with a right peripheral vestibular hypofunction?

    A. Age
    B. A history of migraine
    C. A history of anxiety
    D. A history of strabismus

15. Which of the following is *least* useful when attempting to establish the prognosis for recovery from Bell palsy?

    A. Nerve excitability test
    B. Maximal stimulation test
    C. Electrogustometry
    D. Electroneuronography
    E. Physical examination

16. A rapidly expanding enhancing mass of the internal auditory canal (IAC) with accompanying progressive seventh and eighth cranial neuropathies is most likely to be caused by:

    A. Lipoma
    B. Facial schwannoma
    C. Metastatic breast cancer
    D. Vestibular schwannoma

17. A child with severe sensorineural hearing loss (SNHL) presents with fever, headache, nausea and vomiting, and photophobia a day after being diagnosed with acute otitis media (AOM). Temporal bone imaging is most likely to demonstrate:

    A. Dehiscence of the tegmen mastoideum
    B. Patent tympanomeningeal fissure
    C. Mondini malformation
    D. Congenital cholesteatoma
    E. Dehiscence of the jugular bulb

18. Which of the following branches of the facial nerve is most proximal?

    A. Branch to the digastric
    B. Chorda tympani
    C. Branch to platysma
    D. Greater superficial petrosal nerve
    E. Branch to the stapedius

19. Which of the following is a potential inherent shortcoming of ossiculoplasty with a sculpted incus interposition graft?

    A. High risk of graft extrusion
    B. Challenging revision surgery due to fixed integration with stapes head
    C. Established track record of poor-hearing outcomes in the medical literature
    D. Inability to engage the malleus as part of ossicular reconstruction

20. The external auditory canal (EAC) develops from:

    A. The first mesodermal branchial groove between the mandibular (I) hyoid (II) arches
    B. The first ectodermal branchial groove between the mandibular (I) and hyoid (II) arches
    C. The second pharyngeal pouch joining the first pharyngeal groove
    D. The second branchial groove joining the second pharyngeal pouch
    E. Entirely from the third ectodermal branchial groove

21. The mammalian cochlea contains hair cells, supporting cells, and spiral ganglia neurons. Which cell types are required for normal hearing function?

    A. Hair cells
    B. Supporting cells
    C. Spiral ganglia neurons
    D. A and C
    E. All of the above

22. Active middle-ear implants are appropriate in all of the follow conditions except:

    A. Speech discrimination greater that 40%
    B. Absence of middle ear disease
    C. Bilateral moderate to severe conductive hearing loss
    D. Limited performance with conventional amplification
    E. Bilateral moderate to severe sensorineural hearing loss

23. **Brain hernia associated with cholesteatoma is usually the result of:**

    A. Earlier surgical injury to the tegmen
    B. Infectious osteitis with bone resorption
    C. Direct extension of cholesteatoma through the dura
    D. Propagation of venous thrombophlebitis
    E. Hydrocephalus

24. **Which of the following embryonic layers contribute to the tympanic membrane?**

    A. Ectoderm
    B. Mesoderm
    C. Endoderm
    D. A and C
    E. All of the above

25. **Which of the following patients will have difficulty performing the eye/head exercises that are commonly used in vestibular rehabilitation?**

    A. Patients with a history of migraine
    B. Patients with a history of anxiety
    C. Patients who are afraid of falling
    D. A and C
    E. All of the above

26. **On temporal bone computerized tomography in patients with congenital SNHL, morphologic abnormalities of the bony labyrinth are identified in what percentage of cases?**

    A. 0% to 20%
    B. 20% to 40%
    C. 40% to 60%
    D. 60% to 80%

27. **Reasonable diagnostic investigations for necrotizing external otitis (NEO) would include** *all* **of which of the tests listed below?**

    A. Culture of the external canal secretions, positron emission tomography-computerized tomography of the petrous temporal bones, and technetium Tc 99m methylene diphosphonate scanning.

    B. Culture of the external canal secretions, CT of the petrous temporal bones, technetium Tc 99m scanning, gallium-67 scanning, and indium-111-labeled leukocyte planar scintigraphy.

    C. Culture of the external canal secretions, CT of the petrous temporal bones, gallium-67 scanning, and MRI/MRA of the skull base.

    D. Culture of the external canal secretions MRI/MRA of the skull base, technetium Tc 99m methylene diphosphonate scanning, and indium-111-labeled leukocyte planar scintigraphy.

    E. Culture of the external canal secretions, indium-111-labeled leukocyte planar scintigraphy, gallium-67 scanning, and MRI/MRA of the skull base.

28. **Lymphoscintigraphy and sentinel lymph node biopsy should be performed for patients when:**

    A. A biopsy demonstrates a Breslow depth > 2 mm
    B. A biopsy demonstrates a Breslow depth > 0.76 mm but < 2 mm
    C. The surgeon believes the procedure will offer a survival benefit
    D. There is clinical or radiographic evidence of neck metastasis

29. **Which of the following is true regarding intact canal wall tympanomastoidectomy for cholesteatoma?**

    A. The rate of recurrent cholesteatoma is high.
    B. Attic reconstruction is not necessary.
    C. It provides long-term visualization of the mastoid antrum.
    D. It has worse hearing results than canal-wall-down tympanomastoidectomy.
    E. It is not advisable in children.

30. **A patient with petrous apicitis and diplopia usually has a deficit in which cranial nerve?**

    A. III
    B. IV
    C. VI
    D. VII

31. **Which of the following is characteristic of right posterior semicircular canal BPPV (benign paroxysmal positional vertigo)?**

   A. With the right ear positioned toward the ground in the Dix–Hallpike maneuver, the resulting nystagmus is pure horizontal geotropic.
   B. With the right ear positioned toward the ground in the Dix–Hallpike maneuver, the resulting nystagmus is downbeating, geotropic, and torsional.
   C. With the right ear positioned toward the ground in the Dix–Hallpike maneuver, the resulting nystagmus is downbeating, ageotropic, and torsional.
   D. With the right ear positioned toward the ground in the Dix–Hallpike maneuver, the resulting nystagmus is upbeating, geotropic, and torsional.
   E. With the right ear positioned toward the ground in the Dix–Hallpike maneuver, the resulting nystagmus is upbeating, ageotropic, and torsional.

32. **Measures for preventing postcochlear implantation meningitis include all of the following except for:**

   A. Vaccination against *Pneumococcus*
   B. Avoiding a separate intracochlear electrode positioner
   C. Coating the array with antibiotic solutions
   D. Sealing the cochleostomy

33. **Hearing loss in adults may lead to:**

   A. Social isolation
   B. Communication impairment
   C. Compromised overall health
   D. Withdrawal from social situations
   E. All of the above

34. **Which of the following would be considered a type II tympanoplasty reconstruction technique using the modified Wullstein/Zollner criteria?**

   A. Placement of a composite perichondrium-cartilage island graft directly upon the stapes capitulum.
   B. Use of an Applebaum prosthesis between an eroded incus long process and stapes capitulum.
   C. Titanium TORP (total ossicular replacement prosthesis) set between the stapes footplate and reconstructed tympanic membrane.
   D. Sculpted incus interposition graft placed between the malleus neck and stapes capitulum.
   E. Placement of a composite HA-titanium PORP on the stapes capitulum to the tympanic membrane.

35. A 72-year-old woman presents with an asymmetric sensorineural hearing loss. What is the most important step in her evaluation and treatment?

    A. MRI
    B. Hearing aid evaluation
    C. CT
    D. Laboratory evaluation
    E. Auditory Brainstem Responses

36. Which objective finding is most reassuring for recovery when evaluating a patient with temporal bone fracture and facial paralysis?

    A. Maximal stimulation threshold on fractured side is greater than 3.5 mA in comparison to nonfractured side.
    B. Evoked electromyography compound muscle action potential demonstrates decline of 92% 5 days after injury.
    C. Facial nerve stimulation threshold on fractured side is 2 mA higher than on nonfractured side 1 week after injury.
    D. Facial nerve stimulation threshold on fractured side is equal to that on nonfractured side 1 day after injury.
    E. Evoked electromyography compound muscle action potential demonstrates decline of 74% 2 days after injury.

37. A 6-year-old child sustains a mild concussion and reports new hearing loss and positional dizziness. An audiogram shows a unilateral flat 70-dB sensorineural hearing loss, and CT scan demonstrates a Mondini deformity. The most likely diagnosis is:

    A. Benign paroxysmal positional vertigo (BPPV)
    B. Labyrinthine concussion
    C. Posttraumatic Ménière syndrome
    D. Perilymph fistula
    E. Tympanometry

38. A patient presents with a low-frequency conductive right-sided hearing loss. Stapedial reflexes are present. Which of the following is the next step in management?

    A. Hearing aid
    B. Stapes surgery
    C. Temporal bone CT
    D. Observation
    E. Intralabyrinthine hemorrhage

39. Which one of the following is the most common facial nerve abnormality in congenital aural atresia?

    A. Horizontal segment of facial nerve displaced inferior to oval window
    B. Vertical segment of facial nerve displaced anteriorly/laterally
    C. More obtuse angle of facial nerve at second genu
    D. Dehiscent vertical segment of facial nerve
    E. Enlarged geniculate ganglion

40. Which of the following agents has a potential role in the etiology of otosclerosis (OS)?

    A. Influenza virus
    B. Measles virus
    C. Mumps virus
    D. Ebstein-Barr virus

41. The purpose of a large portion of the laboratory studies for vertigo, dizziness, and unsteadiness is to:

    A. Render a diagnosis
    B. Determine the extent and site of lesion
    C. Determine functionality and disability
    D. Determine the optimal treatment path

42. Which of the following is a far-field monitoring technique used for intraoperative monitoring of the auditory system during vestibular schwannoma resections?

    A. Electrocochleography
    B. Continuous noninvasive arterial pressure monitoring
    C. Auditory brainstem response (ABR)
    D. Intraoperative facial nerve monitoring

43. Which of the following best monitors and/or best measures the integrity of cochlear blood supply?

    A. Electrocochleography (ECochG)
    B. Continuous noninvasive arterial pressure monitoring
    C. Auditory brainstem response
    D. Intraoperative facial nerve monitoring

44. **Which of the following can be inferred from the type of fracture present on CT scan?**

    A. Patients with otic capsule-sparing fractures are less likely to have cerebrospinal fluid (CSF) fistula.
    B. Facial nerve injury is more likely when the otic capsule is not involved.
    C. Sensorineural hearing loss is not related to the type of fracture present.
    D. Otic capsule-sparing fractures typically result from a blow to the occipital region.

45. **All of the following are characteristic of peripheral vestibular pathology *except*:**

    A. Nystagmus is suppressed with visual fixation.
    B. Nystagmus is enhanced with visual fixation.
    C. Nystagmus is generally horizontal-rotary jerk nystagmus.
    D. Has a positive postheadshake nystagmus.
    E. Has normal oculomotor tests.

46. **The initial treatment of patients presenting within 72 hours of onset of Bell palsy should include:**

    A. Steroids, antivirals and eye care
    B. Steroids and eye care
    C. Antivirals and eye care
    D. Eye care, no further treatment (prognosis not improved)
    E. No further treatment (prognosis not improved)

47. **Where is the most common site for a dehiscent facial nerve?**

    A. Mental segment
    B. Tympanic segment
    C. Labyrinthine segment
    D. Mastoid segment

48. **What is the only intraoperative electromyography (EMG) pattern that corresponds to deterioration of facial nerve function?**

    A. Prolonged, audible activity in the EMG patterns
    B. C train
    C. A train
    D. Burst activity

49. A 42-year-old man is seen in the clinic for evaluation of headaches and diplopia. His physical examination reveals a midline submucosal nasopharyngeal mass. Further diagnostic evaluation would most likely show:

    A. Chronic sphenoid sinusitis on a sinus CT scan
    B. Vacuolated physaliphorous cells in a deep nasopharyngeal biopsy
    C. Internal carotid aneurysm on a CT angiogram
    D. Antoni A cells with Verocay bodies on a deep nasopharyngeal biopsy

50. Which of the following best describes the cochlear modifier or amplifier?

    A. A passive process within the cochlea due to the stiffness of the tectorial membrane
    B. An active process involving the inner hair cell system to tune the basilar membrane
    C. Affected by distortions due to large signal-to-noise ratios
    D. Dependent on outer hair cell motility and the mechanical properties of the stereocilia and tectorial membrane
    E. Allows sound coming in to be tuned across a wide spectral frequency band so that every frequency is stimulated equally

51. Children learning language ideally would have audibility out to which bandwidth?

    A. 2,000 Hz
    B. 3,000 Hz
    C. 4,000 Hz
    D. 6,000 Hz
    E. 8,000 Hz

52. Where is the most common site of origin of congenital cholesteatoma?

    A. Epitympanum
    B. Posterior–superior quadrant of the middle ear
    C. Anterior–superior quadrant of the middle ear
    D. Mastoid antrum

53. A patient presents with left-sided fluctuating hearing loss, aural fullness, and episodic vertigo. Which of the following tests results is most consistent with the following symptoms:

    A. Normal caloric testing
    B. Summating potential/Action potential (SP/AP) ratio > 0.5
    C. Low-frequency left conductive hearing loss
    D. Lowered left cervical vestibular-evoked-myogenic potential (VEMP) threshold

54. Which of the following patient groups would *most likely* benefit from an SSRI (selective serotonin reuptake inhibitor) for control of their dizziness symptoms?

    A. Persons with Ménière disease
    B. Persons with neuritis
    C. Persons with labyrinthitis
    D. Persons with anxiety and dizziness

55. During a revision stapedectomy, the previously placed piston prosthesis is noted to be displaced out of the stapedotomy and the lenticular and distal long process are absent, but a majority of the long process is still present. What is the best way to proceed?

    A. Use a notched bucket-handle prosthesis between the incus long process and the stapedotomy
    B. Use a total ossicular replacement prosthesis between the stapes footplate and the malleus
    C. Use a partial ossicular replacement prosthesis between the stapes footplate and the incus
    D. Place a piston on the malleus neck down to the stapes footplate
    E. Use a shorter piston from the distal incus to the stapedotomy

56. Which of the following is *true* regarding otosyphilis?

    A. The otic capsule is not involved during the secondary and/or tertiary stages of infection.
    B. Physical examination will reveal signs consistent with sensorineural hearing loss (SNHL) and a peripheral vestibular loss.
    C. Hearing loss is always present in congenital syphilis and rarely present in patients with neurosyphilis.
    D. Hearing loss secondary to syphilis is reversible with proper antimicrobial treatment.

57. Which of these are the most common drugs causing ototoxicity?

    A. Loop diuretics
    B. Aminoglycosides
    C. Cisplatin
    D. Vancomycin
    E. B and C

58. A 78-year-old woman presents with chronic imbalance, recurrent falls, and difficulty walking in the dark. She was treated with intravenous antibiotics for a hip fracture one year ago. What is her most likely diagnosis?

    A. Vestibular neuritis
    B. Vertebrobasilar insufficiency
    C. Bilateral vestibulopathy
    D. Migraine-associated vertigo

59. Which of the following causes of acute facial paralysis carries the best prognosis for recovery?

    A. Acute otitis media (AOM)
    B. Penetrating trauma
    C. Temporal bone fracture due to blunt trauma
    D. Metastatic cancer
    E. Ramsay Hunt syndrome

60. Acute bilateral facial paralysis is uncommon, but which of the following is not a potential cause?

    A. Lyme disease
    B. Metastatic carcinoma
    C. Skull base osteomyelitis
    D. Guillain–Barré syndrome
    E. Stroke

61. A 35-year-old man is presenting with spontaneous events of external vertigo lasting 1 to 2 hours associated with photophobia, without any auditory symptoms and well-diagnosed migraine headaches. He is put through laboratory testing. The results show clinically significant right-beating positional nystagmus with all other studies normal. What would be the most likely integrated interpretation of the above information?

    A. Peripheral vestibular system involvement cannot be ruled out, but migraine-related dizziness most probable diagnosis
    B. Developing labyrinthine lesion on the left given the fixed direction of the positional nystagmus
    C. Peripheral vestibular system involvement as either an irritative lesion on the right or paretic lesion on the left, source of the lesion undetermined
    D. The positional nystagmus with photophobia during the spells would be highly suggestive of central vestibular system involvement

62. Rotational chair testing provides for which of these situations?

    A. An expansion of the investigation of peripheral vestibular system involvement
    B. Allows for the isolated assessment of the horizontal semicircular canals on the left and the right
    C. A dedicated investigation of the central vestibular system function
    D. Localization of a peripheral vestibular system lesion to the left or the right

63. If hearing in noise is essential for your patient, which of the following would be good suggestions?

    A. Using a hearing aid full-time
    B. Using two hearing aids with bilateral hearing loss
    C. Directional microphones
    D. Assistive listening devices
    E. All of the above

64. Spontaneous hearing recovery after a sudden sensorineural hearing loss, if it is to occur, occurs within what time frame?

    A. 3 days
    B. 2 weeks
    C. 2 months
    D. 6 months

65. The sensory organization test (SOT) of posturography allows:

    A. An additional site-of-lesion study to separate peripheral vestibular from central vestibular involvement
    B. An evaluation to determine the involvement of the vertical semicircular canals
    C. Assessment of the interaction between the semicircular canals and the otolith organs
    D. A dedicated function evaluation of the patient's integrated use of vision, foot support surface cues, and the peripheral and central vestibular system cues

66. Which of the following statements about interaural attenuation is *incorrect*?

    A. It is frequency dependent.
    B. It is independent of the nature of the hearing loss.
    C. It is dependent on the type of earphone.
    D. It is greater for bone than for air conduction.
    E. It must be considered with audiometric testing of asymmetric hearing loss.

67. Which cochlear potential is not generated by sound stimuli?

    A. Endocochlear potential
    B. Summating potential
    C. Whole-nerve action potential
    D. Cochlear microphonic potential
    E. None of the above

68. **What is the most common change seen on vestibular-evoked myogenic potential (VEMP) testing in the elderly?**

    A. Decreased thresholds
    B. Decreased amplitude
    C. Decreased latency
    D. Increased amplitude

69. **Which of the following is a true statement regarding facial paralysis and chronic otitis media (COM)?**

    A. Facial paralysis associated with COM is usually due to *Hemophilus influenzae* type B.
    B. Facial paralysis associated with COM has a poor prognosis even with proper treatment.
    C. Facial paralysis associated with COM is usually due to cholesteatoma and involves the tympanic segment of the nerve.
    D. Facial paralysis associated with COM is usually due to cholesteatoma and involves the geniculate ganglion.
    E. B and C.

70. **Which statement is *incorrect* regarding otoacoustic emissions (OAEs)?**

    A. They are a comprehensive test of hearing.
    B. They reflect outer hair cell function.
    C. They are often normal in auditory neuropathy.
    D. They may be used to monitor ototoxicity.
    E. They can differentiate cochlear from retrocochlear pathology.

71. **You have just completed the canalith repositioning maneuver on a patient with long-standing posterior canal BPPV (benign paroxysmal positional vertigo). Which of the following would you tell your patient after the maneuver?**

    A. Their perception of earth vertical may be off for a few days.
    B. They will be able to see better.
    C. They may have balance deficits for a few days up to a few months after repositioning.
    D. A and C.
    E. All of the above.

72. A 34-year-old woman with insulin-dependent type I diabetes has a 2-day history of left-sided flat moderate-to-severe sensorineural hearing loss (SNHL). Blood glucose levels have been well controlled preceding the hearing loss. Which of the following represents the best treatment option?

    A. Transtympanic dexamethasone
    B. Valacyclovir
    C. Medrol dose pack
    D. Carbogen inhalation

73. Otoacoustic emissions (OAEs) can be described best as which of these?

    A. Proof that the cochlea is a passive system
    B. Spontaneous when measured without sound stimuli and this occurs in 80% to 90% of individuals
    C. Used to provide frequency-specific hearing levels when elicited in the transient and/or distortion product mode
    D. Sounds that can be heard with the stethoscope, correlating with objective tinnitus
    E. Sounds detected by a middle-ear probe in response to sound stimuli and do not require an intact tympanic membrane or ossicular chain

74. **Real-ear probe microphone measures are:**

    A. An unreliable way to verify the hearing aid fitting
    B. Best utilized for hearing aid programming using published adult and pediatric hearing aid guidelines
    C. Extremely time-consuming
    D. Impossible to complete in young children
    E. None of the above

75. What is the greatest average bone-conduction threshold for which osseointegrated implantation is still possible?

    A. 35 dB HL
    B. 45 dB HL
    C. 55 dB HL
    D. 65 dB HL

76. **Which is the most common ossicular abnormality in congenital aural atresia?:**

    A. Fixed stapes footplate
    B. Fused incus–stapes
    C. Fused malleus–incus
    D. Absent incus–long process

77. Which of the following statements regarding the anatomy of the vestibular system is true?

    A. The bilateral anterior semicircular canals respond to the same angular rotations, but just 180 degrees out of phase.

    B. The saccular and anterior and lateral canal nerves run in the anterior branch of the vestibular nerve.

    C. The cell bodies of vestibular afferent nerve fibers are located near the genu of the seventh nerve.

    D. Vestibular afferent nerve fibers project to the vestibular nuclei, cerebellar cortex, and cerebellar nuclei.

    E. The polarities of the hair cells in all of the semicircular canals are arranged such that ampullofugal rotation is excitatory.

78. Sensory hair cells are characterized by which of these?

    A. Express *Atoh1*

    B. Responsive to mechanical stimulation

    C. Form synaptic connections with neurites from spiral ganglia neurons

    D. Contain staircase-like stereocilia

    E. All of the above

79. What is the most common cause of dizziness in elderly patients?

    A. Ménière disease

    B. Benign paroxysmal positional vertigo (BPPV)

    C. Cerebrovascular accident (CVA)

    D. Central neurologic disorder

80. Posterior canal benign paroxysmal positional vertigo (BPPV), provoked by the Dix–Hallpike maneuver, produces nystagmus with the following features *except*:

    A. Delayed onset, appearing several seconds after head positioning

    B. Vertical downbeating nystagmus

    C. Fatigable, becoming weaker with repetitions of the maneuver

    D. Transience, usually lasting 40 seconds or less

81. A person subjected to prolonged constant-velocity rotation in the dark will eventually not perceive that he is rotating. This effect is due to:

    A. The physics of the semicircular canals

    B. Efferent modulation of vestibular hair cells

    C. Depletion of neurotransmitter in the vestibular hair cells

    D. Adaptation of the vestibular nerve fibers

    E. Central nervous system adaptation

82. A 65-year-old man without a significant past medical history presents with a 6-week history of ataxia with progressive worsening. His speech, walking, and eye movements are involved. He has a downbeat nystagmus. Social history is significant for tobacco and ethanol abuse. There is no family history of problems with balance. Which diagnosis should be high on the differential?

    A. Friedreich ataxia
    B. Multiple sclerosis (MS) with a lesion at the root-entry zone
    C. Migraine-associated ataxia
    D. Paraneoplastic antineuronal antibody cerebellar degeneration
    E. Benign paroxysmal positional vertigo (BPPV), horizontal-canal variant

83. Which of the following statements best describes evaluation of nonpulsatile tinnitus?

    A. It should always include an auditory brainstem response (ABR).
    B. It never includes an MRI.
    C. It always includes a temporal bone CT and ABR.
    D. It should always include an audiogram and other testing as indicated by history and physical examination.

84. Which principle measure is used to determine cochlear-implant candidacy?

    A. Three-frequency pure-tone average
    B. Four-frequency pure-tone average
    C. Hearing in noise test (HINT)
    D. Speech discrimination score in the better hearing ear
    E. Speech discrimination score with binaural amplification

85. All of the following may show physical findings in a patient with third-window pathology *except*?

    A. Fistula sign
    B. Tragal compression
    C. Closed-glottis Valsalva maneuver
    D. Hyperventilation
    E. Tullio phenomenon

86. Which of the following indications in congenital aural atresia is the most important determinant of surgical candidacy by CT scan?

    A. Degree of mastoid pneumatization
    B. Size and position of ossicles
    C. Thickness of atretic bone
    D. Size of middle ear

87. **Spontaneous downbeating nystagmus typically localizes to:**

    A. Unilateral posterior semicircular canal crista ampullaris
    B. Uvula or flocculonodular lobes of the cerebellum
    C. Frontal eye fields on the ipsilateral side of the nystagmus
    D. Dorsolateral medullary brainstem (Wallenberg syndrome)
    E. Utricular or saccular maculae (otolithic organs)

88. **Which of the following best describes hearing loss associated with Paget disease?**

    A. Only conductive, secondary to destruction of the ossicles
    B. Only sensorineural, secondary to changes in bone density and geometry in the inner ear
    C. Both conductive and sensorineural, secondary to destruction of the ossicles and compression of the cochlear nerve
    D. Both conductive and sensorineural, secondary to changes in bone density of geometry in the middle and inner ear

89. **Diagnosis of autoimmune inner ear disease (AIED) is made based on:**

    A. Clinical pattern and treatment response consistent with the disease
    B. Serologic testing
    C. History and physical examination findings
    D. Clinical history and positron emission tomography (PET) imaging

90. **Which of the following patients is *not* a good cochlear-implant candidate for developing open-set speech perception?**

    A. Adult patient with bilateral profound hearing loss, patent cochlea, and a recent history of meningitis
    B. 25-year-old man with congenital profound sensorineural hearing loss (SNHL) and lack of spoken language
    C. 1-year-old child with proven connexin-26 mutations and profound SNHL
    D. 80-year-old man with progressive, moderate sloping to profound SNHL, and lack of benefit from conventional amplification via hearing aids

91. Which of the following is true regarding the presence of semicircular canal fistula from erosion by cholesteatoma?

    A. Most patients complain of vertigo.
    B. The majority involve the posterior semicircular canal.
    C. Removal of the matrix from a fistula inevitably results in an anacoustic ear.
    D. It is best managed with topical neomycin.
    E. In an extensive fistula with a contacted mastoid, a canal-wall-down (CWD) procedure is best.

92. The organ of Corti is located in which of the following fluid compartment?

    A. Scala vestibuli
    B. Scala media
    C. Scala tympani
    D. Middle-ear space

93. Which of the following would be the strongest indicator of a central vestibular disorder?

    A. An upbeat, torsional nystagmus that beats down toward the ground (geotropic) in the head-hanging position
    B. Autonomic signs accompanying the vertigo: nausea, vomiting, pallor of the skin, and clamminess
    C. Ocular tilt, skew deviation with diplopia, and a split image vertically
    D. An abrupt onset complete inability to walk, even with assistance, when the patient can normally could ambulate alone
    E. A positive Romberg test, with tilting toward one side repeatedly upon eye closure

94. Which of the following is a shortcoming associated with cartilage-graft tympanoplasty?

    A. Always results in poor hearing outcomes compared with fascia grafting due to thickness and rigidity
    B. Opaqueness may complicate postoperative otoscopic surveillance
    C. Not suitable for use with hostile middle-ear environment
    D. Cannot be utilized for total tympanic-membrane repair

95. Which of the following solutions may be appropriate for an individual with single-sided deafness?

    A. Bone-anchored hearing aid
    B. Contralateral routing of offside signals aid
    C. Frequency modulation system with signal to the good ear
    D. A, B, and C
    E. None of the above

96. Which of the following is the most common site of dehiscence of the Fallopian canal?

    A. Superior to the oval window
    B. At the stylomastoid foramen
    C. At the second genu
    D. Within the facial recess

97. Enhanced nystagmus with gaze in the direction of the fast phase describes:

    A. Ewald law
    B. Posterior semicircular canal (SCC) benign paroxysmal positional vertigo (BPPV)
    C. Horizontal SCC BPPV
    D. Alexander law
    E. A positive head-impulse test

98. A 20-year-old woman presents with episodes of spontaneous vertigo. She has also noted diplopia when looking to the right side, and she has a history of losing the vision in her right eye. On examination, she has internuclear ophthalmoplegia and optic-disc atrophy on the right side. Which of the following studies is most important to diagnose her condition?

    A. A CT scan with contrast of the brain
    B. An MRI with FLAIR (fluid-attenuated inversion recovery) imaging
    C. An audiogram with tympanometry
    D. Vestibular-evoked-myogenic potentials
    E. Vestibular electronystagmogram

99. Which of the following paralytic agents is acceptable during induction when intraoperative facial nerve monitoring is being utilized?

    A. Succinylcholine
    B. Vecuronium
    C. Gallamine
    D. Atracurium

100. In contrast to an intact canal-wall mastoidectomy, the canal-wall-down procedure requires:

    A. Meticulous identification of the fallopian canal
    B. "Blue-lining" the sigmoid sinus
    C. Saucerization of the margins of the mastoidectomy
    D. Thinning of the bone of the tegmen mastoideum

101. Which of the following is *not* a category of presbycusis described by Schuknecht?

   A. Neural
   B. Conductive
   C. Strial
   D. Central

102. Which branchial arches contribute to the development of the auricle?

   A. First and second
   B. Second and third
   C. Third and fourth
   D. First, second, and third

103. In the external auditory canal, the *apopilosebaceous unit* is composed of:

   A. Hair follicles and sebaceous and endocrine glands
   B. Hair follicles sloughed squamous epithelium, and apocrine glands
   C. Hair follicles and sebaceous and apocrine glands
   D. Exfoliated cerumen, hair follicles and sebaceous glands
   E. Glandular secretions, cerumen, and desquamated epithelium

104. Occupational noise exposure is responsible for what percentage of hearing impairment in American adults (all ages, both sexes)?

   A. 5% to 10%
   B. 10% to 20%
   C. 20% to 40%
   D. 40% to 60%
   E. More than 60%

105. Which of the following best describes idiopathic intracranial hypertension?

   A. It can be treated with diuretics.
   B. It will not resolve following cerebrospinal (CSF) diversionary procedures.
   C. It is improved following weight gain.
   D. It cannot be diagnosed with lumbar puncture.

106. A 74-year-old healthy man experienced the onset of sudden right-sided moderate high-frequency sensorineural hearing loss (SNHL) 2 days prior to evaluation and audiometry. The best positive predictor of prognosis for spontaneous hearing recovery in this patient is:

    A. Absence of vestibular symptoms
    B. High frequency hearing loss
    C. Patient age
    D. Lack of systemic comorbidities

107. A patient presents with a conductive hearing loss (CHL) with intact acoustic reflexes. A stapedectomy is performed with no improvement in hearing. What is the most likely cause of this poor result?

    A. Prosthesis displacement
    B. Prosthesis is too short
    C. Undiagnosed lateral chain fixation
    D. Inner-ear third window

108. Which of the following has been or still is associated with vestibular disorders?

    A. An increased prevalence of falls
    B. Dizziness with movement
    C. Anxiety with movement
    D. B and C
    E. All of the above

109. What characteristics are more common in acquired cholesteatoma than in congenital cholesteatoma?

    A. Extension into the cranial cavity
    B. Origin in the anterosuperior mesotympanum
    C. Thickness of epithelial matrix and proliferation of peripheral inflammatory cells
    D. High signal intensity on T2-weighted images

110. **Which are the four fundamental principles of treating external otitis in all stages?**

    A. Application of appropriate medicated drops, control of pain, avoidance of manipulating the ear, and avoiding water exposure

    B. Application of appropriate medicated drops, a broad spectrum oral antibiotic, pain control, and avoiding water exposure

    C. Application of at least two medicated drops, each from separate classes of antibiotics, treatment of associated inflammation and pain, and recommendations for avoidance of future infection

    D. Thorough and meticulous cleaning of the ear, use of appropriate topical and/or oral antibiotics, treatment of pain, avoidance of manipulating the ear, and avoiding water exposure

    E. Cleaning of the ear, acidification of the ear, redebridement of the ear, use of an appropriate long-term drop

111. **Which of the following anatomical relationships is key to surgical identification of the endolymphatic sac?**

    A. Posterior to the lateral semicircular canal

    B. Posterior and inferior to the posterior semicircular canal

    C. Inferior to the round window

    D. Posterior to the round window

112. **Which of the following best describes the head-impulse test?**

    A. Detects utricular abnormalities

    B. Involves linear movement of the head

    C. Requires movement less than 2,000 degrees/second^2

    D. Involves rotational head movements

    E. Head movement is directed in the plane perpendicular to the semicircular canal being tested

113. **Salient clinical features supporting the diagnosis of necrotizing external otitis (NEO) include:**

    A. Persistent otalgia for more than 1 month, solitary polyp in otherwise dry external canal, nondiabetic patient

    B. Persistent otalgia for more than 1 month, persistent purulence, perforation of the tympanic membrane, younger patient

    C. Acute, exquisite otalgia for 24 to 48 hours, purulent discharge from the external canal, swollen external canal, shoddy periauricular lymphadenopathy

    D. Acute, exquisite otalgia for 1 week, purulent discharge from the external canal, swollen external canal, older patient

    E. Persistent otalgia for more than 1 month, persistent purulent granulation tissue, diabetes mellitus, advanced age, immunocompromised state

114. **Radiographically, meningioma of the cerebellopontine angle can be distinguished from acoustic neuroma most reliable by the finding of:**

    A. Enhancement during injection with intravenous contrast
    B. Tumor extension into the internal auditory canal
    C. Salt and pepper pattern on enhanced MRI
    D. Hyperostosis of the adjacent petrous bone

115. **The process of lateral inhibition regulates cell fates between hair cells and supporting cells in the developing cochlea, and is mainly regulated by:**

    A. Brain-derived growth factor
    B. Wnt signaling
    C. Notch signaling
    D. *Atoh1*

116. **What is the stimulation site for an auditory brainstem implant?**

    A. Dorsal cochlear nucleus
    B. Superior olivary complex
    C. Central nucleus of the inferior colliculus
    D. Cochlear nerve
    E. Nucleus solitarius

117. **Auditory steady-state responses (ASSR) differ from auditory brainstem response (ABR) as described by which of the statements below?**

    A. ABRs are better technique for evaluating hearing aid performance.
    B. ABRs can be used for cochlear-implant candidacy for children and adults, whereas ASSR is only indicated for adults.
    C. ASSR can be used to measure frequency-specific information for sound > 120 dB.
    D. ABR is more time efficient (more thresholds measured in a shorter time period).
    E. ABRs are provoked by providing a steady continuous stream of sound to the inner ear.

118. **Noise-induced hearing loss (NIHL) and age-related hearing loss (ARHL) share all of these general characteristics *except*:**

    A. Sensorineural
    B. Accelerating
    C. Symmetrical
    D. High-frequency
    E. Male predominance

119. Congenital aural atresia involves all the following embryonic structures *except*:

    A. Otic capsule
    B. First branchial grove
    C. First branchial arch
    D. Second branchial arch

120. A patient with a long history of unilateral hearing loss and intermittent otorrhea complains of vertigo when exposed to loud sounds and whenever manipulating his auricle. The most likely explanation of these symptoms is:

    A. Superior semicircular canal dehiscence syndrome
    B. Endolymphatic hydrops related to prior serous labyrinthitis
    C. Postinflammatory Ménière disease
    D. Semicircular canal fistula due to cholesteatoma
    E. Suppurative labyrinthitis

121. Abnormalities in pursuit tracking and/or saccade testing are representative of:

    A. Mixed peripheral and central vestibular involvement
    B. An indication of possible peripheral vestibular involvement
    C. Definite lesion in the central vestibular system pathways
    D. An indication of possible central vestibular system involvement

122. During the initial evaluation of a patient with suspected temporal bone fracture, which of the following is *not* indicated?

    A. Bedside hearing evaluation
    B. Evaluate ear canal after irrigating away any debris
    C. Assessment of facial nerve function
    D. Eye examination to check for nystagmus

123. "Real-world" use of hearing protection devices will usually provide at least which degree of effective attenuation (in dB)?

    A. 0
    B. 10
    C. 20
    D. 30
    E. 40

124. In evaluating a patient with a temporal bone fracture, which presentation is most indicative of a facial nerve paralysis due to anatomical discontinuity of the nerve?

    A. A patient with initial presentation of decreased facial movement

    B. A patient with initial presentation of no voluntary facial movement

    C. A patient with initial Glasgow Coma scale of 3

    D. A patient who initially had facial movement, but progresses to no facial movement over the next several days

125. A 30-year-old patient presents with chronic disequilibrium, and a contrasted MRI of the brain reveals an enhancing lesion 2 cm in greatest dimension that fills the left internal auditory canal (IAC) with extension in the cerebellopontine angle (CPA). The pure-tone average on the right is 5 dB and on the left 75 dB, and word recognition scores were 100% on the right and 30% on the left. This patient would benefit most from:

    A. Combined translabyrinthine and suboccipital approach

    B. Translabyrinthine resection of the mass

    C. Middle-cranial fossa approach with division of the superior petrosal sinus and complete tumor resection

    D. Retrolabyrinthine approach to the CPA

126. Which of the following signs is often present in the anterior inferior cerebellar infarct (AICA), but not in the posterior inferior cerebellar infarct (PICA) or Wallenberg syndrome?

    A. Spontaneous, rotational vertigo with nystagmus

    B. Facial paralysis

    C. Profound hearing loss

    D. Truncal ataxia with difficulty or inability to ambulate

    E. Horner syndrome (miosis of the ipsilateral pupil)

127. Vestibular schwannomas most commonly originate from:

    A. The neural components of the vestibular nerves

    B. The Schwann cells medial to the Obersteiner–Redlich zone

    C. The neural components of the cochlear nerve

    D. Intracanalicular vestibular nerves and may extend into the cerebellopontine angle

128. Where is the most common site of origin of acquired cholesteatoma?

    A. Anterior epitympanum
    B. Posterior epitympanum
    C. Posterior mesotympanum
    D. Anterior mesotympanum
    E. Inferior mesotympanum

129. All of the following pathogens can cause sensorineural hearing loss *except*:

    A. Human immunodeficiency virus (HIV)
    B. Cytomegalovirus
    C. Coxsackie virus
    D. Varicella zoster virus

130. During a routine stapedectomy, the facial nerve is found to completely cover the stapes footplate. What is the best option in this setting?

    A. Decompress the facial nerve and perform a stapedotomy
    B. Decompress the facial nerve and perform a stapedectomy
    C. Amplification with a hearing aid
    D. Stapedotomy between the facial nerve and the round window

131. A 46-year-old woman reports with a 9-year history of progressive hearing loss in the right ear. An audiogram shows mild to moderate sensorineural hearing loss in the right ear, and an MRI of the brain shows an enhancing mass on the right that erodes the posterior face of the petrous bone. What other diagnostic studies would be appropriate in this patient?

    A. Echocardiogram
    B. Genetic testing to evaluate for mutation on chromosome 22
    C. Renal ultrasound
    D. Vestibular-evoked myogenic potential testing

132. Autoimmune inner ear disease (AIED) is defined as:

    A. A progressive unilateral sensorineural hearing loss (SNHL) that responds to immunosuppressant therapy
    B. A progressive bilateral SHNL that responds to immunosuppressant therapy
    C. A progressive bilateral SNHL that does not respond to immunosuppressant therapy
    D. A sudden bilateral SNHL that responds to immunosuppressant therapy

133. Stem cells are characterized by:

    A. Asymmetric division
    B. Ability to self-renew
    C. Pluripotency
    D. All of the above

134. Which of the following statements best describes treatments for nonpulsatile tinnitus?

    A. They are a waste of time and money.
    B. They should never be attempted in the setting of psychiatric disease.
    C. They may include acupuncture, meditation, and massage.
    D. They may worsen tinnitus.

135. A 13-year-old girl presents with generalized headache, neck stiffness, and diplopia 2 weeks after a course of amoxicillin for acute otitis media. Gadolinium-enhanced MRI with MRV is most likely to demonstrate:

    A. Sigmoid sinus occlusion with ventricular dilatation
    B. Sigmoid sinus occlusion without ventricular dilatation
    C. Petrous apex abscess
    D. Epidural abscess
    E. Brain abscess

136. Mutations in which of the following gene have been identified to be associated with Pendred syndrome?

    A. *GJB2*
    B. *COCH*
    C. *SLC26A4*
    D. *PAX3*

137. Which is *not* a function of the middle-ear muscles?

    A. Protect from loud sound
    B. Contribute to the blood supply of the ossicular chain
    C. Decrease the dynamic range of the middle ear
    D. Reduce noise caused by chewing and vocalization
    E. Improve signal-to-noise ratio for high-frequency signals

138. A patient presents with a conductive hearing loss and negative Rinne tuning fork test (BC>AC). They also report episodic vertigo, low-pitched tinnitus, and ear fullness. What is the best management option for their hearing loss?

    A. Stapedotomy

    B. Amplification with a hearing aid

    C. Partial stapedectomy

    D. Stapes mobilization

139. Which of the following maneuvers may require reestablishment of an intraoperative baseline auditory brainstem response (ABR) prior to manipulation of the auditory system?

    A. Retraction of the cerebellum

    B. Opening of the dura

    C. Irrigation

    D. Acoustic masking from drilling noise

140. Which of the following platinum-containing chemotherapy drugs causes the least ototoxicity?

    A. Cisplatin

    B. Oxaliplatin

    C. Nedaplatin

    D. Carboplatin

141. Which complication would be expected to occur more often with overlay as compared to underlay tympanoplasty techniques?

    A. Malleus fixation to the anterior canal wall by scar tissue

    B. Graft failure due to medial displacement

    C. Excessive postoperative middle-ear adhesions

    D. Postoperative middle-ear effusion

142. The preferred series of radiographies for the initial evaluation of a suspected paraganglioma is:

    A. High-resolution CT and MRI

    B. High-resolution CT and MR angiography

    C. High-resolution CT and arteriography

    D. MRI and octreotide scintigraphy

143. Risk factors for nonpulsatile tinnitus include:

    A. Psychiatric disease
    B. Fenestral otosclerosis (OS)
    C. Sensorineural hearing loss (SNHL)
    D. All of the above

144. Which of the following electrocochleographic responses is atypical for the associated pathology?

    A. Reduced summating potential/action potential (SP/AP) ratio in superior semicircular canal dehiscence
    B. Increased SP/AP ratio in Ménière disease
    C. Increased SP/AP ratio in perilymph fistula
    D. Absent in profound sensorineural hearing loss

145. A 7-year-old, otherwise healthy child with a normal otologic examination experiences a unilateral sudden mixed hearing loss documented by pure-tone audiometry. The most appropriate additional study is:

    A. Auditory brainstem-response audiometry
    B. Distortion product otoacoustic emissions
    C. MRI
    D. Ultrasound
    E. Exploratory tympanotomy

146. Which of these factors is nearly as important as occupational noise exposure as a cause of adult hearing loss in America?

    A. Use of MP3 players
    B. Ototoxicity
    C. Head injury
    D. Recreational shooting
    E. Acoustic tumors

147. A 65-year-old patient has a 1-year history of left pulsatile tinnitus. An MRI reveals a brightly enhancing diffuse lesion in the left jugular foramen with multiple flow voids. During surgical resection of this mass, proximal and distal venous control is obtained. Which vessel is most likely to complicate surgical resection of this mass?

    A. Cavernous sinus
    B. Basilar artery
    C. Inferior petrosal sinus
    D. Superior petrosal sinus

148. Aminoglycoside susceptibility is affected by which of the following genetic inheritance pathways?

    A. Autosomal dominant
    B. Autosomal recessive
    C. X-linked
    D. Mitochondrial
    E. None of the above

149. In congenital malformation of the ear canal and middle ear, compared to normal course, the facial nerve course is typically:

    A. More anteriorly displaced only
    B. More anteriorly and laterally (superficially) displaced
    C. More posteriorly displaced only
    D. More posteriorly and medially (deeply) displaced

150. Which of these best describes pulsatile tinnitus during pregnancy?

    A. It will not resolve postpartum.
    B. It indicates preeclampsia.
    C. It occurs due to a high-flow state.
    D. It can be treated by plasmapheresis.

151. A 31-year-old man with chronic otitis media resulting in cholesteatoma. Which complication is depicted on this image?

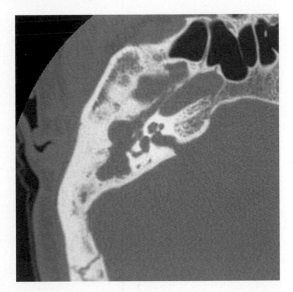

   A. Lateral semicircular canal fistula
   B. Tegmen tympani erosion
   C. Tegmen mastoideum erosion
   D. Fallopian canal erosion
   E. Cerebral abscess

152. A young adult with microtia. What surgically important structure is depicted by the arrow?

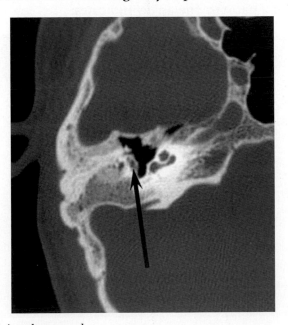

   A. Posterior semicircular canal
   B. Lateralized facial nerve
   C. Dysmorphic ossicles
   D. Enlarged vestibular aqueduct
   E. Stapes footplate sclerosis

153. A 60-year-old with hearing loss. What pattern of hearing loss would be expected with this CT appearance?

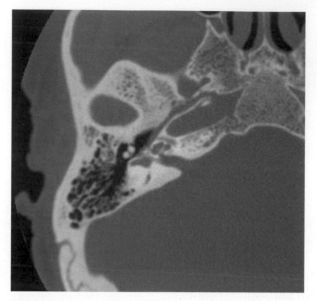

    A. Conductive hearing loss

    B. Sensorineural hearing loss

    C. Mixed hearing loss

    D. Intact hearing

    E. Tullio phenomenon

154. An 8-year-old trauma patient. The arrow indicates:

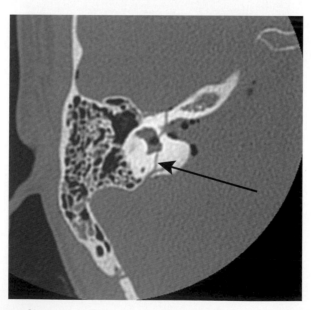

    A. A normal suture line

    B. The vestibular aqueduct

    C. The superior petrosal vein

    D. The subarcuate canal

    E. A capsule-violating temporal bone fracture

155. **An 89-year-old man in motor vehicle accident. What is the most likely cause for his hearing loss?**

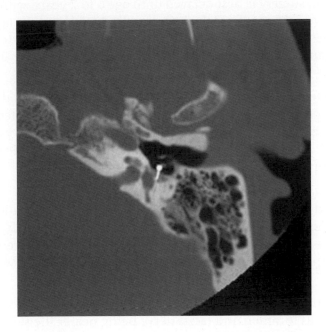

A. Recurrent cholesteatoma

B. Capsule-violating temporal bone fracture

C. Displaced stapes prosthesis

D. Otosclerosis

E. Perilymphatic fistula

Chapter 9 Answers

1. **Answer: B.** Atresia surgery is best delayed until age 6 to 7 years, with use of a bone-vibrator hearing aid before this age is reached. Currently, the minimum age for BAHA implantation is 5 years per FDA guidelines. A "soft band" that holds an external BAHA sound processor firmly against the skull can be worn by infants. PAGES 2389 AND 2396

2. **Answer: C.** The lesion being described is most likely an arachnoid cyst. This is characterized as being hypointense in T1 and hyperintense on T2. Other lesions with those signal characteristics are chordoma and chondrosarcoma. However, they are destructive infiltrative tumors and do not appear as a smooth nonenhancing lesion. MRI with FLAIR sequencing will appear hypointense in arachnoid cysts. PAGE 2577

3. **Answer: E.** Based on the morphology of their peripheral terminations, vestibular afferent neurons are classified as one of three distinct types: bouton, calyx, or dimorphic. Calyx afferent neurons with their calyceal endings terminate exclusively on type I hair cells, where they can innervate anywhere from one to five hair cells. PAGE 2295

4. **Answer: B.** The mastoid and the tympanic bones are poorly developed in infants, resulting in the stylomastoid foramen and facial nerve being nearer the skin surface than in adults. PAGE 2451 AND FIGURES 152.1 AND 152.5

5. **Answer: D.** One oft-neglected aspect of neotympanic membrane creation in a canal wall down situation is that exteriorization of the epitympanum usually involves opening the communication of the anterior epitympanum with the supratubal recess. If this opening, located anterior and superior to the tensor tympani tendon is not recognized and separated by the accounted for with graft material the barrier separation between the moist middle-ear mucosa and the epithelialized open-mastoid cavity will not occur. This often results in a tympanic membrane perforation and mucosalization from the middle ear to the mastoid cavity causing weeping and more frequent chronic cavity care. PAGE 2477

6. **Answer: D.** The incidence of meningitis in patients with CSF leaks ranges from 2% to 88%. The wide range in incidence is a result of multiple factors, the most significant of which is the duration of leakage. PAGE 2424

7. **Answer: C.** This is an established threshold of 85 dBA where a hearing conservation program must be initiated when time-weighted average of noise exposure over an 8-hour shift is at or exceeds that level. PAGE 2538

8. **Answer: B.** Sigmoid sinus thrombosis may present with the rapid onset of prominent otologic symptoms (otorrhea, otalgia, and postauricular pain/erythema), severe headache, torticollis, and the classic high-spiking "picket fence" fever of sepsis with leukocytosis. PAGE 2406

9. **Answer: C.** Experimental studies suggest that the mechanism of toxicity from lead poisoning is neurogenic and is not within the organ of Corti. PAGE 2544

10. **Answer: C.** The initial primary treatment for presumed autoimmune inner-ear disease is oral steroids modified by the patient's weight and response to treatment. The other methods of immunosuppression for breakthrough or salvage include cyclophosphamide, methotrexate, etanercept, and intratympanic steroids. PAGES 2525, 2526

11. **Answer: D.** All three audiometric tests can be used to monitor potential ototoxicity. High-frequency loss occurs initially. OAEs reflect the integrity of the outer hair cells, which are more susceptible to ototoxicity. PAGE 2547

12. **Answer: E.** The first step is to determine the degree of sensorineural hearing loss for four test frequencies (500, 1,000, 2,000, and 3,000 Hz) from the audiogram. Though functionally important word recognition scores are not considered in the calculation of hearing impairment. PAGE 2277

13. **Answer: D.** Approximately 10% to 15% of cases are due to an identifiable etiology. (PAGE 2589). Patients are directed to have an MRI, which is routinely normal. Metabolic blood tests are of limited utility. The pathophysiology of SSNHL includes a vascular (ischemic) source, inner-ear membrane break, and viral infection. These sources cannot be verified with existing diagnostic tools.

14. **Answer: A.** Migraine, anxiety, and strabismus may compound problems with recovery from a peripheral vestibular insult. Age, alone, does not affect compensation. (PAGE 2739) It would have to be accompanied by other disorders such as cerebellar dysfunction, peripheral hypoesthesia (altered proprioception), or compromised vision.

15. **Answer: C.** Electrogustometry, though conveying information along the chorda tympani nerve, is an insensitive measure of facial nerve function and recovery. Nerve excitability, maximum stimulation, and electroneuronography provide evidence of nerve integrity and function. Physical examination showing evidence of residual facial muscular motion is a good prognostic sign. PAGE 2507

16. **Answer: C.** Lipoma and facial and vestibular schwannomas are all slowly growing tumors of the IAC. Metastatic breast cancer has a more aggressive growth pattern and presentation. PAGE 2578

17. **Answer: C.** The rapid onset of meningitis with AOM in a child with SNHL may indicate the presence of an inner-ear malformation that allows communication through the oval or round windows to the vestibule, cochlea, and internal auditory canal. Accordingly, temporal bone imaging may reveal Mondini malformation, enlarged vestibular aqueduct, common cavity malformation, or congenital stapes footplate fixation. PAGE 2405

18. **Answer: D.** The greater superficial petrosal nerve is most proximal, followed by branch to the stapedius, chorda tympani, branch to the digastric, and branch to platysma. PAGES 2503–2504

19. **Answer: B.** The disadvantages (of incus interposition) are that there is a low possibility of continued necrosis, the incus may not be available in all cases, and autologous ossicular grafts tend to fuse strongly to engaged native ossicles or to other adjacent structures such that revision surgery can be challenging. PAGES 2479–2480

20. **Answer: B.** The EAC is derived from the first ectodermal branchial groove between the mandibular (I) and hyoid (II) arches. PAGE 2333

21. **Answer: E.** Hair cells (inner and outer) and spiral ganglion neurons provide the auditory pathway for electrical sound transmission. Supporting cells are critical to homeostasis of the structural environment of the organ of Corti. The supporting cells may be capable of differentiating into hair cells. PAGES 2747, 2749

22. **Answer: C.** Middle ear implants are an appropriate option for patients with bilateral non-progressive symmetric moderated to severe sensorineural hearing loss with speech discrimination greater that 40%, no evidence of middle ear disease, and having had limited benefit from conventional hearing aids. At present, they are contraindicated by FDA guidelines in patients with conductive hearing loss. At the time of this writing there are current trials investigating whether round window placement of the SoundBridge device is of benefit for conductive hearing loss not amenable to other surgery or hearing aid. PAGES 2641–46

23. **Answer: A.** Brain herniation may develop following previous mastoid procedures, presenting as an encephalocele or meningoencephalocele through a defect in the tegmen tympani or tegmen mastoideum. The etiology is thought secondary to aggressive drilling that exposes and traumatizes the dura during previous mastoid surgery. PAGE 2444

24. **Answer: E.** The tympanic membrane has a trilaminar origin of ectoderm from the floor of the first branchial cleft laterally as the epidermal layer, endoderm of the first pharyngeal pouch medially as the mucosal layer, and neural crest mesenchyme with cephalic mesoderm interposed as the fibrous layer. PAGE 2241

25. **Answer: E.** All are correct. Patients with migraine often are intolerant of activities with increased visual motion in their peripheral vision. Anxiety and fear of falling impede their ability to participate in challenging eye and motion exercises. PAGE 2736

26. **Answer: A.** A practical categorization divides inner-ear anomalies into those affecting the osseous and membranous labyrinth and those affecting the membranous labyrinth alone. As many as 20% of patients with congenital sensorineural hearing loss fall into the first category, which can be identified with radiologic techniques. PAGE 2248

27. **Answer: B.** Tc-99m bone scanning and Ga-67 scanning have been advocated in the evaluation of SBO. Their sensitivity for the presence of infection is far greater than their specificity for the cause. Tc-99m scanning gives excellent information about bone function but poor information about bone structure. PAGE 2341

28. **Answer: B.** Lymphoscintigraphy with sentinel node biopsy has been recommended in appropriate surgical candidates with Breslow depth ≥0.76 mm, and is becoming established as the standard of care. PAGE 2368

29. **Answer: A.** With high rates of recurrence or recidivistic disease, especially with canal-wall-up or canal-wall-reconstruction procedures, monitoring the mastoid for cholesteatoma has become extremely important. PAGE 2437

30. **Answer: C.** Petrous apicitis is classically characterized by deep retroorbital pain, abducens nerve palsy, and otorrhea (Gradenigo syndrome). Pain is likely carried by cranial nerve V but this is not a provided option (PAGE 2458)

31. **Answer: D.** The direction of nystagmus with *right* posterior canal BPPV is upbeating (toward the forehead), geotropic (beating toward the ground), and torsional (counter-clockwise). PAGE 2693

32. **Answer: C.** The Centers for Disease Control and Prevention provides guidelines updated for pneumococcal vaccination in patients who are to receive or have received a cochlear implant. (Page 2637 discusses *S. pneumoniae* and the FDA.) The entry into the cochlea via round window or separate cochleostomy should be sealed with an autograft. Coating the array with antibiotics does not protect an infection from subsequently occurring. There was a high rate of meningitis infections when a separate positioner was used to push the electrode closer to the modiolus. (PAGES 2625, 2637; 2625 – REF 49) (Page 2637 discusses "best outcomes from cochlear implants" in the section Clinical Results [right-hand column].)

33. **Answer: E.** Hearing loss can add to problems of social isolation, impaired communication, and compromised medical health. (PAGE 2654) Withdrawal from social settings may exacerbate the symptoms of dementia and Alzheimer disease.

34. **Answer: B.** Applebaum prosthesis is a type II ossicular chain repair. The other options are Type III repairs. The reader is encourage to review this modified classification as it has change from the original classification system which was based on reconstruction methods that were not available at that time. PAGE 2479

35. **Answer: A.** The answer to this question is fundamental to the evaluation of unexplained asymmetric SNHL. Support for the correct response is given on page 2611. Radiologic studies may be ordered as deemed necessary, especially with asymmetric otologic complaints. MRI is the most sensitive test for determining retrocochlear hearing loss. Laboratory evaluation has a low yield. CT would be able to show retrocochlear pathology of a large tumor. Hearing aid evaluation is premature in the management plan. ABR is not a sensitive as a MRI.

36. **Answer: C.** In nerve excitability testing, the branches of the facial nerve are stimulated on both the injured side and the contralateral side, which serves as a control. The current used is incrementally increased just until threshold is reached, manifested by facial twitching, and this threshold level is recorded for each side individually. A threshold difference of 3.5 mA or greater between the affected and nonaffected sides of the face suggests significant neural degeneration. 92% in decline of response at 5 days ofter the uinjury has a poorer prognosis for complete recovery. A 74% reduction in the response at 2 days is premature to estimate the degree of injury. PAGE 2418

37. **Answer: D.** Mondini deformity has a higher likelihood of trauma causing leakage of CSF and perilymph from the inner to middle ear. (PAGE 2706) BPPV and labyrinthine concussion do not entail hearing loss. Cochlea concussion, an option not offered, describes hearing loss from trauma.

38. **Answer: C.** Conductive hearing loss from the middle ear (fluid or ossicular disorder) has absent reflexes. The presence of an intact stapedial reflex suggests a third-window disorder. Thin-cut bone window CT imaging should identify the pathology. Since the patient likely came to you with a complaint, observation is not appropriate and evaluation warranted. PAGES 2710, 2711

39. **Answer: B.** Facial nerve abnormalities are common in major atresia patients. The anticipated abnormalities include complete dehiscence of the tympanic segment, inferior displacement of the tympanic segment, and anterior and lateral displacement of the mastoid segment. PAGE 2394

40. **Answer: B.** A number of findings point toward a viral etiology for OS. Measles antigens and RNA, as well as nucleocapsid structures identical to measles virus have all been identified in OS lesions. Increased levels of measles-specific IgG have also been detected in the perilymph of OS patients undergoing stapedectomy. It is not yet certain that the measles virus is involved in the development of OS, and the pathogenesis is yet to be elucidated. PAGE 2488

41. **Answer: B.** Determination of extent and site of lesion within the peripheral and central vestibular system. PAGE 2303

42. **Answer: C.** Several studies have attempted to evaluate the prognostic value of intraoperative ABR although their significance is unclear, but certain intraoperative ABR patterns are associated with postoperative hearing outcomes. Persistence of wave V at the conclusion of the procedure has been associated with serviceable hearing. Similarly, complete elimination or irreversible and progressive loss of wave V indicates a high likelihood of postoperative hearing loss. PAGE 2317

43. **Answer: A.** Clinically, ECochG may be used to predict postoperative audition and is sensitive to changes in cochlear blood supply. PAGE 2318

44. **Answer: A.** There is a two- to tenfold increase in CSF fistula in otic capsule-disrupting fractures as well as a much greater risk of intracranial injuries, compared to otic capsule-sparing fractures. PAGE 2412

45. **Answer: B.** Peripheral vestibular nystagmus is suppressed with visual fixation, is generally horizontal-rotary, can be more easily detected after headshaking, and has normal oculomotor tests. (Page 2694, Table 165.5 nicely summarizes the symptoms and physical examination findings of peripheral vestibular versus central nervous system disease.)

46. **Answer: A.** Eye care is important to prevent cornea/conjunctiva problems from dryness and exposure. Early intervention with oral steroids and antiviral medication has been shown to provide better opportunity for recovery if given within the first 72 hours. Beyond this time, it is not clear that antiviral medications provide benefit. PAGE 2512

47. **Answer: B.** Treat the facial nerve as if it is dehiscent until proven otherwise, especially in the tympanic segment. This is important in middle ear and stapes surgery. PAGE 2327

48. **Answer: C.** The A train has been shown to be the only intraoperative EMG pattern associated with deterioration of facial nerve function. PAGE 2327

49. **Answer: B.** Chordomas are divided into histologic subtypes, but the main microscopic features are stellate, intermediate, and vacuolated physaliphorous or soap-bubble cells in a mucoid matrix growing in nests, cords, or trabeculae. Immunohistochemical staining is positive for cytokeratin and epithelial membrane antigen, which helps to distinguish chordoma from chondrosarcoma. PAGE 2374

50. **Answer: D.** Factors that may contribute to the cochlear amplifier include motility of outer hair cells and the mechanical properties of the stereocilia and tectorial membrane. PAGE 2258

51. **Answer: E.** Bandwidth out to 8,000 to 9,000 Hz is necessary for correct perception of sound(s) for young children. PAGE 2664

52. **Answer: C.** Two-thirds of the middle-ear congenital cholesteatomas are seen as a white mass in the anterior–superior quadrant PAGE 2433

53. **Answer: B.** A positive response on electrocochleography is an elevated SP/AP ratio > 0.5. Caloric testing often identifies a reduced caloric response on the involved side and demonstrates elevated VEMP thresholds. Early endolymphatic hydrops may present with a low-frequency conductive loss, but the more likely finding is ipsilateral low-frequency up-sloping sensorineural hearing loss. PAGE 2703

54. **Answer: D.** SSRI medications are antidepressants and can offer relief to those with anxiety and dizziness. There may be benefit for patients with migraine variants, but that was not an option. Patients with visual vertigo and space and motion discomfort respond well to this class of medications. (PAGE 2740) They provide no significant help to those with Ménière disease, neuritis, or labyrinthitis.

55. **Answer: A.** Assuming the original procedure was successful, the question suggests the prosthesis has migrated out of the oval window opening and eroded the distal incus. If enough incus remains a crimp on piston could be used again (E) however the length should be longer, not shorter. Of the options given a notched-bucket handle would be best suited though the stapedotomy opening may need to be made larger and a tissue graft obtained. The other options are incorrect since they indicated repair to the residual footplate. Since there was otosclerosis initially repair must be to the vestibule. PAGE 2499

56. **Answer: B.** Given the presentation of otosyphilis, hearing loss and peripheral vestibular loss can be identified. SNHL is common in both congenital syphilis and late-acquired syphilis. The otic capsule may be involved with secondary and/or tertiary stages of infection. Hearing loss may not be present in congenital syphilis. Hearing loss may be stabilized with antibiotic treatment, but was reported to improve in less than one-third of treated patients. PAGE 2521

57. **Answer: E.** Aminoglycosides and cisplatin are well known to cause sensorineural hearing loss, predominately in the high frequencies. (PAGE 2543) Loop diuretics are a rare cause of hearing loss but can be enhanced with impaired renal function, prematurity, and concomitant use of aminoglycosides. PAGE 2544

58. **Answer: C.** Chronic imbalance defines an ongoing dysfunction likely from the vestibular system. Vestibular neuritis, vertebrobasilar insufficiency, and migraine-associated vertigo are short-lived acute events that may be recurrent. Bilateral vestibulopathy is chronic and possibly from ototoxic medication. PAGE 2620

59. **Answer: A.** Facial paralysis from AOM typically responds to drainage and antibiotics. Delayed facial paralysis following temporal bone trauma also has a favorable prognosis. Penetrating trauma and metastatic cancer are unlikely to resolve. The prognosis for Ramsay Hunt syndrome is poor for good to normal recovery. PAGE 2513

60. **Answer: E.** Stroke affects one side of the brain and the contralateral side of the face. Lyme disease, metastatic carcinoma, skull base osteomyelitis, and Guillain–Barré syndrome can cause bilateral facial paralysis. Other disease processes that can have bilateral facial paralysis include severe trauma causing bilateral temporal bone fractures, sarcoid, and intracranial infection. PAGE 2507–TABLE 155.3

61. **Answer: A.** See the analogous case history on page 2311. PAGE 2311

62. **Answer: A.** On-axis total body rotation—rotational chair: The purpose of the test is to expand the investigation of the peripheral vestibular system by applying natural head movements and using three outcome parameters to characterize the peripheral vestibular system. PAGE 2307

63. **Answer: E.** Hearing in the midst of noise can be challenging. People comfortable with hearing aid use in all settings, those using bilateral hearing aids fitted with directional microphones, or those using assistive listening devices (infrared or FM systems) can facilitate better function in noisy situations. PAGES 2665, 2670

64. **Answer: B.** Patients in whom there is no audiometric improvement within 2 weeks of presentation are unlikely to demonstrate much recovery. PAGE 2594

65. **Answer: D.** The purpose of the SOT is to determine the individual's ability to utilize visual, proprioceptive/somatosensory, and vestibular cues for maintaining quiet stance. PAGE 2309

66. **Answer: D.** With bone-conduction stimulation, interaural attenuation is <10 dB. PAGE 2276

67. **Answer: A.** Unlike the other cochlear potentials, the endocochlear potential is not generated in response to acoustic stimulation. PAGE 2262

68. **Answer: B.** The changes in vestibular function in the elderly assessed by VEMP testing reveal decrease in amplitude. PAGE 2618 The thresholds and latency are not characteristically altered.

69. **Answer: C.** When facial paralysis occurs due to cholesteatoma, the site of lesion depends on the anatomy of the cholesteatoma. Most commonly, the nerve is compromised in the tympanic segment, due to bone erosion by the cholesteatoma. PAGE 2404

70. **Answer: A.** OAEs are generally not detected in patients with middle-ear pathology and conductive hearing loss. PAGE 2284

71. **Answer: D.** Repositioning otoconia from the posterior semicircular canal back into the vestibule may still incur space and motion disorientation. This can be manifested by altering the perception of earth vertical and problems with navigation. PAGE 2737

72. **Answer: A.** Of the choices offered, transtympanic steroid injection is the best choice. A medrol dose pack may not provide sufficient dosing for body weight if the patient is insulin-dependent. Antiviral medications have not been shown to be effective in idiopathic sudden SNHL. (PAGE 2593) Carbogen (5% carbon dioxide and 95% oxygen) is considered a vasodilator and increases perilymph oxygen tension. Support for hyperbaric oxygen is limited. PAGES 2592–2593

73. **Answer: C.** OAEs also are used widely in clinical situations. The responses are generated by sound stimulation. The transient-evoked otoacoustic emission and distortion product otoacoustic emission techniques complement each other. PAGE 2269

74. **Answer: B.** Real-ear probe measurement provides an objective and reliable means of programming a hearing aid, is a relatively quick procedure, and is most useful in young children. PAGE 2667

75. **Answer: D.** Currently each manufacturer defines his own thresholds for an osseointegrated implant. At the time of this writing, the Cordell (body-worn BAHA processor) can be used with a 65-dB average bone threshold. PAGE 2639

76. **Answer: C.** In major atresia cases, the expected finding is a fused and deformed malleus–incus complex. PAGE 2394

77. **Answer: D.** Central axonal branches of primary afferent neurons ramify in the vestibular nuclei. Afferent terminals from the different end organs primarily innervate the various divisions of the vestibular nuclei, although vestibular afferent terminations are seen in the cerebellum and other brainstem nuclei as well. PAGE 2299

78. **Answer: E.** Sensory hair cells possess all of the attributes provided by the four choices in the question. They have staircase-like stereocilia with a single kinocilium, connect to proximal neurites from spiral ganglion cells, are responsive to mechanical stimulation, and express *Atoh1*. PAGES 2747, 2749

79. **Answer: B.** BPPV is considered to be the most common cause of dizziness in the elderly. Idiopathic vestibulopathy, migraine dizziness, and Ménière disease are close behind. CVA is relatively rare. PAGE 2615

80. **Answer: B.** The direction of nystagmus with posterior canal BPPV is upbeating (toward the forehead), geotropic (beating toward the ground), and torsional. It is delayed in onset, fatigable, and of brief duration. Vertical downbeating nystagmus suggests a disorder in the brainstem. PAGES 2708, 2709

81. **Answer: A.** Steinhausen torsion-pendulum model predicts that deflection of the cupula is proportional to head velocity so long as the frequency of head velocity falls between 0.1 and 10 Hz. Beyond the boundaries of this frequency range, however, the sensitivity of the semicircular canal to velocity decreases as cupular deflection under these conditions is not as great. At 0 Hz, which corresponds to constant-velocity rotation, the torsion-pendulum model predicts there will be no response. PAGES 2297–2298

82. **Answer: D.** The presentation should raise suspicion of a paraneoplastic process triggering subacute cerebellar ataxia (PAGE 2729) . Given the smoking history, small cell carcinoma of the lung should be considered. Friedreich ataxia is seen in the young population in the first three decades. (PAGE 2729) The history and neurologic findings of this patient are not consistent with a root-entry zone lesion from MS. This is not a manifestation of BPPV from any canal.

83. **Answer: D.** The evaluation of tinnitus begins with a thorough history and physical examination. An audiogram is necessary to provide important insight into the function of the auditory system. Subsequent workup, including imaging, is determined by the information gathered. PAGE 2601

84. **Answer: C.** HINT is a key measure of auditory performance used to screen hearing-impaired individuals for cochlear-implant candidates. PAGE 2278

85. **Answer: D.** Tragal compression and Tullio phenomenon (increased sound wave compression on the tympanic membrane) both increase the pressure to the middle and inner ear. Valsalva maneuver increases intracranial pressure, as does cough or heavy-weight lifting, causing ampullopetal stimulation of a dehiscent superior semicircular canal. (PAGES 2697, 2698) Hyperventilation does not enhance a third-window problem, but does affect cerebral perfusion with a drop in CO_2, vasoconstriction, and decreased intracranial pressure. It may induce dizziness in patients with anxiety or demyelinating disease. PAGE 2698

86. **Answer: D.** Hypoplasia of the middle-ear space, ranging from mild to severe, occurs in most cases of congenital atresia, and ossicular development can be expected to correlate directly with middle-ear size. The risk of surgical complications will be minimized, and the chances for a successful hearing result are increased if the middle ear and mastoid size are at least two-thirds of the normal size and if all three ossicles, although deformed, can be identified. PAGE 2388

87. **Answer: B.** Downbeating nystagmus often localizes to the cervicomedullary junction and midline brain. Pathologies include cerebellar ataxia, vertebrobasilar ischemia, multiple sclerosis, and Arnold–Chiari malformation. The latter creates increased pressure on the flocculonodular region. (PAGES 2720–2721) Wallenberg syndrome may have eye saccades to the side of the dorsolateral medullary stroke. PAGES 2725–2726

88. **Answer: D.** Paget disease affects the otic capsule creating bone remodeling and causes both sensorineural and conductive hearing loss. Bony overgrowth encroaching on the middle-ear ossicles may contribute to a conductive loss. The cochlear nerve is not compressed and the ossicles are not destroyed. There is demineralization of the otic capsule which causes both types of loss. PAGE 2526

89. **Answer: A.** The diagnosis is construed in the setting of a normal physical examination and progressive bilateral sensorineural hearing loss that responds to immunosuppression. There are no consistent markers for AIED (serologic testing), physical examination, or imaging findings (PET scan). PAGE 2524

90. **Answer: B.** Answers A, C, and D all are appropriate cochlear-implant candidates and should do well. A prelingual deaf adult with no oral language is a poor cochlear-implant candidate. PAGE 2628

91. **Answer: E.** Most patients with canal erosion do not have vertigo. They predominately affect the horizontal semicircular canal. With care the matrix can be removed if the defect is small and localized. Neomycin is ototoxic and should be avoided. If the fistula involves one of the semicircular canals and if the mastoid is small, a CWD mastoidectomy, leaving the matrix on the fistula, is appropriate. PAGE 2443

92. **Answer: B.** The organ of Corti lies within the scala media, which contains endolymph. The scala vestibuli and tympani both contain perilymph and no neural structures. PAGE 2751

93. **Answer: D.** A patient with rapid-onset imbalance and inability to walk suggests an acute central event, such as Wallenberg stroke. (PAGE 2717) Answers A, B, C, and E can all be seen in an acute peripheral vestibular event.

94. **Answer: B.** Postoperative appearance of tympanic membrane after total drum reconstruction using a composite perichondrium–cartilage island graft (shows opaqueness of cartilage-graft tympanoplasty). PAGE 2483, FIGURE 153.10

95. **Answer: D.** All three options are available and appropriate to an individual with single-sided deafness. This holds also for other osseointegrated implantable devices (Pronto, Alpha 2) and SoundBite. (PAGES 2656–2657) There will likely be other brand name implants and devices available in the future.

96. **Answer: A.** The facial nerve is dehiscent approximately 50% of the time just superior to the oval window in its tympanic segment. PAGE 2453

97. **Answer: D.** Enhanced nystagmus is the definition of Alexander law. (PAGE 2685) Ewald's three laws describe the effect of nystagmus relative to stimulation of the SCC. (PAGE 2687) Posterior and horizontal BPPV is nystagmus elicited by position change if otoconia are free floating or adherent to the crista ampullaris. A positive-impulse test is also brought on by head movement (assessing the SCC) and does not entail direction of gaze.

98. **Answer: B.** The symptoms and signs are suggestive of multiple sclerosis. MRI with FLAIR sequences is the most sensitive test listed amongst the options provided. (PAGE 2728) A contrast CT, audiogram, or other vestibular tests do not provide specific answers to identify the source of pathology.

99. **Answer: A.** Succinylcholine is used for induction because of its short duration of effect with complete recovery from neuromuscular blockade within 15 minutes. Atracurium and vecuronium typically induce paralysis for up to 30 minutes. (PAGE 2326)

100. **Answer: C.** Saucerization makes the cavity shallow by allowing surrounding soft tissues to prolapse inward. PAGE 2455

101. **Answer: D.** Schuknecht identified four categories of presbycusis based on clinical and histopathologic changes within the cochlea. They are sensory, conductive, strial, and neural. He did not define central presbycusis. PAGE 2617

102. **Answer: A.** From the fifth week of gestation, three hillocks arise on the first branchial (mandibular) arch (hillocks 1–3) and three arise on the second branchial (hyoid) arch (hillocks 4–6) on either side of the first branchial cleft. PAGE 2239

103. **Answer: C.** The skin of the cartilaginous canal contains many hair cells and sebaceous and apocrine glands such as cerumen glands. Together, these three adnexal structures provide a protective function and are termed the *apopilosebaceous unit.* PAGE 2333

104. **Answer: A.** Occupational and nonoccupational noise have *each* been estimated to cause 5% to 10% of the adult hearing burden in the United States. PAGE 2534

105. **Answer: A.** Intracranial hypertension resolves with measures taken to lower the production source or presence of elevated CSF pressure. It is often seen in overweight women and can be helped with weight loss. It is diagnosed by lumbar puncture and can be managed with diuretics. If not successful, a ventriculoperitoneal shunt will lower the pressure. PAGE 2610

106. **Answer: A.** The association of vestibular symptoms with sudden idiopathic SNHL suggests greater insult to the inner ear and is less likely to recover. He is elderly, which may work against his recovery. The best positive predictor in this setting would be the absence of vestibular symptoms. PAGE 2594

107. **Answer: D.** The presence of stapedial reflexes with a significant CHL warrants evaluation for an inner-ear third window (i.e., superior semicircular canal dehiscence). PAGE 2490

108. **Answer: E.** This question emphasizes the overlapping relationship between vestibular disorders and motion intolerance, anxiety, and tendency to fall. All of the mentioned disorders are aggravated by underlying vestibular dysfunction. PAGE 2738

109. **Answer: C.** Congenital cholesteatoma arise in the anterosuperior mesotympanum, while acquired cholesteatoma arise in the epitympanum or posterior mesotympanum. PAGE 2363

110. **Answer: D.** The four fundamental principles in the treatment of external otitis in all stages are frequent and thorough cleaning, judicious use of appropriate antibiotics, treatment of associated inflammation and pain, and recommendations regarding the prevention of future infections. PAGES 2337–2338

111. **Answer: B.** As the posterior fossa plate is thinned, the endolymphatic sac comes into view just posteroinferior to the posterior semicircular canal. PAGE 2457

112. **Answer: D.** The head-impulse test is a means to detect unilateral or bilateral vestibular hypofunction. The movements are in the plane parallel to the semicircular canals. The semicircular canals are stimulated with angular acceleration. The movement must accelerate faster than 2,000 degrees per square second. (PAGES 2687–2688) Utricular function detects gravitational and linear movement and is not involved with the impulse test.

113. **Answer: E.** Skull base osteomyelitis usually begins as an acute external otitis that does not resolve despite medical therapy. The history is significant for a long-standing infection of the external canal accompanied by aural discharge and severe deep-seated pain. The disease is usually found in elderly diabetic patients in poor metabolic control, although it may be found in any chronically ill, debilitated, or immunocompromised patient. The HIV status of the patient should be known. PAGE 2341

114. **Answer: D.** Calcification within the tumor or associated hyperostosis supports the diagnosis of meningioma. Vestibular schwannomas are isodense or hypodense to brain and they exhibit inhomogeneous enhancement and lack of calcification or hyperostosis. MRI of vestibular schwannoma is more likely to show erosion of the internal auditory canal where the tumor originates and pronounced enhancement with injection of intravenous contrast. PAGE 2380

115. **Answer: C.** Developing hair cells express Notch ligands and activate Notch signaling. *Atoh1* promotes hair cell development. Notch controls *Atoh1* expression and thus regulates the development/regeneration of hair cells. (PAGE 2749) Wnt signaling proteins are important in cell-to-cell communication in embryologic development.

116. **Answer: A.** The auditory brainstem implant makes direct contact with the dorsal cochlear nucleus. The superior olivary nucleus, inferior colliculus, and cochlear nerve are part of the auditory pathway but not the sites of contact with this device. The nucleus solitarius receives input from the taste fibers (cranial nerves 7, 9, and 10) and viscera (carotid body, pharynx, and abdomen). PAGE 2648

117. **Answer: C.** ASSR can provide threshold information in a frequency-specific manner at intensity levels of 120 dB or greater. PAGES 2270–2271

118. **Answer: B.** NIHL is not accelerating and does not progress once exposure has been terminated. The majority of loss occurs within the first 10 years of exposure. ARHL is high-frequency sensorineural, more common in men, and accelerates with age. PAGE 2539

119. **Answer: A.** The embryology of the otic capsule is separate from that of the branchial arch-derived external and middle ear. PAGE 2384

120. **Answer: D.** If symptoms are present, they consist of vertigo with Valsalva or straining, motion- or position-provoked vertigo, Tullio phenomenon (vertigo secondary to auditory stimuli), vertigo with manipulation of the auricle or external auditory canal, and varying degrees of hearing loss. PAGE 2403

121. **Answer: D.** Saccade testing, along with gaze-stability evaluation, can be used to suggest localization of lesions within the central vestibular system. PAGES 2304–2305 and 2312

122. **Answer: B.** The ear is examined as aseptically as possible. Blood and cerumen in the ear canal should never be debrided with irrigation. PAGE 2413

123. **Answer: B.** The proper use of ear protection can provide over 20 dB of protection, especially when plugs and muffs are used together. In a practical sense, the usual amount of protection afforded is closer to 10 dB. PAGE 2538

124. **Answer: B.** Immediate onset facial paralysis (no voluntary movement) indicates an acute severe injury. This suggests possible disruption of the nerve. Options A and D describe residual function at onset and delayed onset paralysis, respectively. The Glasgow Coma score has no predictive impact on facial nerve status or recovery. It addresses gross motor function and response to pain. PAGE 2413

125. **Answer: B.** A translabyrinthine approach is the most direct for resecting the tumor. A middle-fossa approach is not appropriate due to the large size and poor hearing. A retrolabyrinthine approach provides limited access to the IAC and CPA. A retrosigmoid approach provides good access, but this is not one of the options. PAGE 2564

126. **Answer: C.** Wallenberg syndrome does not affect the inner ear (internal auditory artery) or cochlear nuclei. Hearing loss and prolonged vertigo are characteristic of an AICA stroke. Facial weakness and vertigo can occur in both. PAGE 2725

127. **Answer: D.** The most common site of origin is within the lateral internal auditory canal near Scarpa ganglion. There is a misconception that tumors develop at the glial–Schwann cell junction (Obersteiner–Redlich zone). PAGE 2558

128. **Answer: B.** The most common locations of origin of cholesteatomas in decreasing frequency are the posterior epitympanum, the posterior mesotympanum, and the anterior epitympanum. PAGE 2436

129. **Answer: C.** Coxsackie virus type A causes oral ulcerations and hand, foot, and mouth disease. Type B viruses cause pleurodynia. Both types A and B viruses can affect the meninges and myocardium. There is no compelling evidence of Coxsackie virus causing hearing loss, unlike HIV, cytomegalovirus, and varicella zoster virus. PAGES 2519–2520

130. **Answer: C.** A dehiscent or inferiorly displaced fallopian canal with or without a prolapsed facial nerve can at times obscure the oval window. If footplate removal and prosthesis placement can be achieved safely, surgery should continue. If the surgeon believes the nerve is in jeopardy, the procedure should be aborted. PAGE 2499

131. **Answer: C.** Aggressive papillary adenocarcinoma of the endolymphatic sac may erode the posterior face of the petrous bone and may be associated with von Hippel–Lindau disease and renal cyst or tumors. PAGE 2371

132. **Answer: B.** In order to consider the diagnosis of AIED, there must be bilateral involvement and should be progressive, responding to immunosuppression. It is not a unilateral disease. Progressive loss that does *not* respond to immunosuppression does *not* meet the definition of AIED. PAGE 2523

133. **Answer: D.** Stem cells are unspecialized cells capable of renewing themselves. They can also differentiate to become any specialized cells of organs, blood, nerve, brain, bone, or other specific tissue. Stem cells may undergo asymmetric division. In the case of the organ of Corti, supporting cells can divide and differentiate into hair cells. PAGE 2750

134. **Answer: C.** Effective measures are available for modifying tinnitus. Addressing psychiatric disease may alleviate the burden of tinnitus. It is not common to aggravate tinnitus. Acupuncture, meditation, and massage have a place in managing tinnitus. (A diagnosis and treatment algorithm for nonpulsatile tinnitus is presented on page 2601, Figure 161.3. page 2604 discusses therapies such as neurofeedback and transcranial magnetic and transcranial direct stimulation.)

135. **Answer: B.** MRI with MRV/MRA is more sensitive in detecting sigmoid sinus thrombosis, and delineates the extent of the thrombus and the integrity of collateral circulation while also identifying other intracranial complications. PAGE 2407

136. **Answer: C.** As part of the genetic Pendred syndrome, large vestibular aqueduct can be associated with disturbance of thyroid organification resulting from mutations in *SLC26A4*, a chloride–iodide transporter gene. PAGE 2249

137. **Answer: C.** One function of the middle-ear muscles is to protect the cochlea from loud sounds. The following functions have been attributed to the middle-ear muscles. Some of these functions include providing strength and rigidity to the ossicular chain; contributing to the blood supply of the ossicular chain; reducing physiologic noise caused by chewing and vocalization; improving the signal-to-noise ratio for high-frequency signals, especially high-frequency speech sounds such as voiceless fricatives, by means of attenuating high-level, low-frequency background noise; functioning as an automatic gain control and increasing the dynamic range of the ear; and smoothing out irregularities in the middle-ear transfer function. PAGE 2256

138. **Answer: B.** Ménière disease is an absolute contraindication for stapedectomy/stapedotomy. When the endolymphatic space is dilated (endolymphatic hydrops), the saccule may be enlarged to the point that it adheres to the undersurface of the stapes footplate. A stapes procedure can injure the saccule and result in profound sensorineural hearing loss. PAGE 2489

139. **Answer: B.** Nontraumatic maneuvers such as opening the dura alter the conduction patterns of the ABR appearing as changes on the monitor; in these situations, an intraoperative baseline may need to be reestablished prior to further manipulation of the auditory system. PAGE 2316

140. **Answer: B.** Oxaliplatin is a third-generation cisplatin analogue that is not associated with nephrotoxicity or ototoxicity. PAGE 2543

141. **Answer: A.** In overlay repair, blunting can be functionally understood as dense scarring of the anterior tympanic membrane that results in reduction of the functional surface area of the drumhead and "pseudo-malleus fixation" caused by adhesion between the manubrium and the anterior canal wall. PAGE 2476

142. **Answer: A.** CT characterizes the bony changes, and MRI the soft tissue aspects as well as cervical and intracranial extension. PAGE 2362

143. **Answer: D.** Hearing loss is the most prevalent risk factor for tinnitus. Tinnitus is associated with psychiatric disease and SNHL. (PAGE 2598) Fenestral OS may incur pulsatile or nonpulsatile tinnitus. Cochlear OS may cause tinnitus. PAGE 2611

144. **Answer: A.** Similar elevations in the SP/AP ratio have, however, been reported in perilymph fistula, autoimmune inner ear disease, and superior semicircular canal dehiscence. PAGE 2283

145. **Answer: C.** An MRI scan would be appropriate in an adult. MRI as high resolution T2 images are excellent in detecting inner ear malformations and have the advantage of also showing the VIIIth nerve and brainstem. It also has no ionizing radiation. One consideration for choosing CT may be the need for general anesthetic in a younger child for MRI. PAGE 2591

146. **Answer: D.** Adults do not use MP3 players as much as youth and adolescents. There is insufficient evidence of noise-induced hearing loss (NIHL) from personal stereo systems. The most important nonoccupational source of NIHL is gunfire. (PAGE 2535) Ototoxicity and acoustic neuroma are relatively rare.

147. **Answer: C.** The tumor likely describes a glomus jugulare. Proximal control isolates the sigmoid sinus and would include the superior petrosal sinus. The cavernous sinus is remote from this area. The inferior petrosal sinus provides venous drainage into the medial aspect of the vascular tumor and is encountered during resection of the body of the tumor. PAGES 2580–2581

148. **Answer: D.** Patients having inherited mitochondrial susceptibility can experience sensorineural hearing loss whether it is given intravenously or by transtympanic delivery. The pattern of inheritance is through a maternally transmitted mitochondrial defect, the *A1555G* mutation. PAGE 2545

149. **Answer: B.** In ears with congenital defects of the outer or middle ear, the implication of this pattern of development is that the facial nerve lies more anteriorly and superficially in the lateral temporal bone. PAGE 2444

150. **Answer: C.** Pregnancy is associated with hypervolemia and increased cardiac output. It resolves postpartum and is not an indication of preeclampsia. Plasmapheresis is not advisable. PAGE 2609

151. **Answer A.** The bony covering of the anterior limb of the lateral semicircular canal is eroded by the soft-tissue mass that fills the middle ear. The tegmen is not depicted on this more-inferior axial image. The bony covering of the tympanic segment of the facial nerve is intact.

152. **Answer B.** In aural atresia, the tympanic segment of the facial nerve may be displaced to the lateral side of the middle ear, where it is at risk during surgery. This finding should always be sought preoperatively.

153. **Answer C.** Bone loss surrounding the cochlea and in the region of the fissula ante fenestram indicates a diagnosis of otosclerosis, which classically presents with mixed hearing loss. Tullio phenomenon is more closely associated with superior semicircular canal dehiscence.

154. **Answer E.** There are many normal lucencies that can be seen on CT of the temporal bone and should not be mistaken for fracture. But in this case, there is truly a fracture running anterior–posterior through the otic capsule. Air in the vestibule and internal auditory canal are important secondary signs of fracture.

155. **Answer C.** The stapes prosthesis in this image is displaced posterior to the oval window. There is no evidence of fracture or soft-tissue mass or gas in the inner ear. The density of the otic capsule is normal.

Facial Plastic and Reconstructive Surgery

10

1. What is the name of the area where the septum articulates with the nasal bones?

   A. Bridge
   B. Keystone
   C. Fixter
   D. Crest
   E. Base

2. Where is the hyoid bone ideally located?

   A. At the level of first and second cervical vertebrae
   B. High and anterior in the neck
   C. At the level of third and fourth cervical vertebrae
   D. Low and posterior in the neck

3. Which of the following is true regarding nasofrontal angle (NFA)?

   A. Women tend to have a more acute NFA.
   B. The vertex should lie at a position in line with the superior limbus.
   C. Surgical raising of the position of the sellion superiorly will shorten the length of the nose.
   D. All of the above.

4. A reconstructive surgeon plans on using a tissue expander for the scalp. What is the ideal layer of placement of the tissue expander?

    A. Within the skin, between the epidermis and the dermis
    B. Between the skin and the subcutaneous tissue
    C. Between the subcutaneous tissue and the galea aponeurosis
    D. Between the galea aponeurosis and the pericranium
    E. Between the pericranium and the cranium

5. What is an absolute contraindication to performing chemical peels?

    A. History of hypertrophic scarring or keloid formation
    B. Active smoker
    C. History of cutaneous radiation exposure
    D. Isotretinoin use within the past 6 months

6. Which of the following is the best lighting option for office photography?

    A. Fluorescent office lights with on-camera fill flash
    B. Ambient light from office window
    C. On-camera ring flash
    D. Dual studio lights with soft box

7. The correction of microtia/atresia should begin with:

    A. Skin graft to ear with removal of microtic vestige
    B. Correction of the atresia by an otolaryngologist
    C. Combined procedure in conjunction with the otologist
    D. Autogenous cartilage harvest with framework creation
    E. Wait until the child is 18 years of age to decide for himself or herself

8. Which of the following anatomical features predisposes a rhinoplasty patient to postoperative nasal airway obstruction?

    A. Long nasal bones
    B. Wide upper cartilaginous vault
    C. Convex contour of the lower lateral cartilages
    D. Cephalically positioned lateral crura

9. **Which of the following statements best describes the pogonion?**

   A. It is used to calculate the lower face–throat and mentocervical angle.
   B. It is the anterior-most aspect of the chin.
   C. It should approximate the zero meridian in men.
   D. All of the above.

10. **Structural cartilage grafts are needed to:**

    A. Prevent collapse and airway obstruction
    B. Resist cephalic alar retraction
    C. Provide projection to the tip
    D. All the above

11. **Following Sunderland level IV injury, spontaneous recovery is generally:**

    A. Fair
    B. Not possible
    C. Modest
    D. Poor

12. **The principle of aesthetic subunits serve to:**

    A. Improve scar camouflage
    B. Assist with excision of cutaneous malignancies
    C. Guide the placement of structural batten grafts
    D. Dictate the indication of Mohs surgery

13. **Which of the following three facial mimetic muscles make the exception and run *deep* to the course of the facial nerve?**

    A. Zygomaticus major, zygomaticus minor, and buccinator
    B. Buccinator, mentalis, and levator labii superioris
    C. Masseter, mentalis, and buccinator
    D. Levator anguli oris, mentalis, and buccinator
    E. Masseter, mentalis, and orbicularis oculi

14. In selecting the proper implant for a patient's defect or deformity, which of the following is the most important consideration?

   A. Size of the defect
   B. Patient skin type
   C. Resistance to deformation
   D. Ease of implantation
   E. Tissue biocompatibility

15. The nasofacial angle is the angle formed by the intersection of:

   A. A line drawn from the nasion through the nasal tip-defining point and a second line drawn from the nasion through the alar-facial junction
   B. A line drawn from the nasion through the subnasale and a second line drawn from the nasion through the nasal tip-defining point
   C. A line drawn from the nasion through the nasal tip-defining point and a second line drawn from the glabella through the pogonion
   D. A line drawn from the glabella through the nasal tip and a second line drawn from the glabella through the subnasale

16. Transverse chin asymmetry is often associated with:

   A. Treacher Collins syndrome
   B. Pierre Robin sequence
   C. Van der Woude syndrome
   D. Oculoauricular vertebral (OAV) spectrum

17. Which of the following statements explains how the antihelix can be created?

   A. Securing folded helical cartilage with Mustarde-type horizontal mattress sutures
   B. Scoring the helical cartilage anteriorly
   C. Removing thin strips of helical cartilage from a posterior approach
   D. All of the above

18. A caudally positioned radix (low-radix disproportion) will have which of these effects?

   A. Making the nasofacial angle more acute and thereby making the nasal tip look relatively overprojected
   B. Making the nasofacial angle more obtuse and thereby making the nasal tip look relatively underprojected
   C. Making the nasofacial angle more acute and thereby making the nasal tip look relatively underprojected
   D. Making the nasofacial angle more obtuse and thereby making the nasal tip look relatively overprojected

19. If a cutaneous reaction with erythema, vesicle formation, and exudates forms specifically on all areas treated with the topical ointment being used for wound care, the patient should initially:

    A. Stop the topical ointment
    B. Apply more ointment
    C. Apply ointment and steroid cream
    D. Apply vaseline and moisturizer

20. Which of the following facial anatomic locations is most amenable to healing by secondary intention?

    A. Temple
    B. Medial canthus
    C. Both A and B
    D. None of the above

21. Which of the following single-lens reflex (SLR) lens choices is most appropriate for standardized before and after photography when using a digital SLR camera body?

    A. 60-mm macro
    B. 105-mm macro
    C. 35-mm fixed
    D. 24- to 120-mm zoom

22. Which of the following is not a major tip-support mechanism?

    A. Length and strength of the lower lateral cartilages
    B. Attachment of medial crura to caudal septum
    C. Nasal spine
    D. Attachment of the cephalic margin of the lateral crura to the caudal margin of the upper lateral cartilage

23. A small or posteriorly positioned mandible is referred to as:

    A. Microgenia
    B. Prognathia
    C. Retrognathia
    D. Class II malocclusion

24. **Which is true regarding the fat pads of the upper eyelid?**

    A. The lateral fat pad is deeper than the medial fat pad.
    B. Aggressive removal of the central fat pad always improves aesthetic outcomes.
    C. The fat pads are deep to the orbital septum.
    D. Reflection of the levator aponeurosis exposes the underlying fat pads.

25. **Recovery of function after treatment with botulinum toxin involves:**

    A. Development of new axonal collaterals
    B. Formation of temporary axonal collaterals followed by recovery of transmission through the primary nerve terminal
    C. Recovery of neural transmission through the original nerve terminal
    D. Regeneration of acetylcholine within the presynaptic nerve terminal

26. **Which of the following statements about complications after otoplasty is false?**

    A. Telephone-ear deformity can result from failure to correct a prominent, laterally displaced helical root and lobule.
    B. Infection is the most common complication.
    C. Skin necrosis is a rare complication.
    D. Worsening pain after postoperative day 3 suggests infection.

27. **Dermabrasion techniques resurface the skin until punctate bleeding is appreciated. This corresponds to what depth of skin?**

    A. Directly subdermal
    B. Reticular dermis
    C. Papillary dermis
    D. Subcutaneous tissue

28. **How is microgenia best managed?**

    A. Osteotomy and bony advancement
    B. Suprahyoid myotomy
    C. Orthognathic surgery to correct malocclusion
    D. Alloplastic augmentation

29. Which of the following structures separates the medial and central fat pads of the lower eyelid?

    A. Lateral rectus muscle
    B. Nasolacrimal canal
    C. Inferior oblique muscle
    D. Inferior rectus muscle
    E. Infraorbital nerve

30. Where is the cartilage growth center in the nasal septum?

    A. Perichondrium of anterior bony septum
    B. Maxillary crest
    C. Keystone area
    D. Nasal tip
    E. Bony dorsum

31. What is the amount of skin that should be preserved between the brow and the upper eyelid margin after upper eyelid blepharoplasty?

    A. 15 mm
    B. 20 mm
    C. 25 mm
    D. 30 mm

32. Which of the following techniques has been shown to reduce an implant's preplacement bacterial load?

    A. Immersion in antibiotic solution
    B. Irrigation with povidone-iodine (Betadine)
    C. Suction infiltration of an antimicrobial solution
    D. Preoperative intravenous antibiotics

33. The best technique for camouflaging a thin 5-cm straight scar that runs perpendicular to the relaxed skin-tension lines along the cheek is:

    A. Geometric broken-line closure
    B. Serial Z-plasty
    C. Fusiform excision
    D. Dermabrasion

34. Patients who carry the diagnosis of depression can be described by which of the following?

    A. May safely undergo cosmetic surgery
    B. Demonstrate improvement in the postoperative Beck Depression Inventory score following cosmetic surgery
    C. May initially experience intensification of their depressive symptoms following cosmetic surgery
    D. All of the above

35. Which of the following is characteristic of hemangiomas?

    A. Absence at birth
    B. Increase in size with patient growth
    C. Normal rate of endothelial cell growth
    D. Lack of endothelial hyperplasia

36. What is most helpful in preventing postinflammatory hyperpigmentation following resurfacing?

    A. Pretreatment with topical tretinoin
    B. Pretreatment with hydroquinone
    C. Pretreatment and posttreatment with sunscreen and sun avoidance
    D. All of the above

37. Lasers characteristically produce light which is:

    A. Monochromatic
    B. Pulsed
    C. Collimated
    D. Both A and B
    E. Both A and C

38. Identify the dermal vascular apparatus regulated by the sympathetic nervous system:

    A. Preshunt sphincter
    B. Precapillary sphincter
    C. Reticular vascular arcade
    D. Papillary venous shunts

39. **Which term best describes the stress–strain relationship for skin?**

    A. Linear
    B. Parabolic
    C. Infinite
    D. Nonlinear

40. **At what age does the ear reach nearly its full adult size?**

    A. 3 years old
    B. 5 years old
    C. 7 years old
    D. 10 years old

41. **Cartilage grafts are most likely needed for cutaneous defects involving:**

    A. Lower/lateral half of the nose, i.e., ala and sidewall
    B. Nasal tip
    C. Dorsal subunit
    D. Not needed for skin-only defects as long as cartilage has not been sacrificed

42. **In the facelift patient which of the following might increase the risk of hematoma formation postoperatively?**

    A. Coughing
    B. Uncontrolled blood pressure
    C. Uncontrolled pain
    D. Nausea and vomiting
    E. Excessive movement of the head
    F. All of the above

43. **The dominant cause of failure following free-tissue transfer for facial reanimation is:**

    A. Microvascular failure
    B. Inadequate neural penetration
    C. Inadequate suture inset to atrophied modiolus
    D. Incorrect vector of pull

44. **Which of the following is true regarding the Juri flap for hair restoration?**

    A. The Juri flap is better utilized for crown coverage than for frontal hairline restoration.
    B. The Juri flap can be harvested in one stage if the Doppler ultrasonography reveals a strong arterial supply.
    C. The Juri flap is pedicled off the occipital artery and the superficial temporal artery (STA).
    D. The Juri flap can provide excellent density to the frontal hairline, although the hairs will be oriented posteriorly, resulting in an unnatural appearance.

45. **A patient presenting for surgical evaluation demonstrates excessive concern with a very subtle asymmetry of the nostrils. This is so troubling to her that she wears a mask in public and is not able to maintain employment. This patient may be suffering from:**

    A. Borderline personality disorder
    B. Body dysmorphic disorder (BDD)
    C. Narcissistic personality disorder
    D. Histrionic personality disorder

46. **Which of the following statements regarding tarsorrhaphy for the paralyzed eye is most accurate?**

    A. It protects better than eyelid weight and lower lid tightening.
    B. It yields the most aesthetically pleasing result.
    C. It is technically more difficult to execute than other eyelid reanimation techniques.
    D. The revision rate is comparable to that of the eyelid spring procedure.

47. **Stimulated emission of radiation occurs when:**

    A. Photons in a system strike atoms in the laser medium and raise an electron to a higher energy level
    B. An atom in the excited state reemits a photon and the electron returns to the lower energy level
    C. An atom in the higher energy state is struck by an additional photon with the emission of two photons
    D. Photons in a system strike atoms in the laser medium and lower an electron to a decreased energy level

48. Which of the following incisions is necessary for a delivery approach to the nasal tip?

    A. An intercartilaginous incision coupled with a transcolumellar incision

    B. A marginal incision coupled with an intercartilaginous incision connecting to a full transfixion incision

    C. A retrograde incision coupled with a marginal incision connecting to a hemitransfixion incision

    D. A rim incision coupled with an intercartilaginous incision connecting to a full Killian incision

49. Which nerve is most commonly injured during face-lifting?

    A. Marginal mandibular branch of facial nerve

    B. Frontal branch of facial nerve

    C. Great auricular nerve

    D. Lesser occipital nerve

    E. Greater occipital nerve

50. According to the tripod model of nasal-tip dynamics, which of the following is false?

    A. Shortening the lateral crura increases tip rotation.

    B. Shortening the medial crura decreases tip projection.

    C. Increasing the length of the medial crura increases tip rotation.

    D. Lengthening the medial crura and shortening the lateral crura decrease tip rotation.

51. Solitary neurofibromas can develop and are not associated with any specific syndrome. However, a patient with multiple neurofibromas or a plexiform neurofibroma should be referred for workup of what syndrome?

    A. von Recklinghausen

    B. Peutz–Jeghers

    C. Klippel–Trénaunay

    D. Osler–Rendu–Weber

    E. Cowden

52. The extracellular matrix is critical in binding cells to implants. Which of the following is the most important element for this step in the extracellular matrix?

    A. Triglycerides

    B. Glycosaminoglycans

    C. Amino acids

    D. Polylactide

    E. Polygalactide

53. What is an advantage of using a phenol-based solution over trichloroacetic acid (TCA) for peels?

    A. Lack of cardiac toxicity
    B. Absence of need for sedation
    C. Ease of assessing adequate depth of penetration
    D. Improved healing times

54. When utilized as a soft-tissue augmentation implant, human acellular dermis serves in what capacity to fill a defect?

    A. Scaffold for new tissue ingrowth
    B. Stimulation for dermal thickening
    C. Underlying bone formation
    D. Permanent bulk in the defect
    E. Neuromodulation

55. A 33-year-old woman visits her surgeon in consultation for rhinoplasty. Examination reveals short nasal bones. What is she at particular risk of experiencing as a result of undergoing rhinoplasty?

    A. Nasal airway obstruction
    B. Tip bossae
    C. Saddle nose deformity
    D. Open roof deformity

56. In performing a dorsal-hump reduction, the surgeon must take into account which of the following variations in skin thickness along the dorsum of the nose?

    A. In the upper third of the nose, the skin is thickest at the nasion and thinnest at the rhinion.
    B. In the upper third of the nose, the skin is thickest at the rhinion and thinnest at the nasion.
    C. In the upper third of the nose, the skin has the same thickness between the nasion and the rhinion, then becomes progressively thicker toward the tip.
    D. The skin is the thinnest at the tip.

57. Which of the following statements is true about rapid intraoperative tissue expansion?

    A. It relies on biological creep.
    B. A gain of 3 cm of flap length can be achieved.
    C. The expander is usually inflated and deflated once.
    D. There are minor physiologic and metabolic changes that occur at various levels of the skin.
    E. It is more popular than conventional long-term tissue expansion.

58. The risk of bossae formation is increased in patients with:

    A. Tip bifidity, thin skin, and strong lower lateral cartilages
    B. Tip bifidity, thick skin, and strong lower lateral cartilages
    C. Tip bifidity, thin skin, and weak lower lateral cartilages
    D. Tip bifidity, thick skin, and weak lower lateral cartilages

59. The most common smile pattern among humans is:

    A. Full denture smile
    B. Zygomaticus major smile
    C. Canine smile
    D. Risorius smile

60. The best donor site to obtain high-volume skin paddle in a patient with a low body mass index (BMI) is:

    A. Rectus
    B. Latissumus dorsi
    C. Anterolateral thigh
    D. Lateral arm

61. Appropriate selection of a laser is most highly dependent upon:

    A. Specific wavelength absorption of a given tissue
    B. Coagulation temperature of a given tissue
    C. Water content of a given tissue
    D. Power density of the laser

62. Which of the following cells in the skin is the most sensitive to cold injury when using liquid nitrogen for cryotherapy?

    A. Keratinocyte
    B. Melanocyte
    C. Nerve
    D. Merkel cell
    E. Fibroblast

63. Chin augmentation with an alloplast implant commonly corrects:

    A. Transverse chin asymmetry
    B. Horizontal chin deficiency
    C. Vertical chin excess
    D. A deep labiomental sulcus

64. A 23-year-old man with moderate alopecia of the frontal scalp and crown is seen in consultation for surgical hair restoration. Which of the following statements is best regarding the treatment of this patient?

    A. Surgical hair restoration should be directed first to the crown region of the scalp since transplanting in this area will give the patient the best coverage with appropriate styling.
    B. Medical therapy is contraindicated in this patient because of his age.
    C. Surgical hair restoration should be directed first to the frontal region of the scalp since transplanting in this area will give the patient the best coverage with appropriate styling.
    D. One must be cautious in transplanting in this patient because of the risk and uncertainty of future hair loss.

65. The "double-convexity" deformity is an indication for what procedure during blepharoplasty?

    A. Central fat-pad removal
    B. Skin excision
    C. Canthoplasty
    D. Lower eyelid resurfacing
    E. Fat transposition

66. Which of the following is true about complex revision rhinoplasty?

    A. A failed rhinoplasty is likely to illicit anger and frustration in nearly all patients, including well-adjusted individuals.
    B. Revision rhinoplasty patients often display a surprising familiarity with rhinoplasty jargon and surgical techniques.
    C. Revision surgery within 1 year of previous surgery is contraindicated.
    D. Revision of the ultrathick skinned nose is generally much easier than revision of the ultrathin skinned nose.
    E. A and B only.

67. Prior to definitive use, skin testing is recommended for which of the following fillers?

    A. Hyaluronic acids
    B. Poly-L-lactic acid (Sculptra)
    C. Polymethyl methacrylate (Artefill)
    D. Silicone

68. What is the most common complication from face-lifting?

    A. Satyr ear or Pixie ear deformity
    B. Hematoma
    C. Temporal hair-tuft alopecia
    D. Facial nerve injury
    E. Pulmonary embolus

69. The triad of adenoma sebaceum, mental retardation, and epilepsy is characteristic of which autosomal-dominant syndrome?

    A. Tuberous sclerosis
    B. Neurofibromatosis
    C. Sturge–Weber
    D. Osler–Rendu–Weber
    E. Carney

70. Following an upper eyelid blepharoplasty, a patient has persistent scleral show when she closes her eyes. What is this finding called?

    A. Blepharoptosis
    B. Dermatochalasis
    C. Proptosis
    D. Lagophthalmos

71. Myoplasty is not possible with which of the following methods of forehead lifting?

    A. Coronal forehead lifting
    B. Direct brow lifting
    C. Indirect brow lifting
    D. Endoscopic forehead lifting

72. Patient-specific implants utilize which of the following technologies?

    A. Human leucocyte antigen tissue compatibility tests
    B. Messenger RNA encoding
    C. Positron emission tomography scan
    D. Computer-assisted design and manufacturing
    E. MR scan

73. The donor site that supplies the best quality bone for osseointegrated implants is:

    A. Fibula
    B. Iliac crest
    C. Circumflex scapular artery scapula
    D. Thoracodorsal artery scapular tip (TDAST)

74. The best candidate for a coronal forehead lift or one of its modifications from the following is:

    A. A younger woman with a long forehead/high hairline
    B. An older woman with a short forehead/low hairline
    C. A younger man with a short forehead and a family history of androgenic alopecia
    D. An older man with a long forehead and no history of androgenic alopecia

75. The most prominent anterior point on the chin is known as:

    A. Labrale superioris
    B. Menton
    C. Pogonion
    D. Rhinion

76. The dominant reason for proceeding with nerve grafting soon after injury is:

    A. Biological regenerative potential
    B. Practical/technical aspects of surgery
    C. Functional outcome
    D. All of the above

77. With conventional long-term tissue expansion, biological creep occurs at all levels of the skin. Which of the following is a physiologic phenomenon seen in conventional long-term tissue expansion?

    A. A decrease in mitotic activity in the epidermis
    B. Thickening of all layers of the dermis by 50%
    C. Increase in metabolic activity of fibroblasts
    D. Increase in the number of hair follicles and distortion of the pattern of hair growth
    E. Atrophy of capillaries, venules, and arterioles

78. A Z-plasty designed with 60° angle limbs will increase the length of the scar:

    A. 10%
    B. 25%
    C. 50%
    D. 75%

79. The ideal limb length for geometric broken-line closure is:

    A. 1 mm
    B. 5 mm
    C. 7 mm
    D. 10 mm

80. Proportionate facial features are described by which of these statements?

    A. Fall within normal measured values
    B. Required to achieve an aesthetically pleasing result
    C. More likely to harmonize with one another, producing an aesthetically pleasing result
    D. Both A and C are correct

81. When taking a photograph in manual mode, increased photographic exposure can be obtained by all of the following maneuvers *except*:

    A. Changing aperture from f/8 to f/16
    B. Changing shutter speed from 1/125 to 1/60 of a second
    C. Changing ISO setting from ISO 100 to ISO 200
    D. Increasing the ambient light

82. Deprojecting the nasal tip with a full transfixion incision is not effective with which of the following anatomical variants?

    A. Long, strong medial crura
    B. Small nasal spine
    C. Bulbous tip cartilages
    D. Thin skin

83. Which of the following is the approximate temperature of the bone during drilling to prepare for an osseointegrated implant that has been shown to cause osteoblast death?

    A. 20°C
    B. 30°C
    C. 50°C
    D. 70°C
    E. 80°C

84. Scars that extend beyond the natural borders of the wound edges are most accurately categorized as:

    A. Atrophic scars
    B. Hypertrophic scars
    C. Keloids
    D. Fibroids

85. Lack of platysma decussation can predispose a patient to:

    A. Cobra deformity
    B. Turkey-gobbler deformity
    C. Platysmal banding
    D. Obtuse cervicomental angle

86. Which donor site requires preoperative assessment of vascular supply?

    A. Gastroomental and jejunum
    B. Rectus
    C. Radial forearm and fibula
    D. Anterolateral thigh

87. Which of the following will increase photographic depth of field?

    A. Changing from a 60-mm lens at f/8 to a 300-mm lens at f/8
    B. Moving farther from the subject
    C. Changing shutter speed from 1/60 to 1/125 of a second
    D. Changing aperture from f/16 to f/8

88. Which of the following modifications creates the illusion of decreased nasal-tip rotation?

    A. A dorsal augmentation graft
    B. An increase in nasolabial angle
    C. A reduction of a hanging columella
    D. A lateral crural overlay

89. Which of the following statements is true about chin augmentation with an implant?

    A. Implants commonly cause anterior bony resorption of the mandible.
    B. Implants are preferably placed through an intraoral approach.
    C. The reported incidence of mentalis muscle dyskinesis is 25%.
    D. A small button-style implant aesthetically causes less complications than wider implants.

90. Which of the following factors provide strong justification for declining revision rhinoplasty?

    A. A well-defined and exacting cosmetic goal on behalf of the patient
    B. The demonstration of anger or frustration by the patient during the initial consultation
    C. Patient familiarity with fundamental rhinoplasty terminology and common treatment strategies
    D. Surgical skills of the surgeon that are insufficient to achieve the approximate cosmetic goal
    E. All of the above

91. Studies examining length of time required for adhesion between cranium and overlying periosteum or periosteum with overlying galea have demonstrated that biomechanical strength of the dissected flap matches controls at which time period?

    A. 1 to 2 weeks
    B. 2 to 4 weeks
    C. 4 to 6 weeks
    D. 6 to 8 weeks

92. **What are the anatomic elements of the internal nasal valve?**

    A. The caudal margin of the upper lateral cartilage (ULC), the anterior head of the inferior turbinate, and the adjacent septum.
    B. The cephalic margin of the ULC, the anterior head of the inferior turbinate, and the adjacent septum.
    C. The cephalic margin of the ULC, the medial crus of the lower lateral cartilages, and the posterior septum.
    D. The caudal margin of the ULC, the anterior head of the inferior turbinate, and the alar rim.

93. **Which of the following statements are true regarding body dysmorphic disorder (BDD)?**

    A. BDD sufferers are at significantly increased risk for suicide.
    B. Many BDD patients are delusional and lack awareness regarding their preoccupation with trivial cosmetic imperfections.
    C. Cosmetic surgery is generally contraindicated in patients with BDD.
    D. A and C.
    E. All of the above.

94. **What is the plane of dissection for the preseptal transconjunctival approach in blepharoplasty?**

    A. Between the conjunctiva and the lower eyelid retractors
    B. Between the lower eyelid retractors and the orbital fat
    C. Between the skin and the orbicularis oculi muscle
    D. Between the orbicularis oculi muscle and the orbital septum
    E. Directly through the conjunctiva and the lower eyelid retractors near the conjunctival fornix

95. **What is the minimal amount of cartilage width that should remain for adequate support of the L-strut?**

    A. 15 mm
    B. 20 mm
    C. 10 mm
    D. 30 mm
    E. 25 mm

96. **Examples of pivotal flaps include:**

    A. Rotation, transposition, and interpolation flaps
    B. Rotation, advancement, and island flaps
    C. Bilobe, V-Y, and interpolation flaps
    D. Advancement, hinge, and rhomboid flaps

97. **Full-thickness grafts survive initially by diffusion of nutrition from fluid in the recipient site, a process known as:**

    A. Plasma imbibition
    B. Vascular inosculation
    C. Neovascularization
    D. None of the above

98. **Which of the following is the most appropriate method of stabilizing the nasal base in a patient with a retracted columella?**

    A. Caudal septal extension graft
    B. Columellar strut
    C. Set back medial crura on caudal septum (tongue-in-groove technique)
    D. Extended columellar strut fixed to nasal spine

99. **An overprojected (shallow) radix on nasal appearance will:**

    A. Exaggerate nasal dorsal height, creating the illusion of a "pseudohump"
    B. Make the nose look visually longer
    C. Make the nasal tip look more rotated
    D. Make the nasal tip look more projected

100. **How are contour irregularities that are seen 1 week following cervical liposuction and anterior platysmaplasty best managed?**

    A. Reexploration
    B. Steroid injections
    C. Massage
    D. Reassurance

101. What complication from face-lifting is thought to be significantly more frequent in men than in women?

    A. Hematoma
    B. Nerve injury
    C. Skin necrosis
    D. Hypoesthesia
    E. Pixie ear deformity

102. True or False: The greater the pivot of the flap, the shorter the effective length of the flap?

    A. True
    B. False

103. You are asked to evaluate a newborn with bilateral microtia and atresia. What is your most important recommendation?

    A. High-resolution CT scan
    B. Auditory brainstem response testing
    C. Placement of bone conduction hearing aid
    D. Plan to perform surgical correction at 10 weeks
    E. Molding splints to the microtic vestige

104. Which of the following best characterizes a prominent ear?

    A. Absent antihelical fold
    B. Absent antihelical fold and large conchal bowl
    C. Absent antihelical fold and defect of upper one-thirds of the helix
    D. Absent antihelical fold and purse-string appearance at helix

105. Blepharochalasis refers to:

    A. Excess skin of the lower eyelid
    B. Drooping of the lower eyelid
    C. A rare recurrent inflammatory disorder of the eyelids
    D. Orbital fat pseudoherniation
    E. Scleral show

106. During endoscopic browlift surgery, the temporal branch of the facial nerve can be safely preserved:

    A. With endoscopic-assisted dissection lateral to the orbital rim and zygomatic arch
    B. By dissecting along the undersurface of the temporoparietal fascia
    C. By identifying the "sentinel vein" and staying deep in a plane deep to the temporoparietal fascia
    D. By dissecting medially within a radius of 3 cm from the lateral orbital rim

107. Which of the following statements best describes the Tyndall effect?

    A. It can be treated with α-adrenergic ophthalmic drops to stimulate Mueller's muscle.
    B. It is seen with overly superficial injection of polymethyl methacrylate.
    C. It may require treatment with hyaluronidase.
    D. It results from intra-arterial injection of a dermal filler.

108. Which of the following statements regarding the overresected nose is not correct?

    A. Noncompliant skin does not affect successful revision of the overresected nasal tip.
    B. Reducing dorsal septal height exacerbates the sequela of the overresected tip.
    C. The inverted-V deformity can arise without overresection of the dorsum.
    D. Preserving 6 mm of lateral crural width does not always prevent crural collapse.
    E. All of the above.

109. Which type of lighting best replicated natural sunlight to see deviations in nose shape?

    A. Anterior flash
    B. Overhead flash
    C. Side flash
    D. Inferior flash
    E. Posterior flash

110. What type of total pharyngeal reconstruction provides the best speech and swallowing results?

    A. Gastroomental
    B. Anterolateral thigh
    C. Jejunum
    D. Latissumus dorsi from a patient with a high body mass index

111. In general, composite grafts should be limited in size to:

    A. 2 cm
    B. 5 mm
    C. 1 cm or less from each wound edge
    D. The entire aesthetic unit should be replaced

112. A 27-year-old pregnant woman presents to an urgent care clinic with a 3-week history of a rapidly growing red friable papule that easily bleeds on the lateral commissure of the mouth. As the consulting physician you astutely clinically diagnose:

    A. Fibrous papule
    B. Basal cell carcinoma
    C. Angioma
    D. Pyogenic granuloma
    E. Sebaceous hyperplasia

113. A patient is left with a 10-cm² defect of the scalp after resection of a basal cell carcinoma. A reconstructive surgeon plans on using a tissue expander to reconstruct the defect. What is the ideal surface area of the expander base that should be used?

    A. 5 cm^2
    B. 10 cm^2
    C. 20 cm^2
    D. 30 cm^2
    E. 40 cm^2

114. Which of the following is not a consequence of cephalically positioned lateral crura?

    A. Lateral wall collapse
    B. Parenthesis deformity
    C. Increased middle vault width
    D. Ptotic nasal tip

115. Which of the following muscles is a brow depressor?

    A. The corrugator procerus
    B. The depressor supercilii
    C. The depressor oculi
    D. The oculi supercilii

116. The injectable filler most likely to be seen on CT scan is:

    A. Hyaluronic acid (Juvéderm)
    B. Calcium hydroxylapatite (CaHA) (Radiesse)
    C. Poly-L-lactic acid (Sculptra)
    D. Silicone

117. Which of the following is false for the medical treatment of alopecia?

    A. Finasteride is a type II 5a-reductase inhibitor used for the treatment of androgenetic alopecia.
    B. A side effect of oral minoxidil for the treatment of hypertension is hypertrichosis.
    C. Finasteride has beneficial effects for the treatment of androgenetic alopecia in men and women.
    D. The combination of finasteride and minoxidil is frequently used for the treatment of androgenetic alopecia in men.

118. Which of these structures is part of the external nasal valve?

    A. Lateral crura
    B. Glabella
    C. Dorsum
    D. Middle turbinate
    E. Septum

119. Ear molding techniques can be described by which of these statements?

    A. Most successful in neonates less than 1 week old
    B. Most successful at correcting prominent ears
    C. Should not be performed in infants older than 3 months
    D. Most successful at correcting severely constricted ears

120. The reflection of the orbital septum at the superior orbital rim is called?

    A. Whitnall ligament
    B. The levator palpebrae superioris
    C. The tarsal plate
    D. Arcus marginalis

121. Which of the following is true regarding follicular unit extraction (FUE) techniques for the management of alopecia?

    A. The entire follicular unit is visualized prior to extracting the graft in order to minimize transection.
    B. Sharp and dull 1-mm punches are utilized to extract the follicular units.
    C. The back of the scalp is the only donor area that can be utilized using FUE.
    D. The linear scar that results from FUE tends to be less noticeable than the resultant scars from using the strip method for harvesting donor hair.

122. The inverted-V deformity is created by:

    A. Overnarrowing of the nasal tip from transdomal suture placement
    B. Excessive resection of lateral crura during tip reduction
    C. Ischemic necrosis of the septum due to untreated septal hematoma
    D. Disrupting the connection between the upper lateral cartilages (ULCs) and the septum during dorsal-hump reduction

123. What is the effect of increased concentrations of croton oil to an 88% phenol solution?

    A. More profound epidermolysis
    B. Decreased dermal effect
    C. Increased healing times
    D. Decreased healing times

124. Which of the following is incorrect regarding before and after photographs?

    A. The same camera-to-subject distance should be maintained.
    B. The patient should be placed in the Frankfort horizontal plane.
    C. In the oblique view, the patient's head should be turned 45° while the torso faces the camera.
    D. Hair should be pulled back behind ears and jewelry should be removed.

125. In the event of skin necrosis over the neoauricle, which choice is the best for a 5-mm loss of skin?

    A. Apply ointment daily until closed
    B. Silver nitrate application bid
    C. Wet-to-dry dressings
    D. Temporoparietal fascia flap harvest
    E. Split thickness skin graft to exposed cartilage

126. Which of the following is false in terms of complications from surgical hair restoration?

    A. Infections following surgical hair restoration are common and easily treated with oral antibiotics.
    B. If not properly planned, scalp reductions can result in an unnatural hair direction.
    C. Wide donor scars are more common when harvesting a large segment of tissue in the back of the scalp.
    D. Cysts can occur at the recipient site when grafts are placed under the dermis.

127. Bony genioplasty does not correct:

    A. Vertical microgenia
    B. Mentalis muscle dyskinesis
    C. Transverse chin asymmetries
    D. Horizontal macrogenia

128. During a rhinoplasty, the surgeon initiates a lateral osteotomy too inferiorly (low) on the pyriform aperture. Which outcome might be expected?

    A. Medialization of the head of the inferior turbinate
    B. Loss of tip support
    C. Postoperative epistaxis
    D. External nasal valve stenosis

129. What is the first step in treating a retroorbital hematoma following blepharoplasty?

    A. Administration of 2 L oxygen
    B. Administration of intravenous mannitol
    C. Opening of all incisions and exploration
    D. Lateral canthotomy and cantholysis
    E. Topical β-blockers

130. The osseous donor site that has the most soft-tissue options and has the longest pedicle is:

    A. Fibula
    B. Iliac crest
    C. Circumflex scapular artery scapula
    D. Thoracodorsal artery scapular tip (TDAST)

131. **What is the correct management of a patient with a class II neck and normal chin projection?**

    A. Rhytidectomy
    B. Rhytidectomy and cervical liposuction
    C. Rhytidectomy, cervical liposuction, and anterior platysmaplasty
    D. Rhytidectomy, cervical liposuction, and chin augmentation

132. **Advantages of the endoscopic forehead lift include:**

    A. Avoidance of forehead shortening
    B. Significantly less long-term motor nerve injury
    C. Significantly less long-term sensory nerve injury
    D. Faster recovery of sensory neuropathy

133. **Pedicle division of the interpolated forehead flap:**

    A. Is usually performed after 3 weeks
    B. Is usually performed after 7 to 10 days
    C. Is rarely necessary
    D. Should not be performed in smokers

134. **The blood supply to the forehead flap is from:**

    A. Both the collateral flow of the angular artery and the supratrochlear artery
    B. The supraorbital artery
    C. Both the supraorbital and supratrochlear arteries
    D. The anterior branch of the superficial temporal artery

135. **Which flap involves transfer of a flap pedicle across intervening cutaneous tissue?**

    A. Advancement
    B. Interpolation
    C. Rotation
    D. Rhomboid

136. **What is the effect of decreasing the spot size of a laser beam?**

    A. Energy density decreases
    B. Power density decreases
    C. Power increases
    D. Power density increases

137. **What is the cause of involutional or senile ptosis?**

    A. Dehiscence of the orbicularis oculi from the tarsal plate
    B. Separation of the levator aponeurosis from the tarsal plate
    C. Dehiscence of the orbital septum from the levator aponeurosis
    D. Horner syndrome

138. **Hetter disproved which of Brown's postulates on Baker's classic formula with phenol peeling?**

    A. Increased concentrations of phenol prevent deeper peels by causing an immediate keratocoagulation that prevents its further penetration.
    B. Adding a saponin-like septisol increases the depth of penetration of phenol.
    C. Croton oil acts as a buffer for the solution.
    D. All of the above.

139. **Which of the following statements regarding preoperative surgical evaluation is true?**

    A. Surgical (tissue) intolerance cannot be determined with certainty in any patient.
    B. Computer "imaging" (morphing) software programs can greatly facilitate communication between patient and surgeon.
    C. Nasal palpation is an essential component of the preoperative assessment.
    D. Photographic analysis is not a satisfactory substitute for a thorough physical examination of the nose.
    E. A, B, and C.
    F. All of the above.

140. **A 14-year-old man presents with a 2-cm sharply circumscribed, yellow-orange, verrucous, linear plaque on the vertex scalp that has been present since birth but recently changing. The most common malignancy that may develop is called:**

    A. Melanoma
    B. Basal cell carcinoma
    C. Sebaceous carcinoma
    D. Trichoblastoma
    E. Squamous cell carcinoma

141. **The cartilage used for ear reconstruction is best harvested from:**

    A. The contralateral ear
    B. The mother's ear cartilage
    C. Irradiated cartilage
    D. Costal cartilage
    E. The father's ear cartilage

142. Skin biomechanics play a key role in the understanding of how tissue expansion works. What is the biomechanical property that describes the tendency of a solid material to slowly move or deform permanently under the influence of stresses?

   A. Extensibility
   B. Creep
   C. Viscoelasticity
   D. Tension
   E. Stress relaxation

143. A patient returns to her surgeon's office 15 years after undergoing rhinoplasty, and is diagnosed with an inverted-V deformity. What is the likely surgical etiology?

   A. Disrupted connection between the caudal margin of the nasal bones and the cephalic margin of the upper lateral cartilages (ULCs)
   B. Inadequate lateral osteotomies
   C. Failure to place a radix graft
   D. Inappropriate fixation of her bilateral spreader grafts too inferiorly

144. Who is credited for the first description of subdividing the face for analysis into horizontal thirds and vertical fifths?

   A. Leonardo da Vinci
   B. Powell and Humphreys
   C. Galen
   D. Galileo

145. A 19-year-old girl with facial asymmetry. What is the radiologic diagnosis?

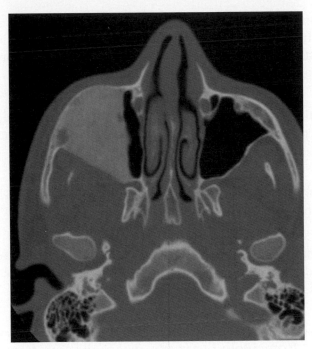

A. Paget disease
B. Fibrous dysplasia
C. Ossifying fibroma
D. Fibrous osteoma
E. Chondrosarcoma

Chapter 10 Answers

1. **Answer: B.** The articulation between the dorsal septum and the nasal bones in the midline is referred to as the "keystone" area. The significance of that area is that sufficient stability and fixation must be maintained or reconstituted at that area to prevent postoperative collapse or settling of the dorsal septum. PAGE 2980

2. **Answer: C.** Ideally, the hyoid bone should be at the level of the third or fourth cervical vertebra. A more posterior and superior hyoid produces a more aesthetic cervical contour. PAGE 3133

3. **Answer: B.** Men tend to have a more acute NFA than do women. The vertex of the NFA lies at the superior limbus of the upper eyelid. PAGE 2762

4. **Answer: D.** Tissue expansion works best in locations where there is solid bony support under the expander balloon device, such as the scalp and forehead. The solid calvarium provides an ideal base for the expander. PAGE 2851

5. **Answer: D.** Postpeel reepithelialization relies upon the epidermis within hair follicles and sebaceous glands. Isotretinoin prevents reepithelialization from these locations. Therefore, isotretinoin use within the last 6 months is an absolute contraindication to chemical peeling. PAGE 3190

6. **Answer D.** Dual lighting with soft boxes or reflective umbrellas placed 45° to the patient provides uniform lighting without harsh shadows and is ideal for standardized photography (PAGES 2775–2776). Fluorescent lights should be avoided since they cast a green hue. Likewise, a single on-camera flash produces harsh shadows and uneven lighting. Ambient window light will vary in intensity and color temperature depending on time of day and weather conditions and is not consistent. A ring flash works well in the intraoperative setting or when photographing intraoral lesions, but is not ideal for studio photography.

7. **Answer: D.** The first stage of auricular reconstruction involves harvest of costal cartilage and creation of an auricular framework. This usually occurs at 6 years of age or later. PAGE 3170

8. **Answer: D.** When the lateral crura are cephalically malpositioned, they provide less support to the nasal ala and alar rim. In such cases, trimming the cephalic border of the lateral crura may diminish that support even further and lead to external valve collapse. Long nasal bones, a wide cartilaginous midvault, and convex lateral crura are all anatomically favorable in terms of support to the nasal airway. PAGE 2932

9. **Answer: D.** The pogonion represents the most anterior projecting point of the chin. It is used to calculate the zero meridian line and multiple other facial angles. PAGE 2767

10. **Answer: D.** Defects involving the nasal ala or sidewall are particularly prone to retraction or collapse with subsequent nasal obstruction. Any defect of sufficient depth

to compromise or remove native structural support will require some form of structural cartilage grafting. Grafts may also be needed to stabilize a reconstructed nasal-tip framework and/or to restore tip projection when compromised. PAGES 2889–2891

11. **Answer: D.** With a level IV injury, there is axonal disruption (disruption of the endoneural sheaths and, by definition, loss of perineural integrity). Only the integrity of the outer epineural sheath separates this from total anatomic disruption of the nerve. Recovery is poor with a level IV injury. PAGE 2905

12. **Answer: A.** Scars that are placed at the border between aesthetic subunits will be less conspicuous. For this reason the reconstructive surgeon may choose to modify the size or shape of the original cutaneous defect to favor a complete subunit reconstruction rather than place scars within or across an aesthetic subunit. PAGES 2874–2875

13. **Answer: D.** The levator anguli oris, buccinator, and mentalis muscles lie in a slightly deeper plane than the remainder of the facial muscles. These muscles are innervated on their superficial surface. PAGE 3106

14. **Answer: E.** There are patient factors and defect issues that guide implant selection, but first and foremost tissue biocompatibility is the most important and essential consideration. PAGE 2789

15. **Answer: C.** The nasofacial angle is formed by the intersection of a line drawn from the nasion through the nasal tip-defining point and a second line drawn from the glabella through the pogonion. The other options do not refer to any named facial angles. PAGE 2943

16. **Answer: D.** OAV spectrum often involves some degree of hemifacial microsomia and includes facial and chin asymmetry. The chin usually deviates to the affected side. PAGE 3177

17. **Answer: D.** Creating an antihelical fold can be performed with a variety of techniques, including scoring and/or excision of cartilage and Mustarde antihelical sutures. PAGE 3148

18. **Answer: D.** A low or caudally positioned radix will make the nasofacial angle more obtuse. In addition, the relative proportions of the nose change, so that the "normal" 3:4:5 ratios (Crumley) are thrown off such that the nasal length from nasion to tip-defining point (the "5") is diminished. In such case, tip projection (the "3") is greater than 60% (3:5) of nasal length, making the tip look overprojected relative to nasal length and "bottom-heavy." PAGE 2949

19. **Answer: A.** Erythema with vesicle formation and exudates in areas treated with a topical ointment are typically signs of an allergic reaction to the ointment. Use of the ointment should be discontinued and the area should be cleansed with soap and water to remove all residual topical medication. PAGE 2819

20. **Answer: C.** Wounds that are superficial and concave are better suited to healing by secondary intention as opposed to deeper wounds or convex surfaces. Superficial wounds of both the temple and medial canthal area are examples of cutaneous defects that heal well by secondary intention. PAGE 2802

21. **Answer A.** The ideal focal length for before and after patient photography is a 60-mm fixed focal length lens with a digital SLR. (PAGE 2779) This is roughly equivalent to a 90- to 105-mm portrait lens with a traditional 35-mm film SLR. A 35-mm wide-angle lens causes distortion of facial features and will make the face appear too narrow. While a 24- to 120-mm zoom lens could be used at a setting of 60 mm, it is much more difficult to maintain consistency with a zoom lens than with a fixed focal length lens.

22. **Answer: C.** The nasal spine is a minor tip-support mechanism. Answers A, B, and D are all major tip-support mechanisms. PAGE 2969

23. **Answer: C.** A retropositioned mandible is referred to as *retrognathia*; this may be associated with a small chin, which is referred to as *microgenia*. *Prognathia* is an anteriorly positioned mandible. PAGES 3180–3181

24. **Answer: C.** The upper eyelid fat pads are deep to the orbital septum and superficial to the levator aponeurosis. Overresection of these fat pads can create a hollowed appearance. PAGE 3076

25. **Answer: B.** Initially, temporary axonal collaterals develop. At about 3 months, however, the collaterals regress as neural transmission through the original nerve terminal is reestablished. PAGE 3241

26. **Answer: B.** Complications such as infection and skin necrosis are very uncommon after otoplasty, but contour abnormalities and malpositions, such as telephone-ear deformity, are more common and are often due to technical errors. PAGE 3152–3156

27. **Answer: C.** With dermabrasion, attention is necessary not to penetrate into the reticular dermis in order to preserve the deeper adnexal structures which serve as the source for reepithelialization. The appearance of fine punctate bleeding during dermabrasion indicates penetration into the papillary dermis, which is desired. PAGE 2867

28. **Answer: D.** Patients with retrognathia are best treated with mandibular advancement, while patients with microgenia can be treated with an alloplast implant. PAGE 3133

29. **Answer: C.** There are three fat pads in the lower eyelid: medial, central, and lateral. The inferior oblique muscle separates the medial and central compartments. PAGE 3085

30. **Answer: A.** Cartilage growth occurs in the perichondrium of the anterior bony septum. Disruption of this process as a result of childhood trauma or surgical intervention can result in loss of vertical growth of the septum. PAGE 2977

31. **Answer: B.** 20 mm of skin (approximately 10 to 12 mm above the incision and 8 to 10 mm below the incision) is required after blepharoplasty to allow good eye closure. PAGE 3081

32. **Answer: C.** Floating in antibiotic solutions, immersion techniques, and antibiotic irrigations have been used to inhibit preimplantation loads, but are typically unproven. On the other hand, suction infiltration of an antibiotic at the time of implantation has been shown to confer a statistically significant advantage in terms of infection prophylaxis. PAGE 2795

33. **Answer: A.** Geometric broken-line closure is a technique that is well suited to relatively long scars and scars oriented 45 degrees or more from the relaxed skin-tension lines. Fusiform excision will do little to diminish scar visibility or to break up/reorient the scar. Serial Z-plasty will add considerably to the overall scar length or number of scars. PAGE 2863

34. **Answer: D.** Although patients who experience depression may safely undergo cosmetic surgery, they are at risk for falling into deeper depression after surgery if the procedure does not fulfill their expectations. PAGE 2758

35. **Answer. A.** Hemangiomas typically appear in the few weeks after birth and grow disproportionately with the infant. Resolution of these lesions is approximately 50% by age 5 years, 70% by age 7 years, and 90% by age 9 years. PAGE 3204

36. **Answer: D.** Avoiding postpeel inflammatory hyperpigmentation includes the use of sunscreen pre- and postpeel and pretreatment with topical tretinoin and skin bleaching agents such as hydroquinone. PAGES 3190–3191

37. **Answer: E.** Laser light is monochromatic, collimated, and coherent. These properties differentiate laser light from ordinary light. PAGE 3200

38. **Answer: A.** The sympathetic nervous system regulates preshunt sphincters located in the deeper subcutaneous tissue, with vasodilation occurring in response to acetylcholine release from sympathetic nerve fibers. PAGE 2799

39. **Answer: D.** This describes the biomechanical property of skin when a deforming stress is applied. Initially, collagen and elastic fibers will stretch in the direction of the force, but beyond a certain point, resistance transitions to eventual inability to deform further with additional force. Hence the stress–strain relationship is nonlinear. PAGE 2798

40. **Answer: B.** The ear generally reaches 85% of its ultimate vertical height, 5 cm, by 3 years of age and is nearly full size, 6 cm, by 5 years of age. PAGE 3143

41. **Answer: A.** Defects located over the alar lobule and cartilaginous nasal sidewall are particularly prone to collapse. Defects in these areas can involve either or both of the internal and external nasal valves. For this reason, poorly supported reconstructions can result in sidewall or alar collapse and symptomatic nasal obstruction. Defects of the nasal tip and dorsal subunit may also require grafts in certain cases, but the highest propensity to airway collapse is over the ala and sidewall. PAGE 2891

42. **Answer: F.** Many factors contribute to the formation of a hematoma. These include postoperative hypertension, coughing, and nausea and vomiting. PAGE 3125

43. **Answer: B.** The most common reason for failure of free-tissue transfer in facial reanimation is thought to be poor neural ingrowth into the transferred muscle. Microvascular failure and improper resting tension of the transferred muscle are less common reasons for failure. PAGE 2916

44. **Answer: D.** The Juri flap is a pedicled transposition flap based on the STA for surgical restoration of the frontal hairline. The Juri flap requires four stages for completion and provides excellent density to the frontal hairline. PAGES 3236–3237

45. **Answer: B.** Patients with BDD exhibit a preoccupation with a real or perceived flaw. This preoccupation negatively affects their life. PAGE 2759

46. **Answer: A.** While a tarsorrhaphy may provide the ultimate in corneal protection, it has the least aesthetic appeal. It is a fairly simple procedure surgically. Eyelid springs are likely the most difficult technically and have a high revision rate. PAGE 2910

47. **Answer: C.** Spontaneous emission occurs when an atom in the excited and unstable state reemits a photon and the electron returns to the lower energy level. If an atom in the higher energy state is struck by an additional photon, two photons are emitted. This process is known as stimulated emission. PAGE 3200

48. **Answer: B.** Delivery of the alar cartilages involves pivoting the alar cartilages from the nose (much like a bucket handle) as a bipedicled chondrocutaneous flap attached medially and laterally. In order to do so, one must release the attachments superiorly and inferiorly. This is done with a marginal incision coupled with an intercartilaginous incision that connects to a full transfixion incision. PAGES 2944, 2946

49. **Answer: C.** Although injuries to facial nerve branches are more devastating complications, they are uncommon. Because of its superficial location, the great auricular nerve (C2 and C3) is the most commonly injured nerve during facelift flap elevation. PAGE 3125

50. **Answer: D.** According to the tripod theory, isolated shortening of the lateral crura will increase tip rotation, while isolated shortening of the medial crura will derotate the nasal tip. The opposite is also true. Lengthening the medial crura and shortening the lateral crura will combine to further increase tip rotation. PAGE 2965

51. **Answer: A.** Multiple neurofibromas are often associated with multiple endocrine neoplasia. Associated conditions include medullary thyroid carcinoma, pheochromocytoma, marfanoid habitus, and kyphoscoliosis. PAGES 3213–3124

52. **Answer: B.** Cells do not adhere directly to the surface of implants. Instead, a substance in the extracellular matrix binds cells to the surface of implants. The most important element in the extracellular matrix for cell adhesion and proliferation is glycosaminoglycans. PAGE 2784

53. **Answer: C.** A benefit of using a phenol-based solution is that the resultant frost is almost immediate, compared to TCA where the practitioner must safely wait 3 to 4 minutes before assessing a peeled area for needed repeated applications. PAGE 3193

54. **Answer: A.** Acellular (cadaveric) dermis resorbs with time and cannot be relied upon for permanent bulk. This resorbable implant can serve as a filler or scaffold for tissue ingrowth or reepithelialization along its surface. It does not directly stimulate dermal thickening or promote bone formation. PAGE 2787

55. **Answer: A.** The upper two-thirds of the nasal dorsum (that portion cephalic to the nasal tip) consists of the nasal bones and dorsal septum together with the paired upper lateral cartilages (ULCs). Shorter nasal bones imply longer ULCs. The longer flexible cartilaginous segment is less well supported on short nasal bones and this puts the patient who undergoes a dorsal reduction at higher risk of midvault/ULC medialization or collapse leading to nasal obstruction. PAGE 2957

56. **Answer: A.** The skin along the nasal dorsum is thinnest at the rhinion and thickest at the nasion. As a result, maintaining slight skeletal height at the rhinion will result in a straight-line profile, while a slight concavity will result if the skeletal profile deep to the skin is level. PAGE 2924

57. **Answer: B.** Rapid intraoperative tissue expansion relies on mechanical creep and a gain of 1 to 3 cm of flap length can be achieved, depending on the site of expansion. PAGE 2854

58. **Answer: A.** The classic triad of tip bifidity, thin skin, and strong lower lateral cartilages increases the risk of postoperative nasal-tip bossae. With thinner skin and strong, divergent (bifid) lower lateral cartilages, overly aggressive excisional techniques can lead to visibility of the thicker cut edge of cartilage as the thinner skin and soft-tissue envelope contracts during the postoperative period. PAGE 2932

59. **Answer: B.** Smile patterns are determined by which muscle groups dominate with smiling. The most common smile pattern (67%) is the zygomaticus major smile which is primarily activated by the zygomaticus muscles and the buccinators. This is followed in frequency by the canine smile (30%) and least commonly the full denture smile (2%). PAGES 2911–2912

60. **Answer: A.** When the BMI is very low, the rectus abdominis affords a high volume skin paddle where there is still ample subcutaneous fat. In patients with a normal BMI, the rectus has been largely replaced by the anterolateral thigh flap for defects with a higher volume soft-tissue deficit. PAGE 2831

61. **Answer: A.** Chromophores are substances that absorb energy at specific wavelengths. The specific absorption patterns of tissues partly determine the most efficacious laser for a given lesion. PAGE 3201

62. **Answer: B.** Cryotherapy (cold therapy) results in tissue destruction by cell membrane damage. Rapid freezing followed by slow thawing is most lethal to cells, with melanocytes being the most susceptible to injury. PAGE 3222

63. **Answer: B.** Alloplast chin implants may correct horizontal microgenia, but do not correct chin asymmetries or vertical discrepancies. Implants also tend to deepen the labiomental sulcus. PAGE 3181

64. **Answer: D.** The younger the patient, the more conservative the physician must be in estimating the donor hair present and establishing a long-term treatment plan. A 23-year-old patient likely will increase his hair loss in the next few years. PAGE 3230

65. **Answer: E.** The double-convexity deformity results from descent of the suborbicularis oculi fat pad and is considered an indication for fat repositioning in lower eyelid blepharoplasty or midface lift. PAGE 3086

66. **Answer: E.** A failed primary rhinoplasty and the prospect of revision surgery can elicit frustration and anger in all patients. (PAGES 2994–2995) Nasal skin quality can affect outcome in revision surgery—thinner or intermediate skin thickness is generally more forgiving and "favorable" than ultrathick or ultrathin skin. (PAGE 2998) In circumstances in which revision surgery is inevitable and soft-tissue contraction might be detrimental (the twisted nose, the overresected nose), revision surgery may be preferable within the first year. PAGE 3003

67. **Answer: C.** Polymethyl methacrylate (Artefill)—PMMA—is suspended in a bovine collagen carrier. The risk of a hypersensitivity reaction to the bovine collagen antigen skin testing for allergic sensitivity is recommended. PAGE 3248

68. **Answer: B.** Hematoma formation is the most common (reported as high as 8.5%) and feared complication during the facelift procedure. PAGE 3125

69. **Answer: A.** Tuberous sclerosis is a congenital syndrome associated with multiple organ hamartomas, mental retardation, seizure disorder, and sebaceous adenomas. Its onset is usually in early childhood to young adult life. (re: Sturge–Weber syndrome, Osler–Rendu–Weber (PAGES 3213, 3216–3217)

70. **Answer: D.** Lagophthalmos after upper eyelid blepharoplasty results from overresection of skin or orbicularis oculi muscle. (PAGE 3084) Dermatochalasis is peripheral loss of vision from excessive eyelid skin. PAGE 3074

71. **Answer: B.** The coronal, endoscopic, and indirect approaches allow myoplasty, while the direct approach does not facilitate muscle resection. PAGE 3066

72. **Answer: D.** Patient-specific implants take advantage of current three-dimensional radiographic modeling and computer-assisted design to customize an implant for a patient's specific needs. PAGE 2787

73. **Answer: B.** Despite having a long bony segment, the fibular flap often lacks the cross-sectional diameter to reliably fix osseointegrated implants. (PAGE 2835) The iliac crest has the largest cross-sectional area as compared to fibular or scapular bone, making it the best choice for retention of osseointegrated implants. PAGE 2838

74. **Answer: B.** In that the coronal approach to brow lifting slightly raises the hairline, patients with a full and low anterior hairline are the best candidates. (PAGE 3059)

75. **Answer: C.** The pogonion is the most anterior or prominent point on the chin, whereas the menton is the lowest midline point on the chin. PAGE 2941

76. **Answer: D.** Within the first 72 hours after nerve transection, the distal nerve segments retain electrical stimulability, making their identification easier. With increasing time lapse between nerve injury and grafting, the biological regenerative potential diminishes and long-term functional outcomes are compromised. PAGES 2906–2907

77. **Answer: C.** Conventional tissue expansion increases the metabolic activity of fibroblasts, thins the dermis, but does not change the number of hair follicles or distribution of hair growth. PAGE 2851

78. **Answer: D.** Proper design of a Z-plasty allows the surgeon to plan both the length and degree of reorientation of the revised scar. Changing the angle produces predictable changes in both variables. A 60° angle will produce a 75% increase in length of the scar. Angles should never be less than 30° because of the risk of necrosis of the narrow flap tips that result. PAGES 2862 AND TABLE 176.4

79. **Answer: B.** The appeal of geometric broken-line closure is the irregular scar that results which favors better scar camouflage. Ideal flap length should fall between 3 and 7 mm (ideally about 5 mm) since larger flaps are more conspicuous or visible, while smaller flaps are difficult to work with and close. PAGE 2863

80. **Answer: D.** Proportionate features are not required to achieve an aesthetic facial appearance. PAGE 2757

81. **Answer A.** Photographic exposure can be increased by one of three methods, including increasing the aperture. Since the f-stop is inversely related to the aperture size, changing from f/8 to f/16 in this answer would decrease exposure. (PAGE 2778) The other ways to increase exposure are slowing the shutter speed, increasing the light sensitivity of the camera by increasing the ISO, or increasing the ambient light when in manual mode.

82. **Answer: A.** Although a full transfixion incision will disrupt the attachment of the medial crura to the caudal septum (a major tip-support mechanism), long and strong medial crura may resist or minimize the effect of a full transfixion incision on deprojecting the nasal tip. In such cases, if deprojection is desired, some direct modification of the crura will need to be undertaken. PAGE 2967

83. **Answer: C.** Heating bone to more than 50°C during drilling can cause osteoblasts to die. Keeping the temperature of the bone down is thus the rationale for irrigation of cooler saline directly onto the bone when drilling. PAGE 2784

84. **Answer: C.** By definition, keloids are fibrous scars that extend beyond the edges of the original wound, while hypertrophic scars are confined within the borders of the original wound. The difference clinically can have implications for treatment and recurrence rates. Atrophic scars are nonhypertrophic scars that are depressed below the level of the normal adjacent skin. PAGE 2860

85. **Answer: B.** The turkey-gobbler deformity is caused by a laxity in the platysma muscle that does not decussate in the midline. (PAGE 3132) Cobra deformity may result from overaggressive fat resection. PAGE 3138

86. **Answer: C.** The radial forearm flap requires a preoperative Allen test to confirm adequate bloodflow to the thumb and index finger through the ulnar artery via the palmar arches to avoid risking ischemia to the hand when the flap is harvested. (PAGE 2826) With the fibular-free flap one must insure that there is adequate blood supply to the foot when the peroneal artery is sacrificed, so preoperative angiography is indicated. PAGE 2836

87. **Answer B.** Depth of field is increased the farther the camera is placed from the subject. (PAGE 2778) Changing from a 60-mm to a 300-mm lens will lessen or compress depth of field. Changes in shutter speed will affect exposure but will not change depth of field. Since aperture is inversely related to f-stop, changing from f/16 to f/8 would decrease depth of field.

88. **Answer: A.** An increase in the nasolabial angle by definition reflects increase nasal-tip rotation. By shortening the lateral limbs of the tip tripod, a lateral crural overlay will also increase tip rotation. A dorsal-hump reduction also creates the illusion of increasing tip rotation. A hanging columella creates the illusion of a more acute nasolabial angle, and therefore, reduction makes the nasolabial angle appear more obtuse, increasing apparent tip rotation. Augmenting the nasal dorsum, on the other hand, is one of many techniques that applies to visually lengthen the nose and visually derotate the tip (i.e., decrease tip rotation). PAGES 2923, 2935

89. **Answer: A.** Chin implants often cause a small amount of resorption of the anterior mandible. This condition is exacerbated by implant mobility. The mandibular resorption is usually not clinically significant. PAGE 3187

90. **Answer: D.** Pinpointing the specific desires of the patient can be a critical aspect of surgical planning and can facilitate communication between the surgeon and prospective patient. The surgeon must however be confident that his/her skills are commensurate with the challenges of revision surgery before agreeing to proceed surgically. PAGE 3001

91. **Answer: D.** Various studies have shown that 6 to 8 weeks are required for adhesion between the cranium and overlying periosteum. PAGE 3069

92. **Answer: A.** Anatomically the internal nasal valve is delimited by the space bounded by the caudal aspect of the ULC, the head of the inferior turbinate, and the dorsal septum. PAGE 2953

93. **Answer: E.** All of the above are features of BDD. BDD is much more common among patients seeking cosmetic surgery than in the general population. Surgical success rates are extremely poor in those suffering from BDD regardless of the cosmetic outcome. Patients with suspected BDD should be referred for psychiatric evaluation and treatment. PAGE 2996

94. **Answer: D.** The preseptal approach involves dissecting inferiorly along the avascular plane between the orbital septum and the orbicularis oculi muscle. The postseptal approach is a more direct approach to the orbital fat through the conjunctiva and the lower lid retractors closer to the conjunctival fornix. PAGE 3091

95. **Answer: C.** The accepted "minimum" width of the dorsal and caudal septal struts that should remain for adequate support of the L-strut is 10 mm. PAGE 2980 .

96. **Answer: A.** Pivotal flaps move around a fixed axis toward the center of the wound. This can include rotation flaps, transposition flaps, and interpolation flaps. Island flaps and V-Y flaps are examples of advancement flaps. Both bilobe and rhomboid flaps are types of transposition flaps. PAGE 2803

97. **Answer: A.** Plasma imbibition, a process whereby nutrients diffuse into the skin graft from fluids in the recipient site, is the first process that is active in the survival of full-thickness skin grafts. This is followed by vascular inosculation and then capillary ingrowth. PAGE 2814

98. **Answer: A.** A columellar strut will stabilize the nasal base when the medial crura are long and the alar–columellar relationship is appropriate. An extended columellar strut may be an option in the patient with poor tip support and a deficient premaxilla. Setting the medial crura back on the caudal septum (tongue-in-groove) is effective when the caudal septum is overly long—the hanging columella. If the columella is short or retracted, a caudal septal extension graft will address the alar–columellar disharmony and restore appropriate length to the septum to allow for stabilization of the medial crura to the extension graft. PAGES 2969–2970

99. **Answer: B.** A shallow (overprojected radix) or a high radix (cephalically malpositioned) will both have the effect of making the nose look visually longer by increasing distance from nasion to tip-defining point. PAGE 2949

100. **Answer: D.** Early contour irregularities following cervical liposuction are the rule rather than the exception. Most resolve as healing progresses and edema lessens. PAGE 3140

101. **Answer: A.** Due to the rich subdermal vascular plexus supplying their hair follicles, hematoma rates are higher in male patients. PAGE 3122

102. **Answer: A.** In general, the greater the degree of rotation or pivot, the shorter the effective length of the flap. This needs to be taken into account with flap design—with increasing degrees of pivot a longer flap must be designed to allow for the loss of effective length. PAGE 2803

103. **Answer: C.** Patients with bilateral microtia/atresia should get a bone conduction hearing aid before their first birthday to maximize their ability to verbally communicate and develop. PAGE 3169

104. **Answer: B.** The prominent ear is a type of deformational auricular anomaly characterized by an absent antihelical fold and a deep conchal bowl. PAGE 3144

105. **Answer: C.** Dermatochalasis refers to excess skin of the eyelids. Dermatochalasis should not be confused with blepharochalasis, which is a rare inflammatory disorder of the eyelids characterized by recurrent edema. PAGE 3086

106. **Answer: C.** The temporal branch of the facial nerve can be reliably found running just superficial to the sentinel vein. The nerve runs in the deep portion of the temporoparietal fascia. PAGE 3054

107. **Answer: C.** The Tyndall effect is a bluish discoloration of the overlying skin seen when hyaluronic acid (HA) fillers are placed too superficially. This can be treated with extrusion of the product through a nick in the overlying skin if seen early. If not noted early, untoward side effects with HA fillers can be treated by dissolving the product with the injection of hyaluronidase. PAGE 3249

108. **Answer: A.** Skeletal reexpansion of the overresected nose in the patient with inelastic skin and a noncompliant skin envelope can jeopardize tissue perfusion and lead to ischemic compromise. Skin stretching exercise may be helpful to improve tissue elasticity. PAGE 3013

109. **Answer: B.** An overhead flash most closely replicates natural overhead sunlight which accentuates deviations in the crooked nose. PAGE 2979

110. **Answer: B.** The anterolateral thigh is a source which is thin, pliable, and affords the surgeon a large skin paddle. Cutaneous donor sites can provide better voice, less dysphagia, and less donor site morbidity. Peristalsis of the jejunal flap can produce functional problems with swallowing and voice issues as well. PAGE 2844

111. **Answer: C.** Survival of composite grafts ultimately depends on ingrowth of capillaries from the wound edges. The farther the center of the graft is from the edge of the defect (i.e., larger grafts), the more likely it becomes that the graft will fail before sufficient capillary ingrowth occurs. Current recommendations are that no portion of the graft should be more than 1 cm from a wound edge. PAGE 2817

112. **Answer: D.** Pyogenic granulomas are the most common acquired hemangiomas. They are often precipitated by minor trauma or pregnancy. PAGE 3216

113. **Answer: D.** The surface area of the expander base should be 2.5 to 3 times as large as the defect size. PAGE 2853

114. **Answer: D.** Cephalically positioned lateral crura offer poor support to the lateral nasal wall/external nasal valve increasing the risk of dynamic collapse. In addition, the cephalic malposition creates a bulbous nasal tip with a "parenthesis" deformity and apparent increase in middle vault width. PAGE 2968

115. **Answer: B.** The depressor supercilii (the fibers of the orbicularis oculi deep to the medial brow) is the only muscle listed that is a brow depressor. The other brow depressors are the corrugator supercilii, the orbicularis oculi, and the procerus. PAGE 3240

116. **Answer: B.** Radiesse is made up of 30% CaHA microspheres suspended in a 70% carrier gel made up of water, glycerin, and carboxymethylcellulose. The CaHA is apparent within the soft tissue on CT imaging. Juvéderm is made up of hyaluronic acid and Sculptra is an injectable poly-L-lactic acid. PAGE 3247

117. **Answer: C.** Finasteride is a competitive and specific inhibitor of type II 5α-reductase. It is not indicated for women and children. Finasteride is often used in combination with minoxidil for the treatment of androgenetic alopecia in men. PAGE 3229

118. **Answer: A.** The structures contributing to the external nasal valve are the lateral crura, the suspensory ligaments of the lateral crura, and the fibrofatty/fibromuscular soft tissue of the nasal ala. Answers B, C, D, and E do not contribute to the external nasal valve. PAGE 2979

119. **Answer: A.** Ear molding techniques are most effective in neonates less than 3 weeks old and lose effectiveness with age and increasing cartilage rigidity. PAGE 3147

120. **Answer: D.** The arcus marginalis is the connective tissue thickening at the orbital margin where the frontal periosteum becomes the orbital septum. PAGE 3076

121. **Answer: B.** Various techniques have been described to harvest donor hair grafts. These include strips harvest with knife blades, and sharp and dull punches (FUE). PAGE 3232

122. **Answer: D.** Inferomedial collapse of the ULCs from lack of support can lead to pinching of the middle third of the nasal vault revealing the V-shaped caudal border of the nasal bones in relief. (PAGE 2929) Overnarrowing of the tip can result in an unnatural pinched appearance to the nasal tip, and excessive resection of the lateral crura may lead to alar collapse or retraction but not an inverted V. Ischemic necrosis of the septum is most likely going to lead to a saddle nose deformity.

123. **Answer: C.** Hetter showed that when added to an 88% phenol solution, increasing concentrations of croton oil increased the healing times. PAGE 3192

124. **Answer C.** When taking an oblique photograph, both the head and torso should be turned 45° to the camera to avoid neck distortion. (PAGE 2775) Every attempt to standardize before and after photographs should be made including standardized camera-to-subject distance, positioning in the Frankfort horizontal plane, and avoiding distracting hairstyles, glasses, and jewelry.

125. **Answer: D.** The temporoparietal fascia flap is a well-vascularized supply of proximate tissue supplied by the superficial temporal artery. It is the tissue of choice for soft-tissue loss over a reconstructed microtic ear. PAGE 3171

126. **Answer: A.** Wide scars may result from large tissue resections, especially in the posterior scalp. Infections after hair transplantation are uncommon. PAGE 3233

127. **Answer: B.** Mentalis muscle dyskinesis is often caused by either a chin implant with an alloplast or a bony genioplasty. The treatment for this condition is an injection with a small amount of botulinum toxin. PAGE 3187

128. **Answer: A.** Lateral osteotomies are generally initiated along the pyriform aperture, *above* the attachment of the inferior turbinate. This maintains stability of the inferior turbinate position and also preserves the suspensory ligamentous attachments between the tail of the lateral crura and the pyriform aperture (minor tip-support mechanism). PAGE 2960

129. **Answer: C.** Retroorbital hematoma is considered to be the most feared complication following blepharoplasty. Treatment should consist of immediate decompression by opening all incisions with exploration to identify and cauterize any offending vessel. PAGE 3101

130. **Answer: D.** The fibular-free flap has a small volume skin paddle and is thus less useful for larger soft-tissue defects. The skin paddle of iliac crest flaps can be difficult to rotate into oral cavity defects. The TDAST combines the advantages of a long vascular pedicle, abundant relatively thin skin, and an independent arc of rotation of the bone and skin paddles, giving it the most versatility for soft-tissue reconstruction among the osseous donor site options. PAGES 2839–2840

131. **Answer: A.** In patients with redundant skin of the cervical region (class II), a standard cervicofacial rhytidectomy is generally considered the treatment of choice. PAGES 3135–3136

132. **Answer: D.** Advantages of the endoscopic approach include smaller incisions, decreased incidence of sensory neuropathy and alopecia, less bleeding, and a faster recovery period. PAGE 3068

133. **Answer: A.** Pedicle division and inset is ultimately necessary in all patients and is typically performed after 3 weeks to allow for sufficient vascular ingrowth, fibroblast development, and flap adherence to the recipient site. PAGE 2889

134. **Answer: A.** The primary blood supply to the forehead flap is through the supratrochlear artery making it an axial pattern vascular flap. In addition, terminal branches from the angular artery provide a blood supply to the base of the flap pedicle. PAGE 2886

135. **Answer: B.** Unlike transposition flaps, the base of interpolated flaps is not contiguous with the defect. Thus, by definition, interpolation flaps involve transfer of the flap over across intervening normal cutaneous tissue. (PAGE 2808) In general, rotation flaps involve transfer of tissue immediately adjacent to the defect and are best used for repair of triangular defects. PAGE 2803

136. **Answer: D.** Power density is a function of the power divided by the cross-sectional area of the laser beam (spot size). As the spot size decreases, the power density increases. PAGE 3201

137. **Answer: B.** Senile ptosis involves a stretching of the levator aponeurosis or a separation of the aponeurosis from the tarsal plate. PAGE 3079

138. **Answer: D.** Hetter proved that the concentration of phenol has little to do with the depth of peel penetration and that increasing concentrations of croton oil increase the healing times. He also noted that multiple coats of peel solution will increase the depth of injury. PAGE 3192

139. **Answer: F.** An unfavorable wound healing response cannot be predicted with certainty in any given patient and may present without any identifying risk factors. (PAGE 2998) Photographic analysis is an essential component of the preoperative assessment, but is not a substitute for direct inspection, palpation, and dynamic observation. (PAGE 2999) Computer imaging can be very beneficial for pinpointing patient expectations and improving communication between the patient and surgeon. PAGE 3001

140. **Answer: B.** Nevus sebaceus is a common benign condition occurring on the scalp of children; it transforms to basal cell carcinoma about 1% of the time. PAGE 3216

141. **Answer: D.** Autologous costal cartilage is the gold standard for auricular reconstruction. Irradiated cartilage has a greater resorption rate than does autologous costal cartilage, and the contralateral ear does not provide a sufficient supply of cartilage to create an adequate framework. PAGE 3170

142. **Answer: B.** *Creep* is defined as a gain in skin surface area that results when a constant load is applied. *Stress relaxation* is defined as a decrease in the amount of force necessary to maintain a fixed amount of skin stretch over time. PAGE 2850

143. **Answer: A.** Disruption of the attachment of the ULCs to the nasal bones brings the caudal aspect of the nasal bones into relief, causing what appears visually as an inverted-V deformity. Correction will generally require spreader grafting in an effort to elevate the collapsed ULC. Inadequate lateral osteotomies can lead to an open roof deformity. PAGE 2961

144. **Answer: A.** Leonardo da Vinci is credited with identifying the equal horizontal thirds and vertical fifths that divide the face. This principle is one of many applied to facial analysis. Powell and Humphreys modified it to serve the basis for modern-day facial analysis. PAGE 2954

145. **Answer B.** This radiograph demonstrates the classic "ground-glass" matrix that is associated with fibrous dysplasia. Fibromas and osteomas should be more exophytic. Chondrosarcoma and Paget disease would have different types of internal calcified matrix.

11 Contemporary Issues in Medical Practice

1. What is the name of the act that the U.S. Congress enacted into law in 2009, which implemented new policies to induce adoption and "meaningful use" of electronic health records (EHRs) by hospitals and physicians?

    A. The Health Information Technology for Economic and Clinical Health (HITECH) Act
    B. The American Electronic Health Records (AEHR) Act
    C. The American Recovery and Health Information Technology (ARHIT) Act
    D. The Health Information Technology and Electronic Health Records (HITEHR) Act

2. Macros may be used compliantly in documentation of which of the following components of evaluation and management services?

    A. Medical history
    B. Physical examination
    C. Medical decision-making (MDM)
    D. Billing and coding

3. The physician specialists of which a larger number of those surveyed in 2007 (latest data available) favor national health insurance than did so in 2002 include:

    A. Anesthesiologists
    B. Surgical subspecialists
    C. Medical subspecialists
    D. A and C
    E. All of the above

4. Which of the following are the characteristics of high-reliability organizations?

    A. Diverse aims
    B. Predictability
    C. Standardization for repetitive processes
    D. No feedback loops as ingenuity drives quality

5. Human error is best described by which of these statements?

    A. The underlying cause of medical mistakes
    B. Due to innate human characteristics
    C. Able to be studied and anticipated
    D. Not preventable, but its effects can be reduced through informed system design
    E. All of the above

6. You are writing a paper on a new and promising medical device. You have stock options in the privately held company which manufactures the device, but have not exercised the options. When submitting the paper, which of the following statements is correct?

    A. You have no responsibility to disclose your potential to invest in the company.
    B. If you exercise the stock option, then you will be required to write a letter to the editor explaining your involvement if the article is published.
    C. You should divest yourself of the potential investment because of the conflict of interest.
    D. You must disclose the information about the potential investment when you submit your paper for publication and review.

7. According to the CIA (Central Intelligence Agency), life expectancy in the United States is longer than in:

    A. Jordan
    B. The United Kingdom
    C. Canada
    D. Bosnia and Herzegovina
    E. None of the above

8. For physicians at teaching hospitals who are providing care in conjunction with residents, when the resident performs and documents a medically indicated comprehensive history and physical examination (H&P) for an admission, CPT (current procedural terminology) code 99223, what is the minimum level of patient care the teaching physician may perform and document, along with appropriate resident teaching, in order to submit a claim for code 99223?

   A. Countersigning the resident's H&P
   B. Problem-focused care (problem-focused history and examination plus straightforward medical decision-making (MDM))
   C. Detailed care (detailed history and examination plus low-complexity MDM)
   D. Comprehensive care (comprehensive history and examination plus high-complexity MDM)

9. A modified wave scheduling technique will promote patient access only if:

   A. patients are made aware of the process.
   B. registration of patients is completed prior to the patients' arrival for their appointment.
   C. room turnover is completed in 2 minutes or less.
   D. appropriate triage of patient is achieved at the time of scheduling.

10. True or False: For-profit insurance companies are limited by U.S. federal law in the amount of money they can spend on "political speech."

   A. False
   B. True

11. Three categories of telemedicine are:

   A. Electronic health record system (EHR), interactive video teleconferencing (VTC), and remote patient monitoring (RPM)
   B. Store and forward (S&F), VTC, and RPM
   C. EHR, S&F, and VTC
   D. Telementoring, VTC, and RPM

12. The end result concept is predicated on the fact that surgeons should examine their results to determine:

   A. The end result of a disease process to better define the most appropriate treatment
   B. The end result of one's intervention to determine its success and potential improvements
   C. What treatment interventions would have ameliorated the outcome
   D. The root cause of a patient's mortality

13. A chief resident is considering a job opportunity where the surgical practice owns a surgicenter and the practice will consider offering a buy-in opportunity to the surgicenter if partnership is offered after year 2 of employment. Which of the following statements is correct?

    A. The chief resident should report the practice to the FBI under the whistle-blower law.
    B. The chief resident will not be able to bring patients with Medicare to this surgicenter.
    C. The chief resident should investigate to make sure that the surgicenter is set up under a "safe harbor" of Stark legislation.
    D. The chief resident should join the practice but should not participate in the surgicenter because of concern of a possible conflict of interest and violate Stark laws if she or he operates on people in this facility.

14. Which features should be added to conventional operative notes to ensure specificity and medical necessity?

    A. Narratives of medical indications and operative findings
    B. Summary of medical indications and preoperative laboratory findings
    C. Narratives of medical indications and postoperative care plan
    D. Narratives of medical indications, operative findings, and postoperative care plan

15. Which two evaluation and management elements must be added to conventional history and physical examination (H&P) documents to promote compliant documentation and coding?

    A. Insurance deductible and copayment
    B. Psychological stability and pain threshold
    C. Three levels of risk and nature of the presenting problem(s)
    D. Data reviewed and tests ordered

16. Responding to a medical mistake should include:

    A. Discussion with department chair
    B. Disclosure to patient and family with apology when appropriate
    C. Reporting to appropriate authorities to enhance study of the system leading to the error
    D. Signing of nondisclosure forms by all involved health care workers
    E. A, B, and C

17. What programming tool is available which allows the researcher to perform clinical data mining from textual data or narrative text records from merging clinical databases?

    A. Ontology semantic Web processing
    B. Textual consolidation processing
    C. Representational difference processing
    D. Natural language processing

18. You are invited to give a lecture at a forum with continuing medical education (CME) credit for learners on a new drug used to treat a rare cancer. In reviewing the literature and background of the drug during the presentation, you will be citing studies that you managed and that were financially supported by a pharmaceutical company. Which of the following steps should the planning committee for the CME activity take?

    A. The planning committee should assign a member to review all of your slides in advance of the lecture to make sure there is no bias present.
    B. The planning committee should revoke your invitation to speak.
    C. The planning committee should trust that you will present in an unbiased manner and poll the audience after the talk to see if they perceived bias.
    D. The planning committee should make certain that marketing materials promoting the drug are available at the podium.

19. Net collection rate is a measure of revenue collections performance and is calculated as:

    A. Total amount collected/Total amount billed
    B. Total amount collected/Total amount billed - Contractual allowances + Refunds and overpayments
    C. Total amount billed/Total allowances
    D. Total amount collected - Contractual allowances/Total amount billed

20. High-reliability organizations share commonalities such as:

    A. Never having an error or adverse event
    B. Minimal economic investments with high yields on such investments
    C. Application of systems science methodologies to drive outcomes
    D. A hierarchical leadership structure to advocate for change

21. Telemedicine otology cases consisting of high-quality images, audiograms and tympanograms, and clinical histories have been shown to be useful for:

    A. Planning chronic ear surgery
    B. Following up pediatric patients post–tympanostomy tube placement
    C. Providing medical clearance for hearing aid fitting
    D. All of the above

22. Which of the following is *not* an advantage of interactive video teleconferencing (VTC)?

    A. Two providers do not need to be simultaneously available.
    B. Patient affect and movement may be assessed.
    C. The consulting provider may have real-time input into the examination and interview.
    D. A "human" connection can be established.

23. Historically, use of telemedicine in otolaryngology was driven by:

    A. The need to serve remote populations
    B. Shortages of available otolaryngologists
    C. Backlogs of patients needing otolaryngology referrals
    D. All of the above

24. Which are the two fundamental coding concepts required for compliant billing?

    A. Compatibility and specificity
    B. Specificity and meaningful use
    C. Medical necessity and specificity
    D. Conversion and compatibility

25. A rhinologist has developed a high-volume practice and is considered to be a leading expert in her community. Two companies which make balloon catheters are vying for her to use their product in the outpatient setting. One company offers to reimburse her 25% of the cost of the balloon for each balloon used if she uses more than five balloons per month. Which of the following responses is most ethical?

    A. The rhinologist should politely refuse the offer, but be flattered that companies are interested in attracting her business.
    B. The rhinologist should politely refuse because the offer is a clear violation of antikickback principles and should write a letter to the chief executive officer of the company explaining the conflict of interest inherent in the offer.
    C. The rhinologist should discuss the offer with the second company and see if they will reimburse 30% of the purchase price.
    D. The rhinologist should refuse the offer but see if the hospital can be given the discount instead of her practice.

26. **High-performance teams that demonstrate highly effective intrateam communication have which of the following characteristics?**

    A. They are led by charismatic leaders who direct all team actions.
    B. All team members are empowered to speak up if they believe the team could be making a mistake.
    C. Team members typically remain quiet until their opinion is sought by the team leader.
    D. Team members participate in simultaneous and competing conversations.
    E. All of the above.

27. **What are the advantages of incorporating "gray literature" when conducting a meta-analysis?**

    A. It allows the incorporation of unpublished data into the meta-analysis.
    B. It allows the incorporation of untranslated foreign language data into the meta-analysis.
    C. It improves the quality of the meta-analysis as it may serve to reduce publication bias.
    D. It increases the study size of the meta-analysis resulting in greater statistical significance.

28. **The HIPAA (Health Insurance Portability and Accountability Act) privacy rules safeguard the confidentiality of protected health information:**

    A. That is transmitted by any electronic means
    B. Obtained by all health care providers regardless of the technology they use
    C. Excluding necessary information contained on billing cards or super bills
    D. Does not apply to patient information used for targeted marketing activities marketing activities

29. **The physician self-referral law, commonly referred to as the Stark law, does which of these?**

    A. Allows referrals for designated health services payable to Medicare/Medicaid as long as the physician himself is not the owner. Immediate family members can be owners.
    B. Covers only clinical laboratory services.
    C. Requires specific proof of intent to violate the law before the law applies.
    D. Covers clinical laboratory services, speech and language pathology, radiology, durable medical equipment, home health services, and inpatient and outpatient hospital services.

30. **Identify the correct statement regarding occurrence or claims-made professional liability insurance policies:**

    A. The occurrence policy will continue to cover those losses for up to 10 years, even if the policy has since expired.
    B. Occurrence policies are typically just as costly as claims-made policies.
    C. Claims-made policies differ from occurrence policies in that they offer protection from claims made during a specific period of time.
    D. Purchasing tail coverage does not reduce the risk of liability exposure to a patient for physicians with claims-made policies.

31. **Medical error is a critical challenge for health care, and accounts for:**

    A. Nearly 18 million deaths in the United States each year
    B. Almost 2 million dollars in excess Medicare costs yearly
    C. Roughly 1 in 20 deaths in the United States annually
    D. One half of the total health care costs in the United States
    F. All of the above

32. **Modifiers are required for payment of two independent procedures on the same date of service for which reason?**

    A. Payers' software has a default setting to pay for only one procedure per day.
    B. Payers are counting the number of procedures performed.
    C. Payers automatically include relative value units for other procedures.
    D. Payers want to review these separately.

33. **The Institute of Medicine's report "To Err Is Human" is a landmark publication as it:**

    A. Reaffirmed human fallibility
    B. Reinvigorated health care's efforts on quality improvement
    C. Was shown to overestimate quality improvement opportunities
    D. Has led to a plethora of organizations that have no demonstrable outcome benefit

34. **With regard to privacy and security, a telemedicine system is:**

    A. Held to the same standards as an electronic health record system (EHR)
    B. Allowed to have a lower level of encryption than an EHR
    C. Safe to use over the Internet with appropriate malware protection software
    D. Safe to use with standard e-mail programs as long as they are password protected

35. Ethical guidelines for expert witness testimony in a medical malpractice action should:

    A. Adopt a position as an advocate or partisan in the legal proceedings

    B. Review all the appropriate medical information in the case and testify to its content so as to best help his side

    C. Limit their testimony to their areas of expertise and should be prepared to state the basis for the testimony presented

    D. Ensure compensation at a rate which reflects the most you can get independent of the time and effort given in the preparation for testimony and ideally should be linked to the outcome of the case

36. The evaluation and management (E/M) coding system takes its origin from:

    A. Administrative calculations developed by insurers, independent of patient care principles

    B. Administrative calculations developed by Medicare personnel, independent of patient care principles

    C. A standard reference text commonly used to instruct medical students in performing and documenting an optimal history and physical examination

    D. A team of physicians and statisticians working at Harvard on the resource-based relative value system

37. A basic strategy practice can be deployed to mitigate the risk of leaking protected patient medical information to

    A. Discuss patient cases openly with all staff to ensure familiarity and reduce the need for staff to access the patient's chart

    B. Secure electronic medical records as paper records are not covered by HIPAA patient privacy regulations

    C. Restrict access to information systems at the appropriate levels, and track individual activity in any system containing protected health information

    D. Assess potential for security weaknesses only in response to an actual breach

38. What is a major obstacle when performing studies with the Veterans Administration (VA) electronic health record (EHR) database?

    A. Most of the clinical information is stored as textual data.

    B. Access to the database is limited by federal legislation.

    C. The search engines associated with these types of databases are not amenable for data mining.

    D. The database is subject to higher selection, analysis, and interpretation biases.

39. What are the major limitations for conducting studies and data mining using insurance databases and most government databases?

    A. Significant portions of the data are recorded as textual data requiring the researcher to manually evaluate each case individually.
    B. They are subject to selection, analysis, and interpretation biases.
    C. The population size is too large to conduct meaningful data analysis.
    D. The search engines associated with these types of databases are not amenable for data mining.

40. Of the several important reasons to retain good employees, which is the most important?

    A. Recruiting costs approximately $2,000 per full-time employee.
    B. Turnover costs range from 0.75 to 2.0 times the salary of the departing individual.
    C. Competitive practices may recruit your employees for lower pay.
    D. Having a low performer on your staff is better than having a vacant position.

41. The main goal for physicians in negotiating managed care contracts is:

    A. Balancing agreed-upon rates with the potential for additional volume of patients
    B. Negotiating rates equal to Medicare
    C. Ensuring the contract includes a no-fault out clause
    D. Agreeing to authorization requirements spanning outpatient services

42. You are a faculty member at the county hospital and the chief resident has privileges to accomplish certain types of basic surgical procedures, like tracheotomy. You are on vacation when the chief resident schedules and accomplishes a tracheotomy on an elderly man with Medicare insurance who has been intubated in the intensive care unit for 3 weeks after a stroke. Upon your return, which of the following is most appropriate?

    A. If the patient had commercial insurance, you could submit a bill for the surgical procedure because you are ultimately responsible for the practice.
    B. Because the patient has Medicare insurance you should submit a bill for the surgical procedure because you are ultimately responsible for the practice.
    C. You are not entitled to bill for the procedure because the chief resident's salary was paid via Medicare Part B funds.
    D. You are not entitled to bill for the procedure because you were not present to supervise the chief resident.

43. Implementation of a "just culture" is a strategy originally instituted in aviation intended to:

    A. Prevent human error
    B. Reduce likelihood of reckless behavior
    C. Relieve individual team members of personal responsibility
    D. Assure effective team communication within high-stress settings
    E. Improve Federal Aviation Administration survey scores

44. Health insurance coverage in the United States, depending on the individual, may be provided by:

    A. A government-run health service, structured like the UK's National Health Service, with physicians employed by the government
    B. A government-financed single-payer health system, like Canada's Medicare system, with physicians in private practice
    C. Private, for-profit health insurance
    D. None of the above
    E. A to D (inclusive)

45. According to the Central Intelligence Agency, infant mortality in the United States is lower than in which of these other industrialized democracies?

    A. Greece
    B. Portugal
    C. Spain
    D. Czech Republic
    E. None of the above

46. Quality in medicine is best defined as:

    A. Delivering the best care possible with the least amount of resources
    B. Achieving a highly reliable system with zero errors
    C. The rigorous measurement of actual outcomes and the use of those data to drive improvement
    D. Application of systems science to drive adverse events to zero

47. For a medical malpractice action, the plaintiff must establish which of the following?

    A. The physician or the health care provider does not owe the patient a duty of care.
    B. The duty of care was breached by conduct that was not in accordance with the standard of care.
    C. The breach in duty of care was not a cause of the plaintiff's injury.
    D. The plaintiff suffered no damages as a result of this breach.

Chapter 11 Answers

1. **Answer: A.** The HITECH Act will result in nearly universal adoption of EHRs in the United States over the next few years. The other choices are not real laws. PAGE 3355

2. **Answer: C.** Macros are a preloaded section that provide detailed structure but initially show all normal results. As such, they are difficult to use compliantly because they often contain information that was not actually obtained by history or examination. They are useful in MDM for importing standard lists of diagnostic tests and/or treatment programs for specific diagnosis. PAGES 3306–3307

3. **Answer: E.** Of the physician specialists listed who support legislation to establish National Health Insurance in the United States, medical subspecialists are highest. PAGE 3346

4. **Answer: C.** High reliability results from standardization. Common aims are essential, as are short feedback loops. Complex systems are unpredictable, which is why standardization is critical. PAGE 3378

5. **Answer: E.** Most medical errors occur because there is a mismatch between human capability and the complexity of the health care system. By focusing on improving both team performance and system design the frequency of injuries can be reduced. PAGES 3257–3258

6. **Answer: D.** Disclosure is one mechanism that is used to minimize the appearance of conflict of interest. By disclosing a potential conflict prior to beginning work on a study, publication, or presentation, an editorial board or meeting organizer is apprised of the relationship of the individual to a technology, drug, or research question. PAGE 3381

7. **Answer: E.** The OECD (Organization for Economic Co-operation and Development) also tracks life expectancies, and the United States does not compare favorably to any of the countries listed in the choices. PAGE 3341

8. **Answer: B.** Attending physicians can use the comprehensive documentation of the resident by attesting to independently performing and documenting problem-focused care. Countersigning the resident's notes alone does not document personal involvement, and detailed or comprehensive repetition of the resident's work is not required. PAGE 3315

9. **Answer: D.** Several scheduling techniques allow physicians to tailor clinic schedules according to patient population served. The success of the modified wave technique depends on appropriate triage of complex and more simple patient problems so clinic hours are balanced between patients with different levels of complexity. PAGE 3334

10. **Answer: A.** The private, for-profit insurance industry uses multimillion-dollar lobbying campaigns and privately financed elections of Congress to block efforts to institute universal coverage in the United States. PAGE 3346

11. **Answer: B.** With advancing technology, the distinctions between areas of telemedicine are blurring, but VTC, RPM, and S&F are the traditional areas. EHR is the standard for collecting and storing health information. Telementoring is a new category using a VTC link. PAGE 3361

12. **Answer: B.** The end result concept was initiated by Codman over 100 years ago and is the basis for morbidity and mortality conference. The end result principle is that physicians must follow the results of their interactions to improve their treatments. PAGES 3372–3373

13. **Answer: C.** Stark legislation aims to prevent physicians and practices from directly referring business to entities in which they have a financial interest. Part II of the Stark legislation addresses medical practice venues and also sets aside exceptions or "safe harbors." Patients referred to a surgicenter by a partner must be fully informed of the surgeon's investment in the ambulatory surgery center. PAGE 3387

14. **Answer: A.** The narrative of medical indications documents medical necessity and the operative findings accurately document the service (specificity). PAGE 3311

15. **Answer: C.** The level of risk to the patients presenting problems, diagnostic procedures, and management options provides support for medical necessity. The nature of the presenting problems helps set the level of care. Data reviewed and tests ordered are elements of the conventional H&P. Insurance deductible and coding are not part of medical documentation. PAGE 3314

16. **Answer: E.** Removing the veil of secrecy that has surrounded medical mistakes places a focus on system errors and preventing errors in the future. An explanation of the events and an apology to the patient allows both the physician and patient to put some sort of closure on the error. PAGE 3264

17. **Answer: D.** Natural language processing has been used in this context. The other choices are distractions that are not applicable. PAGE 3355

18. **Answer: A.** In this case, the meeting planner opted to review the information that would be presented because the author's disclosure statement revealed a close financial and professional relationship between the drug company and the author. PAGE 3381

19. **Answer: B.** See the chart on key measures of practice performance for definition of terms. PAGE 3339

20. **Answer: C.** High-reliability organizations have a number of features, but central to the process is the principle that improved outcomes are driven by application of the principles of systems science. Because systems are unpredictable, errors or adverse events are always possible. Respect for persons and strong, constructive leadership are essential. PAGE 3378

21. **Answer: D.** All of these applications have been published in peer-reviewed literature. PAGES 3364–3366

22. **Answer: A.** The disadvantage of VTC is that it requires a provider on both ends of the video link. The other choices are advantages. PAGE 3361

23. **Answer: D.** Traditionally, use of telemedicine in otolaryngology has thrived in programs with less formidable financial barriers, like the U.S. Public Health Service and Department of Defense. Telemedicine has been used in the field of otolaryngology since the early 1990s. PAGE 3364

24. **Answer: C.** Fundamental to coding compliance is accurately identifying the service performed (specificity) and why they performed it (medical necessity). Meaningful use is the Centers for Medicare and Medicaid Services standard for electronic medical records. Compatibility and conversion are distracters. PAGES 3308–3309

25. **Answer: B.** In this situation, there would be a clear financial advantage to the surgeon for using a particular device and a clear-cut violation of Stark legislation. PAGE 3387

26. **Answer: B.** High-performance teams are characterized by all members being invested in the team's integrity and each being empowered to make a difference. PAGE 3266

27. **Answer: C.** "Gray literature" includes studies that are not available in standard search engines, such as unpublished results, abstracts, proceedings, theses, and book chapters. It may reduce publication bias. However, there are disadvantages, and the gray literature is unlikely to improve the significance of the meta-analysis. Foreign-language articles are available through larger databases. PAGE 3357

28. **Answer: A.** The HIPAA is wide reaching and applies to health care information conveyed by any means (electronics, paper, verbal) for providers who transmit any health care information electronically. It does not apply to all use of protected health information, but does apply to research and marketing uses. PAGES 3294–3295

29. **Answer: D.** The Stark law prohibits referral of patients for a wide range of designated health services (including, but not limited to, clinical lab services) to entities with which the physician or his family has a financial relationship. There is no need for intent to violate the statute to be in violation of the Stark law. PAGE 3282

30. **Answer: C.** Claims-made policies cover for claims made during the coverage period only. Once these policies expire, the physician must buy tail coverage to protect against claims made after the period of coverage for events that occurred during the period of coverage. Occurrence policies cover the physician for incidents during the coverage period, even if the claim is made after the policy is expired, indefinitely and thus generally cost more. PAGES 3276–3277

31. **Answer: E.** Medical errors are the eighth most common cause of death in the United States, and their frequency and overall cost have until recently been underestimated. PAGE 3257

32. **Answer: A.** The other reasons may also apply, but the primary reason is that the default setting is for one procedure per day. PAGE 3320

33. **Answer: B.** This publication organized and synthesized a vast body of literature on medical error. The scale of their estimate that the health care system produces 100,000 potentially preventable deaths annually has been independently supported. The result has been a vigorous, successful effort to improve outcomes for patients and hospitals. PAGE 3373

34. **Answer: A.** The HIPAA (Health Insurance Portability and Accountability Act) applies to all health reformation, regardless of the care delivery model. Mechanisms of collecting, storing, and sharing protected health information that are not acceptable for traditional medicine, such as standard e-mail, are not acceptable in telemedicine. PAGE 3363

35. **Answer: C.** While accountability and repercussions are limited for physicians who serve as expert witnesses, minimal standards of professionalism require that the expert witness should not adopt a position of advocacy, should testify truthfully, should be compensated at a rate that is reasonable and commensurate with time and effort given in preparation for testifying, and should not be paid based on the outcome of the case. PAGE 3275

36. **Answer: C.** The E/M coding system is clearly derived from *Bates' Guide to Physical Examination and History Talking*. The similarities are apparent both conceptually and in wording. PAGE 3304

37. **Answer: C.** The HIPAA (Health Insurance Portability and Accountability Act) sets national standards for patient privacy and protection of their medical data. All choices except C contradict HIPAA regulations. PAGE 3338

38. **Answer: A.** The VA EHR database is massive and has been around longer than most other EHRs. The software system is limited in its abilities for data mining, but data mining can be done. The database is available for retrospective studies and patients are enrolled for prospective studies as well. PAGE 3358

39. **Answer: B.** Databases comprised of insurance claims data or similar data are limited to broad associations because they are incomplete and biased by their purposes for existing. Usually, tools to search these databases are available and automated, and with computers, large databases can be mined. PAGE 3354

40. **Answer: B.** Clinic employee turnover costs are high, making it worthwhile to invest in the right people for the long term. Ensuring salaries are competitive and holding all employees to equal performance standards are practices that will help to retain personnel. PAGE 3333

41. **Answer: A.** Physicians and managed care corporations have many opposing interests in contract negotiations, making it important for physicians to negotiate for maximum allowable rate, minimize authorization requirements, and balance the potential for additional patient volumes. PAGE 3335

42. **Answer: D.** Since Medicare Part A dollars support resident salaries, any further billing for services provided by residents is considered duplicative. Overseeing faculty cannot bill for resident services under Part B of Medicare unless they were actively taking part in direct teaching or supervision of the work. The other choices are false or not permitted under Stark legislation. PAGE 3387

43. **Answer: B.** A "just culture" establishes the balance between system responsibility and individual responsibility by acknowledging recognized boundaries and behaviors that are considered acceptable within that professional community. PAGE 3259

44. **Answer: E.** There are multiple options for health care coverage in the United States and any one of the options is possible depending on the person's employment status, financial resources, medical eligibility, age, health and comorbidity, patient choice, and living situation. PAGE 3347

45. **Answer: E.** The OECD (Organization for Economic Co-operation and Development) is a group of 34 countries that includes most of the world's wealthy industrial democracies. This group compares medical between industrialized nations. For infant mortality, the US rate is much higher than the average rate in OECD countries (as of 2009). PAGE 3341

46. **Answer: C.** Zero errors is a goal, but quality is not equivalent to zero errors. Efficiency is described by the ratio of quality of care to resources used, but quality itself is independent of resources. PAGE 3372

47. **Answer: B.** To sustain an action for medical malpractice, the plaintiff must establish that the physician owed the plaintiff a duty of care, that the duty was breached, that this breach was the cause of injury, and that the plaintiff suffered damages as a result. PAGE 3272

INDEX

A

A1555G mutation, 286
Absorbable suture, examples of, 1, 23
Acellular (cadaveric) dermis, as soft-tissue augmentation implant, 298, 323
Acellular dermal skin substitutes, 16, 30
Acetylcholine neurotransmitter, 101, 117
Acinar cells, for primary salivary secretion, 78, 88
Active middle-ear implants, 240, 274
Acute bacterial rhinosinusitis, pathogens associated with, 41, 63
Acute bacterial sialadenitis, sources of, 74, 86
Acute facial paralysis, prognosis for recovery of, 249, 277
Acute otitis media (AOM)
  bacterial infection and, 156, 175
  for facial paralysis, 249, 277
  pathogens in, 9, 26
  temporal bone imaging for, 239, 273
  vaccines for, 155, 175
  watchful-waiting and, 167, 180
Acute parotitis, bacteria involved in, 74, 86
Acute pharyngitis, in children and adults, 72, 85
Acute retroviral syndrome pharyngitis, 80, 89
Acute rhinosinusitis, 46, 65
Acute sinusitis, 58, 70
  vs. chronic sinusitis, 42, 64
  complication of, 47, 66
  first-line antibiotic for, 39, 62
  indications for imaging in, 45, 65
Adenine, 26
Adenoid cystic carcinoma, management of, 206, 223
Adenoid hypertrophy, anomalies affecting operative intervention, 149, 172
Adenoidal/tonsillar tissue, bacterial infection in, 169, 181
Adenoidectomy
  chronic pediatric rhinosinusitis after, 148, 171
  failure of, 164, 179
Adenoma, 208, 224
Adenotonsillectomy, 227, 232, 233, 235
Adhesion, time length for, between cranium and overlying periosteum, 305, 326

Adjuvant chemoradiation, indications for, 187, 214
Adrenal glands, 15, 29
Adult hearing impairment, in United States
  occupational noise exposure
    cause of, 267, 285
    percentage of, 258, 281
Adults
  acute pharyngitis in, 72, 85
  complementary and alternative medicine among, 6, 25
  hearing loss in, 243, 275
  olfactory dysfunction in, 55, 69
Aesthetic subunits, principle of, 289, 319
Age-related hearing loss (ARHL), 261, 283
Agency for Healthcare Research and Quality (AHRQ), 72, 85
Agger nasi cell, 52, 68
Air embolism, 7, 25
Airway management, requirement of, 133, 143
Airway obstruction, in patients with gunshot wound to mandibular zone, 126, 140
Airway surgery, mitomycin to, 100, 117
Aldosteronism, primary, 15, 29
Allergic disease, environmental control of, 36, 61
Allergic fungal rhinosinusitis, treatment approach for, 35, 61
Allergic fungal sinusitis, 59, 70
Allergic rhinitis
  and asthma, 42, 63
  characteristic of inflammatory response in, 53, 68
  classification of, 47, 66
  diagnosis of, 53, 69
  treatment for, 34, 36, 44, 60, 61, 65
Allergic Rhinitis and its Impact on Asthma (ARIA), 47, 66
Allergy, 33–70, 44, 64
Allocation (susceptibility) bias, 17, 30
Allogenic fibroblasts, 30
Allogenic keratinocytes, 30
Alloplastic augmentation
  for chin, 300, 323
  for microgenia, 292, 320
Alopecia
  follicular unit extraction techniques for, 312, 329
  medical treatment of, 311, 328
Alpha 2, 256, 281

α-adrenergic receptors, 64
Alveolar bone grafting, timing of, 166, 179
American Academy of Pediatrics, postoperative admission for patients, 231, 234
Aminoglycoside-induced hearing loss, genetic testing for, 162, 178
Aminoglycoside-induced ototoxicity, 14, 29
Aminoglycoside susceptibility, genetic inheritance pathways in, 268, 286
Aminoglycosides, 26, 248, 277
Amoxicillin, 39, 62
  group A β-hemolytic streptococcus, 80, 89
Amoxicillin–clavulanate, 87
Amplification with hearing aid, 264, 266, 283, 285
Amyotrophic lateral sclerosis, 15, 29
Androgenetic alopecia, treatment of, 311, 328
Aneurysm, 9, 26
Angiogenesis, proliferative phase of wound healing, 14, 29
Angiosarcoma, 198, 220
Ankylosis, 133, 143
Anterior commissure, laceration of, 141
Anterior ethmoid artery
  location of, 35, 60
  marking posterior limit of frontal recess, 42, 64
Anterior inferior cerebellar artery (AICA)
  occlusion with hearing loss, 10, 27
  stroke, characteristics of, 263, 283
Anterior neuropore
  embryogenesis order of, 163, 178
  to incomplete closure, 147, 171
Anterior septum, 55, 69
Anterior skull base, thinnest part of, 50, 67
Anterior table fracture, 125, 139
  endoscopic repair of, 128, 141
Anterior transmaxillary approach, 43, 44, 64
Anterolateral thigh, 309, 328
Antihelical fold, creation of, 290, 319
Antihistamines, 36, 61
Apert syndrome, diagnostic criteria for, 148, 171
Apopilosebaceous unit, 258, 281
Applebaum prosthesis, 243, 275
Arachnoid cyst, 236, 272
Arcus marginalis, 311, 329